Springhouse Review for

CRITICAL CARE
NURSING CERTIFICATION

FOURTH EDITION

Springhouse Review for
CRITICAL CARE
NURSING CERTIFICATION

FOURTH EDITION

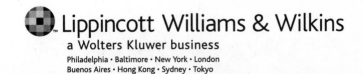
Lippincott Williams & Wilkins
a Wolters Kluwer business
Philadelphia · Baltimore · New York · London
Buenos Aires · Hong Kong · Sydney · Tokyo

STAFF

Executive Publisher
Judith A. Schilling McCann, RN, MSN

Editorial Director
H. Nancy Holmes

Clinical Director
Joan M. Robinson, RN, MSN

Art Director
Mary Ludwicki

Editorial Project Manager
Ann Houska

Clinical Project Manager
Jennifer Meyering, RN, BSN, MS, CCRN

Copy Editor
Linda Hager

Designer
Debra Moloshok (book design)

Digital Composition Services
Diane Paluba (manager), Joyce Rossi Biletz,
Donna S. Morris (project manager)

Manufacturing
Beth J. Welsh

Editorial Assistants
Megan L. Aldinger, Karen J. Kirk, Linda K. Ruhf

Design Assistant
Georg W. Purvis IV

Indexer
Barbara Hodgson

© 2007 by Lippincott Williams & Wilkins. All rights reserved. This book is protected by copyright. No part of it may be reproduced, stored in a retrieval system, or transmitted, in any form or by any means—electronic, mechanical, photocopy, recording, or otherwise—without prior written permission of the publisher, except for brief quotations embodied in critical articles and reviews and testing and evaluation materials provided by publisher to instructors whose schools have adopted its accompanying textbook. Printed in the United States of America. For information, write Lippincott Williams & Wilkins, 323 Norristown Road, Suite 200, Ambler, PA 19002-2756.

CCNC4010906

Library of Congress Cataloging-in-Publication Data

Springhouse review for critical care nursing certification.—4th ed.
    p. ; cm.
    Includes bibliographical references and index.
    1. Intensive care nursing—Examinations, questions, etc. 2. Intensive care nursing. I. Lippincott Williams & Wilkins. II. Title: Review for critical care nursing certification.
    [DNLM: 1. Critical Care--Examination Questions. 2. Critical Care—Outlines. 3. Critical Illness—nursing—Examination Questions.
4. Critical Illness—nursing--Outlines.   WY 18.2 S76952 2007]
RT120.I5C38 2007
616.02'5076—dc22
ISBN 1-58255-506-0 (alk. paper)   2006019521

Contents

Contributors and consultants

Tamara Capik, RN, BSN, CCRN
Registered Nurse—ICU
St. Joseph Hospital
Eureka, Calif.

EM Vitug Garcia, RN, DNS
Chief Nursing Officer/Associate Administrator, PCS
Mission Community Hospital
Panorama City, Calif.
Professor of Nursing Science
Breyer State University
Kamiah, Idaho

Kay Luft, MN, PhD-C, CCRN
Assistant Professor
Saint Luke's College
Kansas City, Mo.

Catherine Pence, RN, MSN, CCRN
Assistant Professor
Northern Kentucky University
Highland Heights

Doris J. Rosenow, RN, PhD, CCRN, CNS-MS
Associate Professor
Texas A&M International University
Laredo

Foreword

For more than 25 years, I have been privileged to write the credential *CCRN* after my name. Earning this certification was an early goal of mine that I have maintained over the course of my career.

In the 1970s, I was an avid critical care nurse, spending most of my time in coronary care units. Being certified as a critical care nurse represented a way to demonstrate my knowledge and offered me many professional opportunities. For example, CCRN certification was recognized in employment applications and annual evaluations. It also was acknowledged on my application for graduate studies. The CCRN credential opened many doors to career advancement that would otherwise have gone unopened for me. As a cardiovascular clinical specialist, I have participated in National Teaching Institutes, including poster presentations, designed critical care internships for new graduates, taught CCRN review courses, and closely followed critically ill patients in multiple clinical settings. These activities and the continuing support I received from the American Association of Critical-Care Nurses and other CCRN colleagues ultimately led to my continued study in nursing. As an academic nurse and outcomes researcher, I was fortunate to be able to direct a critical care clinical nurse specialist program and participate in studies of the critically ill. In essence, the CCRN credential was an early career achievement that gave me the confidence to continue learning.

Today, research is beginning to show relationships between additional preparation and improved patient outcomes. CCRN certification, a valued credential, is one way to demonstrate our expertise and continued professional growth. Not only does the CCRN build confidence and assist in career growth for individual nurses, but it may be related to improved patient outcomes. Isn't this the real essence of critical care nursing?

Taking the CCRN examination is challenging and is often viewed with trepidation. However, with careful planning and preparation, you will be successful. Taking the time to carefully review with specialty texts, such as the *Springhouse Review for Critical Care Nursing Certification*, 4th Edition, will strengthen the knowledge you already have and update you on the most current information in critical care nursing. This approach to preparation will optimize your ability to effectively earn the CCRN credential.

Chapter 1 of *Springhouse Review for Critical Care Nursing Certification*, 4th Edition, is an introduction to the CCRN certification examination. It covers eligibility requirements, application information, a review of the test plan, study tips, and test-taking strategies. The chapter explains the types of questions most likely to appear on the examination and offers effective methods to improve your test performance.

Chapters 2 through 8 are organized by body systems for convenient study. Each chapter reviews anatomy and physiology and then outlines the major pathologies of the body system. These discussions include clinical signs and symptoms and pertinent laboratory values and diagnostic tests. These chapters impart up-to-date information on disorders such as arrhythmias, coronary artery disease, valvular disorders, pulmonary embolism, acute respiratory failure, diabetes, acquired immunodeficiency syndrome, disseminated intravascular coagulation, spinal cord injuries, infectious neurologic diseases, acute gastrointestinal problems such as bowel infarction, and acute renal failure, to name a few. Not only are the diseases described in detail, but also their medical and nursing management and rationales are presented. Review questions at the end of each chapter give you the opportunity to evaluate your newly acquired knowledge.

Chapter 9 is unique because it offers information on multisystem disorders, such as burns and septic shock, that so often plague critical care nurses and their patients. Chapter 10 deals with professional issues of concern to critical care nurses, such as ethical decision-making, caring, collaboration, and continuous learning. This chapter ties the earlier chapters together by providing the context for practice.

Throughout the text, you'll find charts and diagrams that augment the written word. Appendices provide information on drugs used in critical care, care of the bariatric patient, normal aging-related changes, physiologic adaptations to pregnancy, crisis values of laboratory tests, and JCAHO pain management standards. Two posttests offer additional opportunity for self-evaluation before you take the examination. Each contains 50 questions similar to those on the actual examination, followed by the correct answers and rationales. Finally, you'll find a self-diagnostic profile to guide your progress. The reference list is current and allows for further study.

Springhouse Review for Critical Care Nursing Certification, 4th Edition, is a great resource for your successful completion of the CCRN examination. Furthermore, it's a valuable aid for critical care nurses in general and especially for those new to critical care nursing. As you prepare for the examination, remember to study with the assurance that this resource will enhance your growing expertise. Achieving CCRN certification will be a proud moment in your career, one I hope will add to your conviction about the value of critical care nursing. Share your achievement and encourage others to take the examination. Use your new self-confidence to get involved in your professional associations and continue learning. I can think of no greater service to our society than caring for the critically ill.

Joanne R. Duffy PhD, RN, CCRN
Associate Professor
The Catholic University of America
Washington, D.C.

CHAPTER 1

Certification examination

The American Board of Nursing Specialty defines "certification" as formal recognition of the specialized knowledge, skills, and experience demonstrated by the achievement of standards identified by a nursing specialty to promote health outcomes.

Through the critical care registered nurse (CCRN) certification examination, the American Association of Critical-Care Nurses (AACN) recognizes professional nurses who have attained specialized knowledge and expertise in the care of critically ill patients. One of the primary functions of the AACN credentialing process is to define the knowledge and skills required for expert critical care nursing practice. The AACN Certification Corporation administers the examination in cooperation with Applied Measurement Professionals, Inc. (AMP).

As a critical care nurse, you have worked hard to master complex technical skills required for care of critically ill patients, along with the underlying theoretical knowledge. You have developed the ability to make sound nursing judgments in crisis situations that commonly determine whether a patient lives or dies. Despite this advanced education, skill mastery, and decision-making ability, many critical care nurses experience high levels of test-taking anxiety that can prevent them from seeking certification.

The purpose of this book is to alleviate test-taking anxiety by providing a thorough review of the subject matter covered by the CCRN certification examination and pertinent critical care clinical nursing exercises.

Eligibility and application

The AACN establishes criteria for eligibility to take the CCRN certification examination (see *Eligibility requirements for CCRN candidacy*, page 2). Because requirements can change, it's important to review the latest criteria before applying for certification. Contact the AACN for current CCRN eligibility requirements and an examination application booklet at:

American Association of Critical-Care Nurses
101 Columbia
Aliso Viejo, CA 92656-4109
phone: 1-800-899-2226
fax: 949-362-2000
e-mail: *certcorp@aacn.org*
Web site: *www.certcorp.org*

Eligibility requirements for CCRN candidacy

The American Association of Critical-Care Nurses' (AACN) eligibility criteria for certification in adult critical care nursing are as follows:

• Current unrestricted registered nurse (RN) licensure in the United States or any of its territories that use the National Council Licensure Examination as the basis for determining RN licensure. An unrestricted license is one in which there are no provisions or conditions limiting the nurse's practice.

• Critical care nursing practice as an RN for a period of 1,750 hours, in direct bedside care of the critically ill patient during 2 years preceding application, with 875 of those hours accrued in the most recent year preceding application. Clinical practice hours for critical care registered nurse (CCRN) examination or renewal eligibility must take place in a U.S.-based facility or in a facility determined to be comparable by verifiable evidence to the U.S. standard of acute and critical care nursing practice.

• Nurses working as managers, educators (in-service or academic), clinical nurse specialists, or preceptors may apply hours spent supervising nurses or nursing students as the bedside. Nurses in these roles must be actively involved in the care of the patient, such as demonstrating measurement of pulmonary artery pressures or supervising a new employee or student nurse performing a procedure.

• The name and address of a professional associate (such as a clinical supervisor or RN colleague with whom you work) who can verify that you meet the eligibility requirements if you're randomly selected for audit.

• Additional eligibility requirements may be adopted by the AACN Certification Corporation at its sole discretion from time to time. Such requirements will be designed to establish, for the purposes of CCRN certification, the adequacy of a candidate's knowledge and experience in caring for critically ill patients.

To apply for the CCRN examination, you must complete the examination application form and the verification of clinical practice and RN licensure for adult CCRN certification form that come in your application booklet.

Pay careful attention to all steps in the application process, particularly deadlines. The AACN strictly adheres to initial and final postmark deadlines for application. Fees for the computer-based test are $220 (for an AACN member who files by the initial deadline) or $300 (for a non-member). Fees are subject to change without notice and may be more expensive for overseas testing.

AACN Certification Corporation notifies AMP of eligible candidates. AMP then sends an authorization-to-test letter with a toll-free number for the candidate to schedule their examination within a 90-day eligibility period.

The examination may be administered 5 days a week, year-round, at any one of about 100 locations nationwide. Once you have selected a test date and site on your application form, you may reschedule up to 4 business days before the scheduled date by calling the toll-free number in the letter.

No refunds are available for individuals who don't sit for the examination on the date specified in their authorization-to-test letter or who fail to adhere to the rescheduling policy. A $100 rescheduling fee will be charged to any candidate who doesn't schedule an examination within the 90-day eligibility period and needs to obtain a new 90-day eligibility period. All centers are compliant with the Americans with Disabilities Act. Special testing arrangements, such as additional testing time, reader, signer, or amanuensis, can be rescheduled with advanced approval.

Certification test plan

The CCRN examination contains 150 multiple-choice questions, some of which are preceded by a brief clinical situation. Each question carries equal weight toward the final score, and every question must be answered. Candidates have 3 hours to complete the test.

The AACN develops the certification examination based on the task statements identified in its Role Delineation study. This study, completed in 1998, defines the dimensions of critical care practice and determines the skills, knowledge, and experience required by critical care nurses. The CCRN examination tests the critical care nurse's grasp of these skills and concepts.

As of July 1, 1999, the test incorporates the Synergy Model of certified practice, which emphasizes patient characteristics or needs in defining nursing competencies. Nurses are conceptualized to consider the patient in a holistic manner, recognizing that each individual and family have common and unique needs on a continuum of health to illness. By synchronizing the nurse's competencies to these characteristics or needs, a synergistic interaction and optimal patient outcome can occur.

These important dimensions of critical care nursing described by the Synergy Model, collectively referred to as Professional Caring and Ethical Practice, now comprise 20% of the blueprint for the CCRN examination. Components include Advocacy/Moral Agency (2%), Caring Practices (4%), Collaboration (4%), Systems Thinking (2%), Response to Diversity (2%), Clinical Inquiry (2%), and Facilitator of Learning (4%). The remaining 80% of the examination is based on Clinical Judgment, which comprises task and knowledge statements.

While the Synergy Model provides the theoretical framework for the CCRN examination design, the test itself doesn't cover the model's terminology. For more information on the Synergy Model, visit *www.certcorp.org*.

Professional knowledge statements

Clinical Judgment is based, in part, on professional knowledge statements. Knowledge statements are those components of information that a critical care nurse must know to perform a given task. Knowledge statements relate to specific task statements organized around the major body systems affected in a critically ill patient.

About 32% of the test questions on the CCRN examination pertain to the cardiovascular system. The other areas covered are the pulmonary system (17%), neurologic system (5%), renal system (5%), GI system (6%), endocrine system (4%), hematologic and immunologic system (3%), and multisystemic disorders (8%).

Within each of these eight systems, systemwide knowledge is assessed related to anatomy and physiology (including maturational changes), invasive and noninvasive diagnostic tests, pharmacology relevant to the system, and implications of system failure on other systems. In addition, knowledge of specific patient care problems associated with that system is assessed, including: pathophysiology, etiology and risk factors, signs and symptoms, interpretation of invasive and noninvasive diagnostic study results, nursing and collaborative diagnoses, goals and desired patient outcomes, patient care management, and complications.

Items included in patient care management involve: positioning, skin care management, conscious sedation, nutritional management, infection control, transport, discharge planning, pharmacology, psychosocial issues, invasive and noninvasive treatments, and ethical issues.

Systemwide knowledge often involves the assessment and planning phases of tasks in the nursing process, while specific patient care problem knowledge areas emphasize intervention/implementation and evaluation. Multisystem patient care problems are unique, and knowledge and patient care problem statements meld to become indistinguishable.

Levels of cognitive ability

The levels of cognitive ability component measures how knowledge has been learned and how the nurse uses it. Testing at cognitive levels provides a better indication of the professional nurse's ability to identify problems, plan, implement, and evaluate nursing care for the patient and family members. For the CCRN examination, knowledge is tested at three levels and is based on Bloom's taxonomy. The questions are distributed across all levels.

Level 1 consists of knowledge and comprehension questions, involving memory of specific facts and the ability to apply those facts to specific pathophysiologic conditions. Level 1 questions often test knowledge of anatomy and physiology, medication doses and adverse effects, signs and symptoms of diseases, laboratory test results, and the components of certain treatments and interventions.

Here is an example of a level 1 question:

> William Carlton is admitted to the critical care unit (CCU) with acute respiratory failure. What is the normal range for the partial pressure of arterial oxygen (PaO_2) value?
> **A.** 10 to 30 mm Hg
> **B.** 35 to 55 mm Hg
> **C.** 10 to 20 cm H_2O
> **D.** 70 to 100 mm Hg

The correct answer is D. As you can see, this question is designed to test your memory of a specific fact.

Level 2 questions ask you to analyze and apply information to specific patient care situations. *Analysis* involves the ability to separate information into its basic parts and decide which of those parts is important. *Application* involves the ability to use that information in patient care decisions. Level 2 questions may assess your ability to interpret electrocardiogram (ECG) strips and arterial blood gas (ABG) values, make a nursing diagnosis based on a set of symptoms, or decide on a course of treatment.

An example of a level 2 question follows:

> William Carlton is becoming progressively short of breath. The results of his ABG studies include a pH of 7.13, PaO_2 of 48 mm Hg, partial pressure of arterial carbon dioxide ($PaCO_2$) of 53 mm Hg, and bicarbonate of 26 mEq/L. Which problem do these values indicate?

    A. Uncompensated metabolic acidosis with moderate hypoxia

    B. Respiratory alkalosis with hypoxia

    C. Uncompensated respiratory acidosis with severe hypoxia

    D. Compensated respiratory acidosis with normal oxygen

The correct answer is C. Not only must you know the normal values for each of the ABG values given but you must also use that information to determine the underlying condition.

Level 3 questions involve synthesis and evaluation and often ask you to make patient care judgments. Some questions may be followed by more than one appropriate option, but you must choose the *best* option from those listed. Questions at this level ask about the priority of care to be given, the priority of the formulated nursing diagnosis, ways to evaluate the effectiveness of care, and the most appropriate nursing action to take in a given situation.

An example of a level 3 question follows:

    William Carlton has become cyanotic and is experiencing Cheyne-Stokes respiration. What is the *best* action for the nurse to take at this time?

    A. Call a code blue, and begin cardiopulmonary resuscitation.

    B. Call Mr. Carlton's practitioner, and report the condition.

    C. Make sure that Mr. Carlton's airway is open, and begin supplemental oxygen.

    D. Immediately administer the ordered dose of 200 mg I.V. aminophylline by way of push bolus.

The best answer is C. Although answers B and D are also appropriate, opening the airway and oxygenating the patient have the highest priority in this situation. Not only does this type of question require you to know specific facts (definitions of cyanosis and Cheyne-Stokes respiration) but it also requires you to make a decision about the seriousness of the condition (analysis) and to select the type of care to be given from several appropriate options (judgment).

Professional task statement

The professional task statement component encompasses the four steps of the nursing process—assessment, planning, intervention and implementation, and evaluation. All questions on the CCRN examination relate to one of these nursing process steps. Professional task statements provide the framework for the Clinical Judgment portion of the examination.

The assessment step establishes the database on which the rest of the nursing process is built. Components of the assessment phase include subjective and objective data about the patient, significant medical history, history of the current illness, signs and symptoms, environmental elements, laboratory test results, and vital signs. In relationship to the patient's present condition, data from the patient involves gathering psychosocial, cultural, developmental, and spiritual assessment factors.

The ability to analyze the data, collaborate with other health care team members, integrate the data to identify problems and needs, effectively prioritize these problems and needs, and provide continual reassessment as well as documentation and communication of pertinent findings is also involved.

An example of an assessment-phase question follows:

> William Carlton's respiratory status continues to worsen. Which of the following signs and symptoms would best indicate deterioration of his respiratory status?
>
> **A.** Increased restlessness and changes in level of consciousness (LOC)
> **B.** Bradycardia and increased blood pressure
> **C.** Complaints of chest pain and shortness of breath
> **D.** Rapidly dropping $Paco_2$ and pH values

The correct answer is A. The brain is one of the first organs to be affected by decreased oxygenation. Restlessness and changes in LOC reflect this decrease. Choices B, C, and D are signs and symptoms of other conditions.

The planning step of the nursing process involves developing a holistic plan of care. This should reflect the priority of actual and potential problems and the collaboration of other team members. The planning phase integrates the psychosocial, cultural, spiritual, and developmental needs of the patient. Documentation and communication of the collaborative plan of care is also involved.

Here's an example of a planning-phase question:

> William Carlton is diagnosed with acute respiratory failure and connected to a positive pressure, volume-cycled ventilator with positive end-expiratory pressure (PEEP) set at 10 cm H_2O. Which nursing diagnosis would have the highest priority for this patient?
>
> **A.** Impaired skin integrity related to immobility
> **B.** Ineffective cardiopulmonary tissue perfusion related to changes in intrathoracic pressure
> **C.** Ineffective coping related to anxiety
> **D.** Impaired gas exchange related to decreased lung compliance

The correct answer is B. A patient placed on a ventilator with PEEP typically experiences a dramatic decrease in cardiac output due to alterations in normal chest pressure produced by the ventilator. When asked to select the goal or nursing diagnosis with the highest priority, you should remember Maslow's hierarchy of needs—the patient's physiologic and safety needs must be met before higher needs, such as love and belonging, can be fulfilled.

The intervention, or implementation, step of the nursing process involves identifying nursing actions required to meet the goals stated in the planning phase. The intervention phase includes coordination of patient care delivery, implementation of the plan of care, and related documentation and communication.

An example of an intervention-phase question follows:

> William Carlton has been on the ventilator for 3 days. He suddenly becomes extremely restless, and the pressure alarm sounds with each ventilator-initiated inspiration. Which of the following would be an appropriate initial nursing action?
>
> **A.** Disconnect the ventilator and call a code.
> **B.** Disconnect the ventilator and manually oxygenate the patient for a few minutes with a handheld ventilator.
> **C.** Increase the ventilator pressure limit to 50 mm Hg.
> **D.** Remove the endotracheal tube, and reintubate the patient with a tube one size larger.

The correct answer is B. When the pressure alarm sounds, it typically indicates an increase in airway resistance from some cause. Evaluating the amount of airway resistance with a manual ventilator may help determine the source of the problem. Other appropriate nursing actions include suctioning the patient's airway, administering sedatives, assessing ventilator function, and using calming measures to reduce the patient's anxiety. Choices A, C, and D aren't appropriate in this situation.

The evaluation phase of the nursing process determines whether the goals stated in the planning phase were actually met by the nurse's interventions. The evaluation phase also ties the nursing process together. In this phase, data are collected from all pertinent sources for evaluation, including collaboration with other health care team members, and the patient's responses are compared with the desired outcome. If the desired outcome could be achieved more fully by revising the plan of care, a modified plan is made, documented, and communicated.

Questions pertaining to the evaluation phase may include comparison of actual outcomes with expected outcomes, verification of assessment data, evaluation of nursing actions and patient responses, and evaluation of the patient's level of knowledge and understanding.

Here's an example of an evaluation-phase question:

> William Carlton has been extubated and transferred to the step-down unit and is now being prepared for discharge. He needs to take oral theophylline at home for his lung disease. Which response indicates that he has understood the nurse's instructions about how to take theophylline?
>
> **A.** "I can stop taking this medication when I feel better."
> **B.** "If I have difficulty swallowing the timed-release capsules, I can crush or chew them."
> **C.** "If I become very sleepy when I take this medication, I need to cut back on the dosage."
> **D.** "I need to avoid drinking coffee and soft drinks while I'm taking this medication."

The correct answer is D. The patient must be taught to avoid excessive amounts of caffeine because it increases the adverse effects of theophylline. Choices A and C are incorrect because a patient should never suddenly stop taking medication. Choice B is incorrect because timed-release capsules should never be crushed or chewed.

Computerized CCRN examination

The AACN offers the CCRN examination in a computerized format. Candidates with little or no computer experience will be relieved to discover that the test doesn't require extensive computer skills. An optional tutorial is provided before beginning the timed test so that you can familiarize yourself with the computerized format.

The computerized examination is user-driven by way of basic options. You select an answer by using the mouse to click on it or by typing in the response letter. Pressing ENTER advances to the next question. You may mark answered questions for later review or skip questions to revisit. Try to answer each question to the best of your ability. If you're unsure, make an educated guess because unanswered questions are scored as incorrect.

Plan to arrive at least 15 minutes ahead of your scheduled test time for check-in. You'll need two forms of identification with matching names and signatures. One must be a government-issued photo identification, such as a driver's license or passport. The other must show your name and signature, such as an employee identification or credit card. Candidates may also be thumb-printed and photographed to verify identity. In addition, testing sessions may be videotaped.

The examination is graded on a pass-fail basis. A passing score has been set by the AACN Certification Corporation. A preliminary pass or fail score is available to you immediately on completion of the test. A candidate who doesn't pass must retake the entire test. There's no waiting period, and tests may be retaken up to four times in a 12-month period. Official score reports that delineate your performance in each subject area are mailed to you from AMP 4 to 6 weeks after the test.

Study strategies

You can prepare for your certification examination in many ways. Carefully directed study and preparation will significantly increase your chances of passing the test. You may want to use some or all of the following study strategies, depending on your knowledge level, years of experience, and individual learning style.

You have already begun to prepare for certification by purchasing this review book, which covers the key concepts covered on the CCRN examination and closely follows the CCRN test plan. However, a review book is just that—it reviews material you already know to reinforce knowledge and recall old or unused information. Review books aren't designed to present new information. If you're completely unfamiliar with the material in a particular section of this book, you should read a more complete textbook on the subject.

This review book can also pinpoint weak areas in your knowledge base. If you find sections in this book that seem to contain some new material, review that subject in more detail with supplemental resources.

Group study can be an effective method of preparing for the certification examination. To optimize the results of group study sessions, several rules should be followed:

● Be selective about study group members. Everyone should have a similar attitude about preparing for the CCRN examination and commit to meeting once or twice a week for a period of time. An ideal study group has four to six persons; larger groups may become difficult to coordinate. After the group has started, it may be necessary to ask an individual to leave if she doesn't prepare assigned material, disrupts the study process, or displays a negative attitude toward the examination.

● Assign each person a particular section of the study topic to prepare and present to the group. For example, if the next study topic is the endocrine system, ask one group member to discuss the anatomy and physiology of that system, another to review related pathologic conditions, a third to cover medications and treatments, and a fourth to review key elements of nursing care. Each person then presents their section to the group at the next study session. This planned preparation prevents the "What are we going to study tonight?" syndrome that plagues many group study sessions.

● Limit study sessions to 2 hours. Sessions that run longer tend to lose focus and foster a negative attitude toward the examination.

● Avoid turning group study sessions into a party. A few snacks and refreshments may be helpful in maintaining the group's energy level, but a party atmosphere will detract significantly from the effectiveness of the study session.

Even if you participate in a study group, individual preparation for the CCRN examination is essential for success. As you use review or supplemental sources, mentally organize the information into a format similar to that of the CCRN examination. After reading a page, ask yourself, "How might the certification examination test my knowledge of this material?" Try to formulate and answer three or four multiple-choice questions on the information. You can do this in your head or write it out.

An extremely effective method of individual study is to answer practice questions similar to those on the test. You may increase your score by as much as 10% using this study strategy. Answering practice questions helps you become more familiar and comfortable with the test format in addition to reinforcing information you have studied.

Answering practice questions can also quickly identify areas that require further study. It's easy to tell yourself, "I know the renal system pretty well," but much more difficult to correctly answer 10 to 15 questions on that system. If you answer most practice questions on a particular subject correctly, you can move on to the next topic. If you answer a significant number of questions incorrectly, you'll know to review that subject in more detail and try again.

For optimal benefit from practice questions, spend 30 to 45 minutes each day answering 10 to 20 questions, rather than trying to answer 100 questions on your day off. After you answer the questions, compare your response to the correct answers, and review the rationales provided.

After working with multiple-choice questions long enough, you'll begin to organize your knowledge and reviewed concepts in that format. Practice questions are available from various sources. This review book, for example, contains two posttest practice examinations as well as review questions at the end of each chapter. You can also use Internet Web sites, links, and search engines to locate more sources of CCRN-type questions.

Organizations like the AACN offer CD-ROMs of questions from retired CCRN examinations for practice. Other alternatives for review include seminars, audiotapes, in-service training at work, patient care experiences, and review of advanced cardiac life support material through classes or review books.

Although the AACN doesn't directly endorse or sponsor any review courses for the CCRN examination, local chapters of the AACN frequently conduct reviews 1 month or so before an examination date. These reviews range from 2 to 5 days and cover the information found in this review book. Professional review sessions can be expensive—especially if you don't belong to the local AACN chapter—and quality varies, depending on the skills of the instructor presenting the material.

Test-taking strategies

Multiple-choice questions are one of the most commonly used test formats. You may have noticed that some people do well on such tests, whereas others have problems with this format. Those who do well aren't necessarily smarter than those who don't. More likely, they have intuitively mastered some of the strategies needed to do well on multiple-choice tests. Once you understand and apply the following test-taking strategies, you too will be able to score better on multiple-choice examinations.

Read the patient situation, question, and answer choices carefully. Many mistakes are made because the test-taker didn't read all parts of the question carefully. As you read the question and the answer choices, try to determine what kind of knowledge the question is testing.

Treat each question individually. Use only the information provided for that particular question. Avoid reading into a question information that isn't provided. You may have a tendency to think of exceptions or atypical patients encountered in your practice. Most questions on the CCRN examination test textbook-case knowledge of the material.

Be sure to complete the entire examination. Your score is based on the number of questions you answer correctly out of a total of 200 questions. If you have time to finish only 100 questions and answered them all correctly, your score would still be only 50%. Practice answering questions at the rate of one question per minute in your review.

Wear your watch to the test, and monitor the time as you go. You'll have approximately 70 seconds per question. Most test-takers average 45 seconds per question, so you may finish well before the time limit. You should be at least on question 50 by the end of the first hour, question 100 by the end of the second hour, and so on. If you fall behind by 10 or more questions during any hour, make a conscious effort to speed up. If you spend more than 2 minutes on a question, choose an answer and move on.

Keep in mind that there's no penalty for guessing. An educated guess is better than no answer—an unanswered question is scored as incorrect. If you can't decide on the correct answer, select one and move on. You have a one-in-four chance of selecting the right response.

Use the process of elimination to narrow down your choices when possible. One or more answers can usually be identified as incorrect. By eliminating these answers from the possible choices, you can focus your attention on the answers that may be correct and improve your odds of getting the question right. Reread the question and try to determine exactly what type of information is being tested. If you still can't make a decision, select one of the possible correct choices and move on.

Look for the answer that has a broader focus. If you can narrow down the possible correct choices to two, examine the answers to determine whether one answer may include the other. The answer that's broader (that is, the one that includes the other answer) is probably the correct one.

An example of this type of question follows:

> Billy Black is diagnosed with Wolff-Parkinson-White syndrome. When evaluating his ECG, the nurse should note which of the following characteristics of this condition?
>
> **A.** PR interval less than 0.12 second and wide QRS complex
> **B.** PR interval greater than 0.20 second and normal QRS complex
> **C.** Delta wave present in a positively deflected QRS complex in lead V_1 and PR interval less than 0.12 second
> **D.** Delta wave present in a positively deflected QRS complex in lead V_6 and PR interval greater than 0.20 second

The correct answer is C. Answer A may also be correct, but answer C includes the information in answer A and adds more information. Again, reading all the answer choices carefully is essential. Selecting answer A without reading the other answers would have led to an incorrect choice.

You can't change an answer selection after you go on to the next question, unless you marked the answered item for later review. Trust your intuition. The first time you read a question and the answer choices, an intuitive connection is made between the left and right lobes of your brain, with the end result being that your first answer is usually the best one. Studies of test-taking habits have shown that test-takers who change an answer selection on a multiple-choice examination usually change it from a correct answer to an incorrect one, or from one incorrect answer to another incorrect answer. Seldom do they change from an incorrect to a correct answer.

Look for qualifying words in the question. Such words as *first, best, most, initial, better,* and *highest priority* can help you determine the type of information called for in the answer. When you see one of these words, your task is to make a judgment about the priority of the answers and select the one answer with the highest priority.

An example of a judgment question follows:

> Roger Redman, age 62, has a history of coronary heart disease. He's brought to the emergency department (ED) complaining of chest pain. What is the *first* action the nurse should take?
>
> **A.** Give the patient sublingual nitroglycerin grain ¹⁄₁₅₀.
> **B.** Call the patient's cardiologist about his admission.
> **C.** Place the patient in high Fowler's position after loosening his shirt.
> **D.** Check the patient's blood pressure, and note the location and degree of chest pain.

The correct choice is D. When a question asks for a first or an initial action, think of the nursing process. The first step in the nursing process is assessment. If no choice includes the assessment step, look for an answer involving the planning process, and so forth. In this particular situation, the nurse needs to assess the patient's chest pain first to determine whether it's cardiac in nature. Many other conditions also cause chest pain.

Here's another example of a judgment question:

> Mr. Redman is connected to an ECG monitor. He was given sublingual nitroglycerin 5 minutes ago but is still experiencing chest pain. The nurse notices that he's beginning to have frequent premature ventricular contractions (PVCs) and short runs of ventricular tachycardia. What is the *most* appropriate nursing intervention?
>
> A. Administer another dose of nitroglycerin.
> B. Administer an I.V. bolus of amiodarone, and start an amiodarone infusion.
> C. Evaluate the patient's mental and circulatory status.
> D. Notify the ED physician.

The correct answer is B. All four choices should be done at some point, but the most appropriate action at this time is to control the PVCs and tachycardia with amiodarone.

Look for negative words in the question. Negative words or prefixes change how you look for the correct answer. Some common negatives include *not, least, unlikely, inappropriate, unrealistic, lowest priority, contraindicated, false, except, inconsistent, untoward, all but, atypical,* and *incorrect.* In general, when you're asked a negative question, three of the choices are appropriate actions and one isn't appropriate. You're being asked to select the inappropriate choice as your answer. When you see a negative question, ask yourself, "What is it that they don't want me to do in this situation?"

An example of a negative question follows:

> Mr. Redman is admitted to the CCU. He's still experiencing mild chest pain. Which of the following medications would be inappropriate for relieving Mr. Redman's chest pain?
>
> A. diltiazem (Cardizem)
> B. propranolol (Inderal)
> C. digoxin (Lanoxin)
> D. meperidine (Demerol)

The correct answer is C. Digoxin is a positive inotropic drug that increases the heart's contractility and oxygen demands. This medication may increase chest pain in this patient. The other three medications relieve chest pain by means of different mechanisms. If you didn't read the question carefully and missed the *in-* prefix of *inappropriate,* you would not have selected choice C.

Avoid selecting answers that contain "absolute" words, because they're usually incorrect. Such words include *always, every, only, all, never,* and *none.*

Here's an example of this type of question:

> Which of the following is an accurate statement about cardiac chest pain?
>
> A. This pain is always caused by constriction or blockage of the coronary arteries by fatty plaques or blood clots.
> B. True cardiac pain is never relieved without treatment.
> C. This type of pain is relieved only by nitroglycerin.
> D. Patients generally attribute the pain to indigestion.

The correct answer is D. Choice A is incorrect because coronary-type chest pain may also be caused by coronary artery spasm, as in variant (Prinzmetal's) angina. Answer B is incorrect because chest pain sometimes goes away by itself, although it probably will return. A number of other medications also relieve chest pain, thus making choice C incorrect.

Avoid selecting answers that refer the patient to a practitioner. The CCRN examination is for nurses and includes conditions and problems that nurses should be able to solve independently. An answer that refers a patient to the practitioner is usually incorrect and can be eliminated from consideration.

Avoid looking for a pattern in the selection of answers. The questions and answers on the examination are arranged in random order. Treat each question individually, and avoid looking over previous answers for some sort of pattern.

Don't panic if you encounter a question that you don't understand. The CCRN examination is designed so that it's difficult to answer all the questions correctly. As a result, some questions may refer to disease processes, medications, or laboratory tests that you're unfamiliar with.

When test-takers encounter difficult questions about material they don't understand, they have a tendency to select an answer they don't understand. Avoid this practice. Remember that nursing care is similar in many situations, even though the disease processes may be quite different. If you encounter a question you don't understand, select the answer that seems logical and involves general nursing care. Common sense can go a long way in this case.

An example of this type of question follows:

George Green, age 33, is diagnosed as having a pheochromocytoma. Appropriate initial nursing care would involve:

A. administering large doses of xylometazoline to help control the symptoms of the disease.

B. closely monitoring Mr. Green's vital signs, particularly his blood pressure.

C. preparing Mr. Green and his family for imminent death.

D. having the family discuss the condition with the practitioner before informing Mr. Green about the disease due to the protracted recovery period after treatment.

The correct answer is B. A pheochromocytoma is a tumor of the adrenal medulla that causes an increase in the secretion of epinephrine or norepinephrine. This type of tumor can trigger a hypertensive crisis in some patients. Monitoring blood pressure is an important nursing care measure and fits well with the qualifying word *initial* used in the question.

If you don't know what a pheochromocytoma is, you might select choice A if you also don't know what xylometazoline is. This medication is used to relieve nasal congestion. Answer C isn't a good choice because preparing a patient for death usually isn't an initial nursing action. Choice D could be eliminated because it's too long and refers the family to a practitioner for the nursing care measure.

Remember, if you encounter a question like this on the CCRN examination, don't spend a great deal of time on it. You either know the answer or you don't. If you don't know the correct answer, try to eliminate some of the choices using the strategies discussed earlier. If you still have no idea, make an educated guess, and move on to the next question.

When answers are grouped by similar concepts, activities, or situations, select the one that's different. If three of the four choices have a common element, and the fourth answer lacks this element, the different answer is probably correct.

Here's an example of this type of question:

> For several years, Karen Cooper has been treated for severe chronic emphysema with bronchodilating agents and relatively high doses of prednisone (Deltasone). Which activity poses the least risk for triggering an adverse effect of prednisone therapy in this patient?
>
> **A.** Shopping at the mall on a Saturday afternoon
> **B.** Cleaning her two-story house
> **C.** Attending Sunday morning church services
> **D.** Serving refreshments at her 6-year-old son's school play

The correct answer is B. In choices A, C, and D, the common element is that Mrs. Cooper would encounter a group of strangers. Because steroids suppress the immune system, patients taking these medications must avoid exposure to potential infections. Cleaning her house, although strenuous, results in the least exposure to infection.

Think positively about the CCRN examination. People who have a positive attitude score higher than those who are negative. Try repeating these phrases to yourself: "I'm an intelligent person. I'll do well on the CCRN examination. I have prepared for this test and will get a passing score. I deserve to earn certification. I know I can do this!"

Preparing for the certification examination

Being prepared to take the CCRN examination involves not only intellectual preparation but also physical and emotional preparation. Before the day of the examination, drive to the test site to familiarize yourself with the parking facilities and to locate the test room. Knowing where to go will greatly decrease your anxiety on the day of the exam. Try to follow as normal a schedule as possible the day before the examination. If you must travel to the examination site and stay away from home overnight, try to follow your usual nightly routine, and avoid the urge to do something different.

The day before the examination, avoid drinking alcoholic beverages. Alcohol is a central nervous system (CNS) depressant that interferes with your ability to concentrate, particularly with a hangover. Also, avoid eating foods you have never eaten before because these may cause adverse GI activity the day of the test. Avoid taking medications you have never taken before to help you sleep. Like alcohol, most sleep aids are CNS depressants. Some produce a hangover effect, whereas others cause drowsiness for an extended period.

On the eve of the examination, you're probably as prepared as you can be. Don't begin major review efforts now or stay up late studying. Review formulas, charts, or lists of information for no more than 1 hour. Then relax, perhaps by watching television or reading an unrelated magazine or book. These activities help decrease anxiety by giving your mind a break from the test. Go to bed at your usual time.

On the morning of the examination, don't attempt a major review of the material. The likelihood of learning something new at this point is slim, and intensive study may only increase your anxiety.

Also, avoid drinking excessive amounts of coffee, tea, or caffeine-containing beverages before the test. Too much caffeine can increase nervousness and stimulate your renal system. Rest room visits are permitted during the examination, but the testing time limit isn't extended.

Eat breakfast, even if you usually don't, and include foods that are high in glucose and protein. Glucose will help maintain your energy level for 1 to 1½ hours. A protein source is required to maintain your energy level throughout the examination. Don't eat greasy, heavy foods. These tend to form an uncomfortable knot in the stomach that may decrease your concentration. If permitted, bring mints or hard candy into the test room to relieve dry mouth.

Dress in comfortable, layered clothing that can be taken off easily. Many rooms are air-conditioned in the summer and may be cool, even if it's hot outside. Be prepared by taking a sweater or sweatshirt, just in case.

Arrive at the test site at least 15 minutes early, and make sure you have the required papers and documents for admittance to the examination.

Think positively about how you'll do on the test. Taking the CCRN examination demonstrates confidence in your knowledge of critical care nursing. When you receive your passing results, plan to celebrate your success. It's a significant achievement in your life and deserves to be recognized and rewarded.

Cardiovascular disorders

❖ **Anatomy**
- Layers of the heart
  - ◆ Pericardium
    - ▶ The pericardium is a double-walled (fibrous outer wall and serous inner wall) sac that surrounds the heart and roots of the great vessels
    - ▶ It functions as a barrier against infection, holds the heart in a fixed position, and shields the heart from trauma
    - ▶ The pericardium normally contains 10 to 30 ml of pericardial fluid, which serves as a lubricant (It can hold up to 300 ml of fluid without compromising cardiac function, and in chronic disease states, the pericardial space can hold up to 1 L of fluid.)
  - ◆ Epicardium
    - ▶ The epicardium is the outer, visceral layer of the heart
    - ▶ It forms the inner layer of the pericardium and is sometimes called the visceral pericardium
  - ◆ Myocardium
    - ▶ The myocardium is a thick, muscular layer that contains the muscle fibers that contract
    - ▶ Cardiac muscle cells making up the myocardium contain myosin, actin, and sarcoplasmic reticulum
      - • Myosin is a thick contractile protein with tiny projections that interact with actin to form cross-bridges
      - • Actin is a thin contractile protein that's connected to Z bands on one end and the myosin cross-bridges on the other; the Z bands act as an anchor, allowing the muscle fibers to slide over one another
      - • Sarcoplasmic reticulum stores and then releases calcium ions after depolarization; this allows the cross-bridges on the myosin filaments to effect cell contraction
  - ◆ Endocardium
    - ▶ The endocardium is a thin layer of endothelium and connective tissue that lines the heart
    - ▶ It's continuous with the blood vessels, papillary muscles, and valves
    - ▶ Disruptions in the endocardium can predispose the patient to infection
- Position of the heart
  - ◆ The heart lies in the anterior thoracic cavity, just behind the sternum in the mediastinum

- ◆ It's anterior to the esophagus, aorta, vena cava, and vertebral column
- ◆ The right ventricle constitutes the majority of the inferior and anterior surfaces
- ◆ The left ventricle constitutes the anterolateral and posterior surfaces
- ◆ The base of the heart is the superior surface located diagonally at the second intercostal space to the right and left of the sternal border; the apex is the inferior surface located at the fifth intercostal space, left mid-clavicular line
- ■ Normal size and weight
  - ◆ The normal heart is 4.7" (12 cm) long and 3.1" to 3.5" (8 to 9 cm) wide
  - ◆ An adult male heart weighs 10.2 to 11.5 oz (290 to 325 g); an adult female heart weighs 8.1 to 9.3 oz (230 to 264 g)
- ■ Chambers of the heart
  - ◆ Atria
    - ▶ The atria are thin-walled, low-pressure chambers that receive blood from the vena cava and pulmonary veins
    - ▶ Atria act as conduits between the venous system and the ventricles
    - ▶ Atrial contractions contribute up to 30% of ventricular filling; this is known as atrial kick
  - ◆ Ventricles
    - ▶ The right ventricle, which is about 3 mm thick, pumps blood into low-pressured pulmonary circulation
    - ▶ The left ventricle, which is about 10 to 13 mm thick, ejects blood into the high-pressured aorta; it's considered the major pump of the heart
- ■ Cardiac valves
  - ◆ Description
    - ▶ The valves in the heart consist of flexible fibrous tissue thinly covered by endocardium
      - • Chordae tendineae are avascular structures covered by a thin layer of endocardium that connects the papillary muscles to the valve
      - • Papillary muscles connect the chordae tendineae to the floor of the ventricular wall to help prevent the valve cusps from everting during systole
    - ▶ The valves permit unidirectional blood flow; their opening and closing is a passive pressure-driven process
  - ◆ Atrioventricular valves
    - ▶ The atrioventricular (AV) valves are located between the atria and ventricles
    - ▶ AV valves prevent blood backflow into the atria during ventricular contraction
    - ▶ There are two types of AV valves
      - • The tricuspid valve has three cusps and is located between the right atrium and the right ventricle
      - • The mitral (bicuspid) valve has two cusps and is located between the left atrium and the left ventricle
    - ▶ When the mitral and tricuspid valves close, the first heart sound (S_1) is produced

◆ Semilunar valves

  ❱ The semilunar valves have three main cuplike cusps that separate the ventricles from the aorta (aortic valve) and the pulmonary arteries (pulmonic valve)

  ❱ Semilunar valves open during ventricular systole

  ❱ When the aortic and pulmonic valves close, the second heart sound (S_2) is produced

■ Coronary blood supply

  ◆ Coronary veins

    ❱ The coronary veins return deoxygenated blood from the heart to the right atrium via the coronary sinus

    ❱ The thebesian veins empty deoxygenated blood into the right atrium and right ventricle; the great cardiac vein is the main left ventricle venous system; the small and middle cardiac veins form the coronary sinus, which drains the right atrium

  ◆ Coronary arteries

    ❱ The coronary arteries supply the heart with oxygenated blood

    ❱ They arise at the base of the aorta immediately after the aortic valve and run along the outside of the heart in natural grooves called sulci

    ❱ Branches of the main coronary arteries penetrate the muscular wall of the heart to nourish the endocardium

    ❱ During ventricular contraction, no blood flows to cardiac tissue

    ❱ Two major coronary arteries are found in the heart.

      • The right coronary artery supplies blood to the right atrium and right ventricle, the sinoatrial (SA) and AV nodes (in more than 50% of the population), the inferior wall of the left ventricle, the posterior wall of the septum, the posterior papillary muscle, and the posterior (inferior) division of the left bundle branch

        – Occlusion of the right coronary artery can result in posterior or inferior wall myocardial infarction (MI)

      • The left coronary artery branches into the left anterior descending artery and the circumflex artery

        – The left anterior descending coronary artery supplies blood to the anterior portion of the ventricle, the anterior papillary muscle, the anterior division of the septum, the anterior (superior) division of the left bundle branch, and the right bundle branch

        – The circumflex coronary artery supplies blood to the left atrium, posterior surfaces of the left ventricle, and the posterior aspect of the septum

        – Occlusion of the left coronary artery can result in anterior or lateral MI

■ Conduction system

  ◆ Definitions

    ❱ Excitability is the ability of a cell or tissue to depolarize in response to a given stimulus

    ❱ Conductivity is the ability of cardiac cells to transmit a stimulus from cell to cell

    ❱ Automaticity is the ability of certain cells to spontaneously depolarize (these cells have pacemaker potential)

◗ Rhythmicity is automaticity that's generated at a regular rate

◗ Contractility is the ability of the cardiac myofibrils to shorten in response to an electrical stimulus

◗ Refractoriness is the state of a cell or tissue during repolarization when the cell or tissue either can't depolarize (regardless of the intensity of the stimulus) or requires a much greater stimulus than normal

◆ Sinoatrial node

◗ The SA node is the natural pacemaker of the heart and has the highest degree of automaticity of all cardiac cells

◗ Located in the upper portion of the right atrium near the mouth of the superior vena cava, the SA node has an intrinsic rate of 60 to 100 beats/minute

◗ When the SA node depolarizes, atrial depolarization occurs by way of three internodal tracts that carry the electrical impulse from the SA node through the right atrium to the AV node; Bachmann's bundle carries the electrical impulse from the SA node to the left atrium

◆ Atrioventricular node

◗ The AV node is located posteriorly on the right side of the interatrial septum

◗ It conducts all electrical impulses from the atria to the ventricles; its intrinsic rate is 40 to 60 beats/minute

◗ The electrical impulse from the SA node depolarizes the AV node

◗ The AV node then slows conduction of the electrical impulse to allow for optimal ventricular filling from the atrial contraction; the delay is normally 0.04 second

◗ The AV node delay limits the number of impulses that are transmitted to the ventricles

◗ The AV node can also conduct impulses that are initiated in or below the AV node in a retrograde manner, as in junctional ectopic beats and ventricular ectopic beats

◆ Bundle of His

◗ The bundle of His conducts electrical impulses in the ventricles; its intrinsic rate is 40 to 60 beats/minute

◗ The bundle of His is divided into the right and left bundle branches

  • The right bundle branch continues down the right side of the interventricular septum toward the right apex; its conduction velocity is slower than that of the left bundle branch

  • The left bundle branch continues down the left side of the interventricular septum and divides into two branches: the anterior (superior) branch and the posterior (inferior) branch

◗ The Purkinje fibers are the smallest divisions of the right and left bundle branches; they have the fastest conduction velocity of all heart tissue, and their intrinsic rate is 15 to 40 beats/minute

❖ **Physiology**

■ Refractory period

◆ The absolute refractory period is the time during which the myocardium can't respond to even a strong stimulus

◆ The relative refractory period is the time during which the myocardium responds to a strong stimulus or a normal stimulus with delayed conduction
- Cardiac cycle
  ◆ Diastole
    ▶ Diastole is the period during which the chambers of the heart relax
    ▶ Electrical diastole is the resting phase of the electrical cardiac cycle
  ◆ Systole
    ▶ Systole, or ejection, is the period during which the chambers of the heart contract
    ▶ Systole begins as soon as the ventricles fill with blood
    ▶ As the systolic pressure rises, the AV valves are forced to close; this is the source of S_1
    ▶ When the ventricular pressure is greater than the aortic pressure, the semilunar valves open, and blood is ejected into the aorta and the pulmonary artery
    ▶ As the ejection phase ends, the ventricles relax and intraventricular pressure decreases, causing reversal of the blood flow in the aorta and forcing the semilunar valves to close (this is the source of S_2); the end of the ejection phase is reflected by a dicrotic notch on the aorta's pressure waveform (graphic representation of the cardiac cycle when an arterial line is used to monitor hemodynamic variables)
    ▶ Ventricular pressure falls quickly after the semilunar valves close; the atrial tracing on the central venous pressure (CVP) tracing shows a V wave, which denotes the period during which the ventricles relax and blood enters the atria
- Cardiac function
  ◆ Three internal factors influence heart function: preload, afterload, and contractility (see *Factors that influence cardiac workload*)
    ▶ Preload is the volume of blood in the left ventricle coupled with the ability of the ventricle to stretch at the end of diastole; if the intravascular volume exceeds the stretch limit, cardiac output diminishes
      • Preload is best measured hemodynamically by the pulmonary artery wedge pressure (PAWP) in the left side of the heart and the right atrial pressure (RAP) or CVP in the right side of the heart
      • Venous return, total blood volume, and atrial kick affect the volume aspect of preload; the stiffness and thickness of the cardiac muscle wall affect compliance of the ventricle
      • Preload is enhanced through volume administration of crystalloid, colloid, plasma expanders or blood products. It's decreased through the use of diuretics or vasodilators (nitroglycerin or morphine)
    ▶ Afterload is the ventricular wall tension or stress during systolic ejection
      • Afterload is best measured hemodynamically by the systemic vascular resistance in the left side of the heart and the pulmonary vascular resistance in the right side of the heart
      • Afterload is increased by factors that oppose ejection, such as arteriosclerotic disease, hypervolemia, and aortic stenosis

Factors that influence cardiac workload

Drugs, as well as certain conditions, can alter cardiac workload. The table below lists factors that increase and decrease cardiac workload. An alteration in the cardiac workload, in turn, influences stroke volume, stroke volume index, cardiac output, cardiac index, right ventricular stroke work index, and left ventricular stroke work index.

Factors that increase cardiac workload	Factors that decrease cardiac workload
Drugs (increased contractility)	*Drugs (decreased contractility)*
Milrinone	Atenolol
Digitoxin	Metoprolol
Digoxin	Nadolol
Dobutamine	Propranolol
Dopamine	Timolol
Epinephrine	
Isoproterenol	*Abnormal conditions*
	Heart failure
Abnormal conditions	Hypovolemia
Decreased vascular resistance	Increased vascular resistance
Hyperthermia	Myocardial infarction
Hypervolemia	Pulmonary emboli
Septic shock (early stages)	Septic shock (late stages)
	Hyperinflation of lungs
	Continuous positive airway pressure
	Mechanical ventilation
	Positive end-expiratory pressure

- Afterload is reduced through the correction of low preload or with vasodilating agents, such as sodium nitroprusside, morphine, or angiotensin-converting enzyme inhibitors
- Afterload is enhanced through administration of vasopressor agents (dopamine, epinephrine, norepinephrine)
▶ Contractility, or the heart's contractile force, can be increased by the Starling mechanism (in which the heart increases output by increasing preload) and the sympathetic nervous system; sympathomimetic and adrenergic medications can greatly affect contractility
- Contractility is decreased through administration of beta-blocking agents
◆ Heart rate is regulated by nervous control and intrinsic regulation
▶ Nervous control is divided into parasympathetic control and sympathetic control
- Parasympathetic fibers (in the vagus nerve) are concentrated near SA and AV conduction tissue; stimulation of these tissues causes bradycardia
- Sympathetic nerve fibers parallel the coronary circulation before penetrating the myocardium; stimulation of these fibers causes acceleration and increased contractility (known as the fight-or-flight response)

▶ Intrinsic regulation is produced by baroreceptors and chemoreceptors

- Baroreceptors, which are located in the carotid sinus and aortic arch, sense changes in pressure and activate the autonomic nervous system to raise or lower the heart rate accordingly
- Chemoreceptors, which are located in the bifurcation of the aortic arch, sense changes in oxygen tension, pH, and carbon dioxide tension; they trigger increases in respiratory rate and depth

❖ **Cardiovascular assessment**
■ Noninvasive assessment techniques
  ◆ Patient history
    ▶ The patient's presenting symptoms or complaints provide the starting point for obtaining his history
    ▶ The patient history should include the medical history, family history, current medications, and past diagnostic studies
  ◆ Physical examination
    ▶ Inspection focuses on the general appearance of the patient's face, extremities, neck, thorax, and abdomen
      - During the physical examination, note the patient's weight and whether he's overweight or underweight
      - Note the patient's skin color (pale or flushed) and body position; also observe for diaphoresis, confusion, and lethargy
      - Examine the patient's nails for cyanosis, clubbing, and splinter hemorrhages; assess the extremities for hair distribution, skin condition, skin color, varicosities, and edema
      - Check for distention of the external jugular vein by having the patient sit at a 30- to 45-degree angle; assess the fullness of the jugular vein at the end of exhalation
        − Fullness of more than 3 cm above the sternal angle is evidence of increased CVP
        − The higher the sitting angle of the patient when jugular vein distention is discovered, the higher the CVP
      - Assess for right-sided heart failure by checking the hepatojugular reflex
        − Observe the pulsation of the internal jugular vein as you press firmly over the right upper quadrant of the patient's abdomen for 30 seconds
        − The hepatojugular reflex test is considered positive if the amount of distention in the vein is more than 1 cm above baseline after the pressure is removed
      - Check the thorax and abdomen for scars, skeletal deformities, bruises, and wounds
      - Assess for the apical impulse (the point of maximal impulse [PMI]), normally at the fifth intercostal space just left of the midclavicular line in an adult
    ▶ Palpate to assess pulses, capillary refill, presence of edema, and skin temperature

---

Auscultation of the cardiovascular system

Although heart sounds may vary from patient to patient, the ones listed here are the most common. The heart sounds are grouped according to where they can best be heard.

Aortic area
- S_2 loud
- Aortic systolic murmur

Pulmonic area
- S_2 loud and split with inhalation
- Pulmonic valve murmurs

Erb's point
- S_2 split with inhalation
- Aortic diastolic murmur
- Pericardial friction rub

Tricuspid area
- S_1 split
- Right ventricular S_3 and S_4
- Tricuspid valve murmurs
- Murmur of ventricular septal defect

Mitral area
- S_1 loud
- Left ventricular S_3 and S_4
- Mitral valve murmurs

- Assess pulses separately and compare them bilaterally
  - Check the carotid, brachial, radial, ulnar, popliteal, dorsalis pedis, and posterior tibial pulses
  - Use Allen's test to assess adequate blood flow to the hand through the ulnar artery before the radial artery puncture (as in arterial blood gases [ABG] sample draws or insertion of an arterial line)
- To assess capillary refill (which measures arterial circulation to an extremity), compress the nail bed for a few seconds, then quickly release; normal color should return within 3 seconds
- To determine if pitting edema is present (a sign that fluid has accumulated in the extravascular space), press the patient's skin to the underlying bone
  - If an impression remains after pressure is removed, the patient has pitting edema
  - Measure the depth of pitting in millimeters
- Assess for thrombophlebitis using Homans' sign, in which the knee is flexed and the foot abruptly dorsiflexed
  - If the patient experiences pain in the popliteal region or calf, Homans' sign is positive
  - Homans' sign isn't as reliable in identifying thrombophlebitis as the observation of erythema, low-grade fever, edema, and pain in the extremity
- Palpate the PMI, which should be less than 2 cm in diameter
▶ Auscultate to measure blood pressure, detect bruits, and assess heart sounds (see *Auscultation of the cardiovascular system*)
- Listen for bruits (extracardiac, high-pitched "sh-sh" sounds) by placing the bell of the stethoscope over the carotid or femoral artery; the presence of a bruit indicates a tortuous or partially occluded vessel or increased blood flow through the vessel

- Assess heart sounds using the stethoscope
  - S_1 is produced by the rapid deceleration of blood flow when the AV valves close at the start of systole; the S_1 heart sound is best heard over the mitral and tricuspid areas
  - S_2 is produced by the closing of the semilunar valves at the end of systole; it's best heard over the aortic and pulmonic areas
  - S_3 is related to diastolic motion and rapid filling of the ventricles in early diastole; this soft, low-pitched sound is best heard at the apex of the heart; it's normal in patients under age 40 but signals heart failure in older adults
  - S_4 is heard at the end of diastole and is associated with atrial contraction; this soft, low-pitched sound is best heard at the apex of the heart; it's a pathologic condition produced by increased resistance to ventricular filling
  - Summation gallop is heard in mid-diastole and is associated with an S_3 and S_4 being present in tachycardia; this low-pitched sound is best heard at the apex of the heart
- Also listen for murmurs, such as prolonged or extra heart sounds during systole or diastole
  - Murmurs are caused by an increased rate of blood flow through cardiac structures, blood flowing across a partial obstruction or irregularity, shunting of blood through an abnormal passage from a high- to a low-pressure area, or blood backflow through an incompetent valve
  - New murmurs associated with an acute MI may be caused by papillary muscle dysfunction or rupture, ventricular septal defect, or ventricular rupture; these emergency situations may require surgical intervention
  - Assess for pericardial friction rub (a high-pitched sound) at Erb's point; this may occur secondary to pericarditis, following an MI, or after cardiac surgery; occasionally, it's the presenting symptom
  - ❿ Percussion isn't used in cardiovascular assessment
- ■ Noninvasive diagnostic testing
  - ◆ A standard 12-lead electrocardiogram (ECG) shows the heart's electrical activity at 12 locations: 6 on the chest and 6 on the limbs; in addition to detecting abnormal transmission of impulses, the 12-lead ECG provides information on the heart's axis (electrical position) and the size of the cardiac chambers
  - ◆ A Holter monitor is a portable device that produces a continuous ECG and may be used for 12, 24, or 48 hours
    - ❿ The Holter monitor is used to detect arrhythmias, evaluate effectiveness of antiarrhythmic medications, evaluate pacemaker function, and diagnose dizziness, syncope, palpitations, and episodes of chest pain
    - ❿ The patient keeps a diary of activities and symptoms while wearing the Holter monitor, which is correlated with the monitor's data
  - ◆ The exercise stress test evaluates the patient's cardiac response to physical stress; ECG activity, blood pressure, and physical symptoms are monitored during the test
  - ◆ Echocardiography is used to evaluate the internal structures and motions of the heart and great vessels

■ Invasive assessment techniques
  ◆ Cardiac catheterization and angiography are used to visualize the heart's chambers, valves, great vessels, and coronary arteries; these techniques are also useful for obtaining pressure measurements (right and left sides of the heart) to evaluate cardiac function and valve patency
    ❱ In right-sided cardiac catheterization, the catheter is inserted through the brachial or femoral vein; this allows for continuous hemodynamic monitoring, determination of right-side cardiac output and pressures, shunt studies, oximetry, and angiography (of the right atrium, right ventricle, tricuspid and pulmonic valves, and pulmonary artery)
    ❱ In left-sided cardiac catheterization, the catheter is inserted through the femoral or brachial artery; this allows visualization of the coronary arteries, aortic root, and left ventricle; determination of left-side aorta and heart chambers, shunt studies, and angiography (of left ventricular, mitral, and aortic function)
  ◆ Electrophysiologic studies evaluate the heart's electrical conduction system
  ◆ Hemodynamic monitoring requires placement of a multipurpose catheter in the right side of the heart, through the pulmonic valve and into the pulmonary artery (see *Hemodynamic values*, page 26, and *Normal PA waveforms*, page 27)
    ❱ These pressures are used to assess the patient's progress, monitor patient response to fluids and medications, and adjust medication dosages (see *Variations in hemodynamics*, page 28)
  ◆ Intra-arterial pressure monitoring, in which a catheter is placed in a major artery (usually the radial, femoral, or brachial) and connected to a transducer, allows continuous monitoring of blood pressure and provides ready access for arterial blood sampling (see *Troubleshooting hemodynamic monitoring*, page 29)
■ Normal laboratory values
  ◆ Sodium (Na^+): 135 to 145 mEq/L
  ◆ Potassium (K^+): 3.5 to 5.0 mEq/L
  ◆ Calcium (Ca^{+2}): 8.5 to 10.0 mg/dl
  ◆ Magnesium (Mg^{+2}): 1.5 to 2.5 mEq/L
  ◆ Chloride (Cl^-): 98 to 106 mg/dl
  ◆ Cardiac enzymes (see page 42-48)
■ ECG interpretation: components and common abnormalities
  ◆ A normal ECG waveform includes the P wave, PR interval, QRS complex, ST segment, J point, T wave, QT interval and, sometimes, the U wave
  ◆ The P wave is usually rounded, upright, and precedes each QRS complex; the P wave indicates atrial depolarization and impulse origination in the SA node, atria, or AV junctional tissue
    ❱ Peaked P waves are seen in right atrial hypertrophy
    ❱ Broad, notched P waves are seen in left atrial hypertrophy
    ❱ Inverted P waves may be caused by retrograde conduction from the AV node
    ❱ Varying P waves originate from various sites in the atrium wave junction

Hemodynamic values

Hemodynamic parameter	Method of measurement or calculation of value	Normal values
Mean arterial pressure (MAP) Average pressure in aorta during cardiac cycle	[blood pressure [BP] systolic + (BP diastolic $\times$ 2)] $\div$ 3	70 to 105 mm Hg
Cardiac output (CO) Volume of blood ejected from the heart in 1 minute	Measured by thermodilution	4 to 8 L/minute
Cardiac index (CI) Cardiac output indexed for body size	CO / BSA (body surface area)	2.5 to 4 L/minute/m^2
Stroke volume (SV) Volume of blood ejected from the heart with each contraction	CO / HR	60 to 100 ml/beat
Central venous pressure (CVP) or right atrial pressure (RAP) Pressure in right atrium; also indicative of venous return to the heart and preload	Measured at the proximal port of a pulmonary artery catheter	2 to 6 mm Hg
Pulmonary artery pressure (PAP) Pressure in the pulmonary artery with the balloon on the pulmonary artery catheter deflated; pulmonary artery diastolic (PAD) pressure reflects the left atrial pressure and left ventricular end diastolic pressure (LVEDP)	Measured at the distal port of a pulmonary artery catheter with the balloon deflated	PAS 15 to 30 mm Hg PAD 5 to 15 mm Hg
Pulmonary artery wedge pressure (PAWP) Pressure in the pulmonary artery with the balloon inflated; reflects left atrial pressure, LVEDP, and left ventricle preload; a better indicator than the PAP due to decreased blood flow around the catheter	Measured at the distal port of a pulmonary artery catheter with the balloon inflated	6 to 12 mm Hg
Systemic vascular resistance (SVR) The major factor that determines left ventricular afterload	[(MAP − CVP) $\times$ 80] $\div$ CO	900 to 1400 dynes/sec/cm^{-5}
Coronary artery perfusion pressure (CAPP) The pressure in the coronary arteries during diastole	Diastolic BP − PAWP	50 to 80 mm Hg

▶ When at least three different P-wave configurations are present, it's classified as a wandering atrial pacemaker

◆ The PR interval measures electrical activity from the start of atrial depolarization to the start of ventricular depolarization; the duration of the PR interval is normally 0.12 to 0.20 second (measured from the beginning of the P wave to the beginning of the QRS complex)

▶ A PR interval less than 0.12 second indicates that the electrical impulse originated in an area other than the SA node

Normal PA waveforms

During pulmonary artery catheter insertion, the waveforms on the monitor change as the catheter advances through the heart.

Right atrium

When the catheter tip enters the right atrium, the first heart chamber on its route, a waveform like the one shown below appears on the monitor. Note the two small upright waves. The *a* waves represent the right ventricular end-diastolic pressure; the *v* waves, right atrial filling.

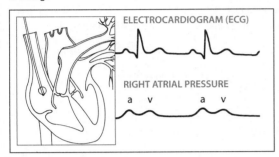

Right ventricle

As the catheter tip reaches the right ventricle, you'll see a waveform with sharp systolic upstrokes and lower diastolic dips, as shown below.

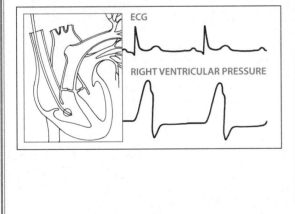

Pulmonary artery

The catheter then floats into the pulmonary artery, causing a pulmonary artery pressure (PAP) waveform such as the one shown below. Note that the upstroke is smoother than on the right ventricle waveform. The dicrotic notch indicates pulmonic valve closure.

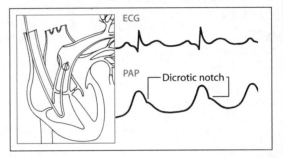

PAWP

Floating into a distal branch of the pulmonary artery, the balloon wedges where the vessel becomes too narrow for it to pass. The monitor now shows a pulmonary artery wedge pressure (PAWP) waveform, with two small upright waves, as shown below. The *a* wave represents left ventricular end-diastolic pressure; the *v* wave, left atrial filling. The balloon is then deflated, and the catheter is left in the pulmonary artery.

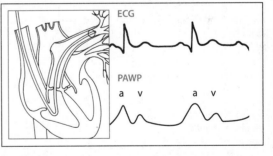

❚ A PR interval greater than 0.20 second indicates that the impulse is delayed as it passes through the AV node

◆ The QRS complex follows the PR interval and reflects ventricular depolarization

❚ The Q wave is the first negative deflection, the R wave is the first positive deflection, and the S wave is the negative deflection after the R wave; the duration of the QRS complex is normally 0.06 to 0.10 second (measured from the beginning of the Q wave to the end of the S wave)

Variations in hemodynamics

Parameter	Causes of increased values	Causes of decreased values
Central venous pressure	• Acute respiratory distress syndrome • Cardiac tamponade • Constrictive pericarditis • Mitral valve stenosis or regurgitation • Positive pressure ventilation • Pulmonary hypertension • Right-sided heart failure • Right ventricular infarction • Tricuspid stenosis or insufficiency • Volume overload	• Reduced circulating blood volume • Vasodilators • Vasodilation caused by shock
Pulmonary artery pressure	• Cardiac tamponade • Constrictive pericarditis • Hypoxia • Left-sided heart failure • Left ventricular failure • Mitral valve stenosis • Pulmonary hypertension • Positive pressure ventilation • Volume overload	• Reduced circulating blood volume • Vasodilation
Pulmonary artery wedge pressure	• Hypervolemia • Left-sided heart failure • Mitral valve stenosis or insufficiency • Pericardial tamponade • Positive pressure ventilation, especially when used with positive end-expiratory pressure • Severe aortic stenosis	• Reduced circulating blood volume • Vasodilators
Cardiac output	• Activation of the sympathetic nervous system (fight-or-flight) • Administration of exogenous catecholamines (dopamine, epinephrine) • Anemia • Early sepsis • Hyperthyroidism • Infection • Positive inotropes	• Decreased contractility • Excessively increased preload • Increased afterload • Increased or decreased heart rate

◗ A widened QRS complex (greater than 0.10 second) can occur when impulse conduction to one ventricle is slowed or when the impulse originates in the ventricles

◗ QRS complexes of varying size and shape may indicate the occurrence of ectopic or aberrantly conducted impulses

◗ A missing QRS complex may denote a block or complete ventricular standstill

◆ The ST segment measures the end of ventricular depolarization and the beginning of ventricular repolarization; it extends from the end of the S wave to the beginning of the T wave; a normal ST segment usually is isoelectric and doesn't vary more than 1 mm

Troubleshooting hemodynamic monitoring

This chart reviews common hemodynamic pressure monitoring problems, their possible causes, and appropriate interventions.

Problem	Possible causes	Interventions
Line fails to flush	• Stopcocks positioned incorrectly	• Make sure the stopcocks are positioned correctly.
	• Inadequate pressure from pressure bag	• Make sure the pressure bag gauge reads 300 mm Hg and the infusion bag isn't empty.
	• Kink in pressure tubing	• Check pressure tubing for kinks.
	• Blood clot in catheter	• Attempt to aspirate clot with a syringe. If the line still won't flush, notify the physician and prepare to replace the line.
Damped waveform	• Air bubbles	• Secure all connections. • Remove air from the lines and the transducer. • Check for and replace cracked equipment.
	• Blood clot in catheter	• Refer to "Line fails to flush" (above).
	• Blood flashback in line	• Make sure stopcock positions are correct; tighten loose connections and replace cracked equipment; flush the line with the fast-flush valve.
	• Incorrect transducer position	• Make sure the transducer is at the level of the right atrium at all times. Improper levels give false-high or false-low pressure readings.
	• Arterial catheter out of blood vessel or pressed against vessel wall	• Reposition the catheter if it's against the vessel wall. • Try to aspirate blood to confirm proper placement in the vessel. If unable to aspirate blood, notify the physician.
Pulmonary artery wedge pressure tracing unobtainable	• Ruptured balloon	• If there is no resistance when injecting air or if blood is leaking from the balloon inflation lumen, stop injecting air and notify the physician. If the catheter is left in, label the inflation lumen with a warning not to inflate.
	• Incorrect amount of air in balloon	• Deflate the balloon. Check the label on the catheter for correct volume. Reinflate slowly with the correct amount. To avoid rupturing the balloon, never use more than the stated volume.
	• Catheter malpositioned	• Notify the physician. Obtain a chest X-ray.

▶ An ST-segment elevation of 2 mm or more above the baseline value may indicate myocardial injury

▶ ST-segment depression may indicate myocardial injury or ischemia

▶ ST-segment changes may occur in patients with pericarditis, myocarditis, left ventricular hypertrophy, pulmonary embolism, or electrolyte disturbances

Normal sinus rhythm

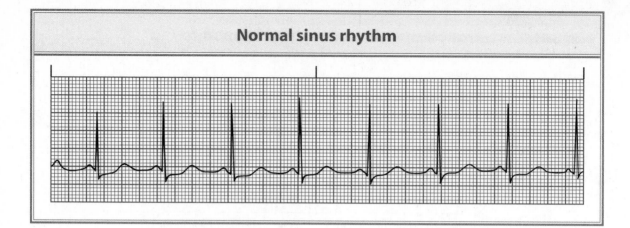

◆ The J point marks the end of the QRS complex and the beginning of the ST segment; it's important in determining ST-segment elevation or depression

◆ The T wave follows the S wave; typically rounded and smooth, the T wave reflects ventricular repolarization

▶ The T wave usually is positive in leads I, II, V_3, V_4, V_5, and V_6

▶ Inverted T waves in leads I, II, V_3, V_4, V_5, or V_6 may indicate myocardial ischemia

▶ Peaked T waves commonly occur in patients with hyperkalemia

▶ Heavily notched T waves may indicate pericarditis in adult patients

▶ Variations in T-wave amplitude may result from an electrolyte imbalance

◆ The QT interval represents the time needed for ventricular depolarization and repolarization; the duration of the QT interval normally is 0.36 to 0.44 second (measured from the beginning of the QRS complex to the end of the T wave)

▶ A prolonged QT interval indicates a prolonged relative refractory period, which may be caused by certain medications or may be congenital

▶ A shortened QT interval may be caused by hypercalcemia or digoxin toxicity

◆ The U wave reflects repolarization of the His-Purkinje system; when present, the U wave follows the T wave and appears as an upright deflection

▶ A prominent U wave may occur in patients with hypokalemia

▶ An inverted U wave may occur in patients with heart disease

■ Normal sinus rhythm

◆ A normal sinus rhythm is the most common rhythm seen on an ECG strip (for a sample ECG rhythm strip, see *Normal sinus rhythm*)

◆ In a normal sinus rhythm, the atrial and ventricular rhythms are regular, and rates are 60 to 100 beats/minute

◆ The P waves are normal, upright, and similar to one another; there's one P wave for each QRS complex

◆ The T waves are normal, and the PR interval, QRS complex, and QT interval are within normal limits

Sinus bradycardia

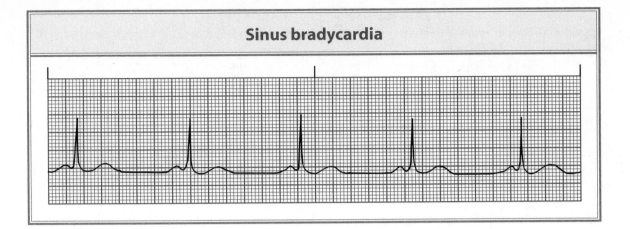

- ◆ No ectopic or aberrantly conducted beats are present
- ■ Step-by-step ECG analysis
  - ◆ Determine the rhythm (regular or irregular)
  - ◆ Determine the rate
  - ◆ Evaluate the P wave
  - ◆ Determine the duration of the PR interval
  - ◆ Determine the duration of the QRS complex
  - ◆ Evaluate the T wave
  - ◆ Determine the duration of the QT interval
  - ◆ Evaluate the other components of the ECG
  - ◆ Consider the clinical significance

- ❖ Arrhythmias
  - ■ Sinus bradycardia
    - ◆ Description
      - ▶ Sinus rhythm, but a rate of less than 60 beats/minute (for a sample ECG strip, see *Sinus bradycardia*)
    - ◆ Clinical signs and symptoms of low cardiac output may be present (hypotension; chest pain; decreased mental status; cool, clammy skin; shortness of breath)
    - ◆ Medical management
      - ▶ Recognize it may be normal during sleep or in athletes
      - ▶ Correct the underlying cause, such as drug toxicity, excess vagal tone, or SA or AV node ischemia
      - ▶ Administer oxygen and prepare for external pacemaker if patient is symptomatic; administer I.V. atropine while waiting for pacing to begin
    - ◆ Nursing management
      - ▶ Assess the patient for signs of low cardiac output and ECG changes
      - ▶ Administer medications as prescribed
  - ■ Sinus tachycardia
    - ◆ Description
      - ▶ Sinus rhythm, but a rate of 100 to 160 beats/minute (for a sample ECG rhythm strip, see *Sinus tachycardia*, page 32)

Sinus tachycardia

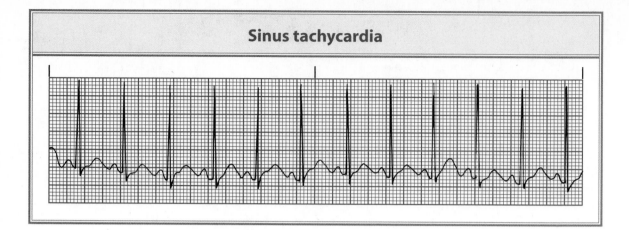

- ◆ Clinical signs and symptoms of low cardiac output may be present at higher rates
- ◆ Medical management
  - ▶ Manage the underlying cause, such as pain, anxiety, exercise, stimulants (caffeine or nicotine), pharmacologic agents, or a compensatory response to other physiologic stressors
  - ▶ Administer oxygen
- ◆ Nursing management
  - ▶ Assess the patient for signs of low cardiac output and ECG changes
  - ▶ Administer medications as prescribed
- ■ Sinus arrest
  - ◆ Description
    - ▶ In sinus arrest, the sinus node fails to generate an impulse and an entire PQRST complex is missing. In contrast, sinus block occurs when the sinus node fires and depolarizes the atria, but the impulse is blocked, resulting in a missing QRST (for a sample ECG rhythm strip, see *Sinus arrest*)
  - ◆ Clinical signs and symptoms of low cardiac output may be present, depending on the number and length of pauses
  - ◆ Medical management

Sinus arrest

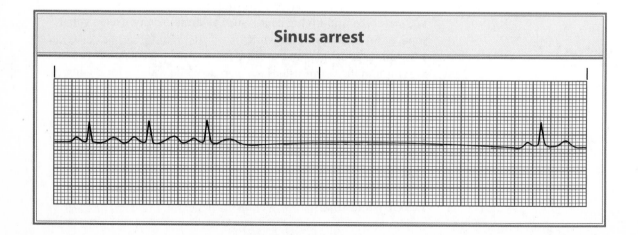

Premature atrial complexes

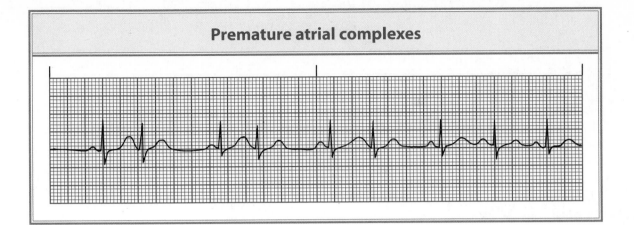

> ▶ Correct the underlying cause, such as drug toxicity, excess vagal tone, SA node ischemia, or sick sinus syndrome

> ▶ Administer oxygen and I.V. atropine if symptomatic; anticipate the potential need for temporary or permanent pacing

- ◆ Nursing management
  - ▶ Assess the patient for signs of low cardiac output and ECG changes
  - ▶ Administer medications as prescribed
- ■ Premature atrial complexes
  - ◆ Description
    - ▶ A premature atrial complex is initiated by irritable atrial tissue, usually not resulting in signs and symptoms, and often normal in some individuals
  - ◆ ECG recognition
    - ▶ The underlying sinus rhythm is interrupted by a premature complex with a nonsinus P wave and a normal QRS (for a sample ECG rhythm strip, see *Premature atrial complexes*)
  - ◆ Medical management
    - ▶ Correct the underlying cause of the irritable atrial tissue, such as ingestion of stimulants, exercise, or postcardiac surgery
    - ▶ Prophylactic treatment with digoxin may be advised in some patients such as postcardiac surgery patients who are at high risk of progression to atrial flutter or atrial fibrillation
  - ◆ Nursing management
    - ▶ Assess the patient for signs of low cardiac output and ECG changes
    - ▶ Administer medications as prescribed
- ■ Atrial tachycardia
  - ◆ Description
    - ▶ Atrial tachycardia (supraventricular tachycardia [SVT]) is a tachycardic rhythm originating above the ventricles; atrial rates run 150 to 250 beats/minute, resulting in shortened diastole, loss of atrial kick, reduced cardiac output, reduced coronary perfusion, and ischemic myocardial changes
  - ◆ ECG recognition
    - ▶ Absent P waves (hidden in T waves); regular, rapid rhythm with rate of 160 to 250 beats/minute; and a narrow QRS; the rapid rate may

Atrial tachycardia

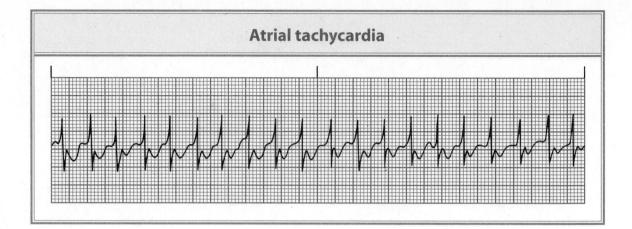

occur regularly or paroxysmally and may result from one irritable focus or multiple foci (for a sample ECG rhythm strip, see *Atrial tachycardia*)

◆ Clinical signs and symptoms depend on the rate and resulting cardiac compromise

◆ Medical management

▶ Correction of the underlying condition that causes atrial tachycardia, such as digoxin toxicity, MI, cardiomyopathy, congenital anomalies, Wolff-Parkinson-White syndrome, valvular heart disease, cor pulmonale, hyperthyroidism, or systemic hypertension

▶ Obtain a 12-lead ECG for differential diagnosis of SVT

▶ If the patient is asymptomatic, consider vagal maneuvers (forceful cough, Valsalva's maneuver, stimulation of dive reflex, carotid sinus massage) or medications, such as adenosine or calcium channel blockers

▶ If the patient has severe symptoms of decreased cardiac output, consider immediate sedation and cardioversion

▶ If the patient doesn't respond to medications or has recurring episodes, radiofrequency ablation may be used to destroy the focus of the arrhythmia or block the conduction pathway

◆ Nursing management

▶ Assess the patient for signs of low cardiac output and ECG changes

▶ Monitor for signs of digoxin toxicity

▶ As vagal maneuvers may result in bradycardia, ventricular arrhythmias, and asystole, keep resuscitative equipment readily available

■ Atrial flutter

◆ Description

▶ Ectopic atrial focus firing 250 to 350 times/minute; AV node should filter out impulses to control ventricular rate

◆ ECG recognition

▶ "Sawtoothed" flutter waves that march throughout rhythm, absence of P waves, no PR interval, normal QRS, and either regular or irregular ventricular rhythm (for a sample ECG rhythm strip, see *Atrial flutter*)

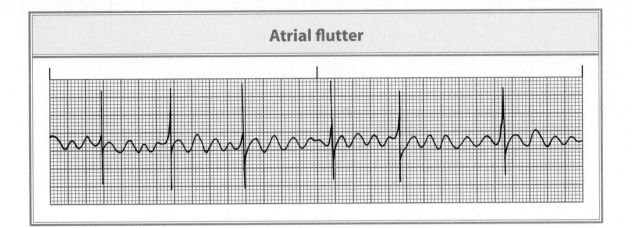

Atrial flutter

◆ Clinical signs and symptoms are dependent primarily upon ventricular rate. As the rate increases, the patient may have signs of low cardiac output
◆ Medical management
  ▶ Correct the underlying cause of the irritable atrial tissue
  ▶ Control the rate with medications, such as digoxin, or calcium channel blockers
  ▶ Convert rhythm through medications or synchronized cardioversion
◆ Nursing management
  ▶ Assess the patient for signs of low cardiac output and ECG changes
  ▶ Administer medications as prescribed
■ Atrial fibrillation
  ◆ Description
    ▶ Multiple irritable ectopic atrial foci firing 350 to 800 times/minute. AV node should filter out impulses to control the ventricular rate
  ◆ ECG recognition
    ▶ No P waves, no PR interval, irregular ventricular rhythm, normal QRS, and sometimes a wavy baseline (for a sample ECG rhythm strip, see *Atrial fibrillation*)
  ◆ Clinical signs and symptoms are dependent upon the ventricular rate

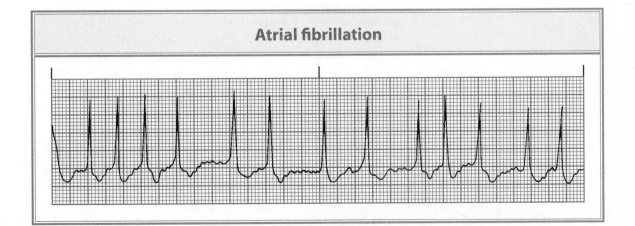

Atrial fibrillation

Premature ventricular contractions

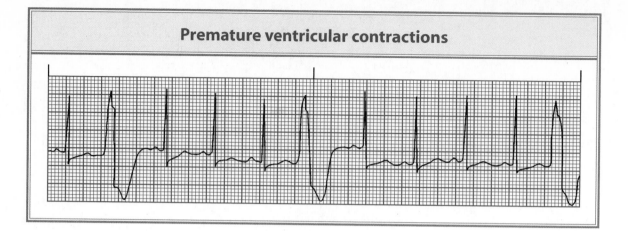

▶ At either rate extreme, the patient may exhibit signs of low cardiac output
◆ Medical management
  ▶ Correct the underlying cause of the irritable atrial tissue
  ▶ Control the rate with medications, such as digoxin, calcium channel blockers, or beta-adrenergic blockers
  ▶ Convert rhythm through medications or synchronized cardioversion
  ▶ Consider anticoagulation for long-term atrial fibrillation to prevent clot formation and embolization
◆ Nursing management
  ▶ Assess the patient for signs of low cardiac output and ECG changes
  ▶ Monitor serum drug levels, and assess for toxicity
  ▶ Provide patient education regarding anticoagulation for those on long-term therapy
■ Premature ventricular contractions
◆ Description
  ▶ Premature ventricular contractions (PVCs) can occur in healthy and diseased hearts; they may occur singly or in pairs, on every second beat (bigeminy), on every third beat (trigeminy), or on the T wave (the R-on-T phenomenon). For a sample ECG rhythm strip, see *Premature ventricular contractions*)
  ▶ PVCs signal danger when two or more occur in a row, if they occur in bigeminy, when they are multiform, or when the R-on-T phenomenon is present
  ▶ PVCs result from the firing of an ectopic focus in the ventricle, which causes the QRS complex to occur early
    • In a patient with PVCs, the duration of the QRS complex is greater than 0.12 second; the configuration is bizarre and usually followed by a compensatory pause
    • The T wave is usually deflected in the opposite direction of the QRS complex
    • Uniform (unifocal) PVCs look alike and originate from the same ectopic focus
  ▶ PVCs may result from drug administration (such as cardiac glycosides and sympathomimetic agents), electrolyte imbalances (hypoka-

lemia and hypocalcemia), stimulants (exercise, caffeine, or tobacco), or other factors (alcohol, hypercapnia, hypoxia, myocardial ischemia, or myocardial irritation by pacemaker electrodes or central venous catheters)
- ◆ Clinical signs and symptoms
  - ❱ Irregular pulse during PVCs
  - ❱ Complaints of palpitations
  - ❱ Hypotension, syncope, and blurred vision if decreased cardiac output is uncompensated
- ◆ Medical management
  - ❱ Correct the underlying cause
  - ❱ Administer I.V. amiodarone or lidocaine if the patient has an underlying cardiac problem
  - ❱ Administer I.V. atropine for symptomatic bradycardia
- ◆ Nursing management
  - ❱ Assess the patient's level of consciousness (LOC), ECG changes, heart rate, and blood pressure; changes in clinical status may indicate low cardiac output
  - ❱ Maintain continuous ECG monitoring to identify arrhythmias
  - ❱ Administer antiarrhythmic medications as prescribed, and monitor the patient's response to maintain therapeutic drug levels and prevent toxicity
  - ❱ Administer oxygen as prescribed for hypoxia to prevent myocardial ischemia and life-threatening arrhythmias
  - ❱ If a life-threatening arrhythmia occurs, initiate prompt treatment, including cardiopulmonary resuscitation (CPR), defibrillation, I.V. drug therapy, and preparation for pacemaker insertion
  - ❱ Maintain a patent I.V. line to ensure access if emergency medications must be given
- ■ Idioventricular rhythm
  - ◆ Description
    - ❱ Bradycardic rhythm originating in the ventricle
    - ❱ ECG recognition: no P waves, no PR interval, regular ventricular rhythm with wide QRS complexes, rate of 20 to 40 beats/minute (for a sample ECG rhythm strip, see *Idioventricular rhythm*)

Idioventricular rhythm

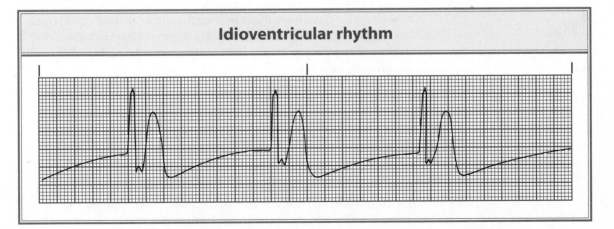

Ventricular tachycardia

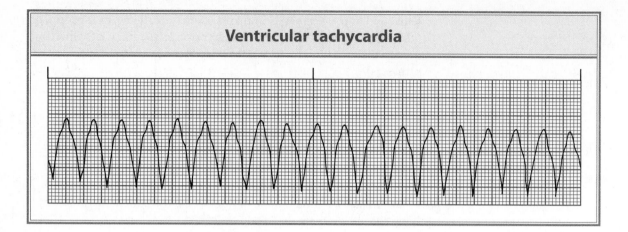

- ◆ Signs and symptoms of low cardiac output are typically present
- ◆ Medical management
  - ▶ Administer oxygen and I.V. atropine if symptomatic
  - ▶ Anticipate potential need for temporary or permanent pacing
  - ▶ Prepare for emergency resuscitative efforts if rhythm doesn't produce pressure of at least 60 mm Hg systolic
- ◆ Nursing management
  - ▶ Assess the patient for signs of low cardiac output and ECG changes
  - ▶ Apply a transcutaneous pacemaker as necessary
  - ▶ Administer medications as prescribed
- ■ Ventricular tachycardia
  - ◆ Description
    - ▶ Ventricular tachycardia is the occurrence of three or more PVCs in a row with a ventricular rate of more than 100 beats/minute; it can be paroxysmal or sustained (for a sample ECG rhythm strip, see *Ventricular tachycardia*)
    - ▶ A rapid ventricular rate without the atrial kick reduces the effective ventricular filling time and decreases cardiac output
    - ▶ Ventricular tachycardia is usually caused by myocardial irritability related to cardiac conditions, including acute MI, coronary artery disease, rheumatic heart disease, mitral valve prolapse, heart failure, and cardiomyopathy; it may also result from the R-on-T phenomenon
    - ▶ Noncardiac conditions that can trigger ventricular tachycardia include pulmonary embolism, hypokalemia, severe hypoxemia, and drug toxicity resulting from digoxin, procainamide, quinidine, or epinephrine therapy
  - ◆ Clinical signs and symptoms
    - ▶ Nonpalpable pulse or palpable with a fast rate
    - ▶ No symptoms or mild symptoms if cardiac output is compensated
    - ▶ Signs and symptoms of decreased cardiac output, and unresponsiveness
  - ◆ Medical and nursing management
    - ▶ Treat the underlying cause
    - ▶ If the patient is conscious and stable, administer amiodarone; if drugs are ineffective, synchronized cardioversion may be necessary

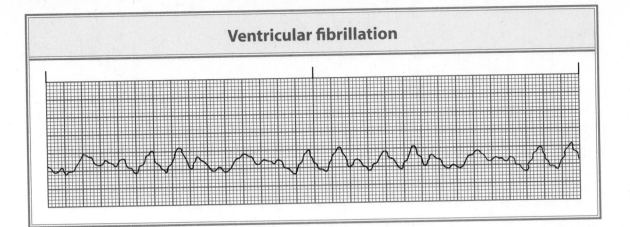

Ventricular fibrillation

▶ If the patient has no pulse, defibrillate once and initiate CPR; initiate CPR if a defibrillator isn't immediately available

■ Ventricular fibrillation
  ◆ Description
    ▶ Ventricular fibrillation is characterized by coarse fibrillating waves on the ECG, which indicate increased electrical activity (for a sample ECG rhythm strip, see *Ventricular fibrillation*); coarse fibrillating waves are easier to convert to a normal sinus rhythm than fine fibrillating waves, which indicate acidosis and hypoxemia
    ▶ During ventricular fibrillation, ventricular muscle fibers rapidly depolarize in a disorganized way; because the ventricles quiver rather than contract, cardiac output is nonexistent
    ▶ Ventricular fibrillation is caused by ischemia secondary to acute MI, untreated ventricular tachycardia, the R-on-T phenomenon, hypokalemia, hyperkalemia, hypercalcemia, severe hypoxemia, acid-base imbalances, epinephrine or quinidine toxicity, electric shock, or hypothermia
  ◆ Clinical signs and symptoms
    ▶ Pulselessness and unresponsiveness
    ▶ Complete cardiopulmonary arrest
  ◆ Medical and nursing management
    ▶ Initiate and continue CPR until a defibrillator is available, as defibrillation is the only definitive treatment
    ▶ Administer epinephrine or one dose of vasopressin and continue CPR
    ▶ Administer antiarrhythmic medications (such as amiodarone, lidocaine, or magnesium)
    ▶ An implanted cardioverter-defibrillator (ICD) may be placed for patients with recurring episodes of ventricular tachycardia or ventricular fibrillation (An ICD is used to interrupt ventricular tachycardia or provide a high energy shock to terminate ventricular fibrillation and return the heart to its normal rhythm)
■ Asystole
  ◆ Description

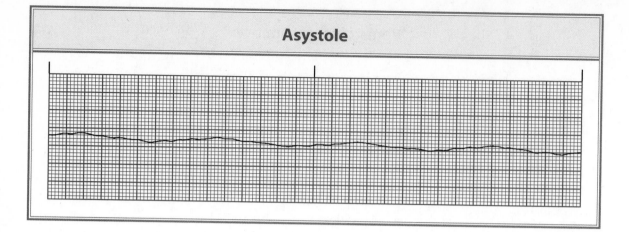

Asystole

- In asystole, there's no electrical activity in the ventricles, no cardiac output, and the ECG shows a flat line; however, if P waves are present on an ECG, it's called ventricular standstill (for a sample ECG rhythm strip, see *Asystole*)
- Asystole can be triggered by any condition that causes inadequate blood flow (such as pulmonary embolism, air embolism, or hemorrhage) or ineffective cardiac contractility (such as heart failure, heart rupture, MI, or cardiac tamponade)
- It can also result from insufficient conduction caused by hypoxemia, hypokalemia, severe acidosis, electric shock, ventricular arrhythmias, AV block, or cocaine overdose and from pulseless electrical activity (separation of the heart's electrical and mechanical activities in which evidence of electrical activity is seen on the monitor but a pulse or blood pressure can't be obtained)
  - ◆ Clinical signs and symptoms
    - Pulseless electrical activity and unresponsiveness
    - Complete cardiopulmonary arrest
  - ◆ Medical and nursing management
    - Check for absence of rhythm in a minimum of two ECG leads
    - Initiate CPR
    - Administer epinephrine (or one dose of vasopressin) and atropine
    - Consider cardiac pacing

❖ **Acute myocardial infarction**
  - ■ Description
    - ◆ An acute MI is a form of acute coronary syndrome that produces zones of infarction, ischemia, and injury (see *Telltale ECG findings: The three I's of an acute MI*)
    - ◆ An infarction is an area of cell death and muscle necrosis
      - Evidence of infarction on the ECG is seen by pathologic Q waves (the Q wave is wider than 0.04 second and its height is between one-fourth and one-third the height of the R wave), which reflect the inability of the dead tissue to depolarize
      - As healing occurs, the necrotic cells are replaced by scar tissue
    - ◆ Injured tissue surrounds the infarcted zone

Telltale ECG findings: The three I's of an acute MI

Ischemia, injury, and infarction (the three I's of an acute myocardial infarction) produce characteristic electrocardiogram (ECG) changes.

Ischemia temporarily interrupts blood supply to myocardial tissue but generally doesn't cause cell death. ECG changes: T-wave inversion resulting from altered tissue repolarization. (See top waveforms.)

Injury results from prolonged blood supply interruption, causing further cell injury. ECG changes: elevated ST segment resulting from altered depolarization. Consider an elevation greater than 1 mm significant. (See middle waveforms.)

Infarction ensues from complete lack of blood flow to the cell, causing myocardial cell death (necrosis). ECG changes: pathologic Q wave resulting from abnormal depolarization or from scar tissue that can't depolarize. Look for Q-wave duration of 0.04 second or longer or an amplitude measuring at least one-third of the QRS complex. (See bottom waveforms.)

CHANGES ON THE OPPOSITE SIDE
(RECIPROCAL CHANGES)

CHANGES ON THE DAMAGED SIDE

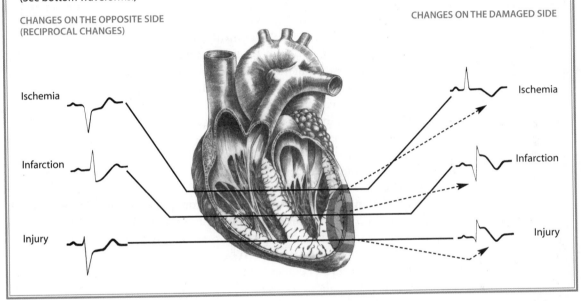

Ischemia

Infarction

Injury

Ischemia

Infarction

Injury

▶ Injured cells don't completely repolarize due to deficient blood supply

▶ An area of injury is recorded on the ECG as an elevated ST segment

◆ Ischemia, an area consisting of viable cells, surrounds the injured zone

▶ Repolarization in the ischemic area is impaired but eventually returns to normal

▶ An area of ischemia is recorded on the ECG as a T-wave inversion

▶ An ischemic zone is the point of origin of many arrhythmias associated with acute MI that are caused by impaired repolarization

■ Classification

◆ A transmural acute MI affects all three muscle layers of the heart and is associated with a higher incidence of left ventricular dysfunction

▶ During depolarization, the ECG typically shows the appearance of new Q waves

▶ In the acute phase of repolarization, the ST segment is elevated in the leads overlying the involved surface, with reciprocal ST changes in the leads overlying the surface opposite the involved site

◆ A subendocardial acute MI affects the endocardium and myocardium

> ◗ It's the most common nontransmural infarction
> ◗ The ECG shows ST-segment depression and T-wave inversion

■ Location

◆ The location and extent of damage caused by an acute MI depends on the site and severity of coronary artery narrowing; the presence, site, and severity of coronary artery spasm; the size of the vascular bed perfused by the compromised vessels; the extent of the collateral blood vessels; and the oxygen needs of the poorly perfused myocardium (see *Identifying the myocardial infarction damage site*, page 43)

◆ Anterior wall infarctions are classified as true anterior, anteroseptal, or anterolateral

> ◗ A true anterior infarction results from occlusion of the left anterior descending coronary artery, resulting in serious left ventricular dysfunction; ECG changes include loss of positive R-wave progression in leads V_1 through V_6, ST-segment elevation in leads V_1 through V_4, and T-wave inversion in leads I, aV_L, and V_3 through V_5
> ◗ An anteroseptal infarction results from occlusion of the left anterior descending coronary artery, resulting in serious left ventricular dysfunction; ECG changes include loss of R-wave progression in leads V_1 and V_2, the presence of Q waves in leads V_2 through V_4, and ST-segment elevation and T-wave inversion (usually without reciprocal changes) in leads V_4 and V_5
> ◗ An anterolateral infarction results from occlusion of the circumflex coronary artery; ECG changes include the presence of Q waves, ST-segment changes, and T-wave changes in leads I, aV_L, and V_4 through V_6 as well as reciprocal changes in leads I and aV_L

◆ Inferior wall infarctions result from occlusion of the right coronary artery; ECG changes include ST-segment elevation in leads II, III, and aV_F; reciprocal ST-segment depression in leads I and aV_L; and abnormal Q waves in leads II, III, and aV_F

◆ Posterior wall infarctions result from occlusion of the right coronary artery or circumflex branch of the left coronary artery; ECG changes include tall R waves and ST-segment depression in leads V_1 and V_2

■ Clinical signs and symptoms

◆ Prolonged, severe chest pain lasting 30 minutes or more and usually located in the substernal or left precordial area

> ◗ The patient may describe the pain as a heaviness or tightness
> ◗ The pain may radiate to the back, jaw, neck, or left arm and isn't relieved by rest or nitrates

◆ Changes in cardiac enzyme levels, especially creatine kinase (CK)

> ◗ CK, a sensitive indicator of acute MI, can be detected 4 hours after an acute MI occurs, peaks at 12 to 24 hours, and returns to the baseline value in 72 to 96 hours; the CK-MB isoenzyme is specific to cardiac tissue

◆ Changes in cardiac biomarker levels

> ◗ Myoglobin, a serum biomarker, rises 2 to 3 hours after myocardial damage, peaks at 6 to 9 hours, and returns to the baseline value in about 12 hours

Identifying the myocardial infarction damage site

Use this chart to identify the location of myocardial infarction damage. Remember that myocardial damage may spread to other areas.

Wall affected	Leads	Possible coronary artery involved	Possible reciprocal changes
Anterior	V_1, V_2, V_3, V_4	Left coronary artery, left anterior descending artery	II, III, aV_F
Anterolateral	$V_1, V_2, V_3, V_4, V_5, V_6$	Left anterior descending artery, circumflex artery	II, III, aV_F
Anteroseptal	V_1, V_2, V_3	Left anterior descending artery	None
Inferior	II, III, aV_F	Right coronary artery	I, aV_L
Lateral	I, aV_L	Circumflex artery, branch of left anterior descending artery	V_1, V_3
Posterior	V_1, V_2	Right coronary artery, circumflex artery	V_1, V_2, V_3, V_4 (R greater than S in V_1 and V_2, ST-segment depression, elevated T wave)
Right ventricular	V_{4r} to V_{6r}	Right coronary artery	None

▶ Troponin T and Troponin I serum biomarkers rise 4 to 6 hours after myocardial damage, peak at 10 to 24 hours, and return to normal values in 10 to 15 days

▶ Ischemia modified albumin rises within 6 to 10 minutes of myocardial ischemia and returns to baseline 6 to 12 hours after the ischemic event stops

■ Medical management

◆ Relieve pain with morphine sulfate (morphine also decreases anxiety, restlessness, autonomic nervous system activity, and cardiac preload)

◆ Administer I.V. beta-blocking drugs to reduce infarct size and decrease mortality

◆ Unless contraindicated, initiate thrombolytic therapy during the early stage of an acute MI (0 to 6 hours after onset of chest pain) to prevent or limit myocardial necrosis

◆ Consider a revascularization procedure (see *Cardiac procedures*, page 44)

▶ Coronary angioplasty—balloon dilation of the coronary artery

▶ Coronary stenting—expandable metal mesh is introduced into the coronary artery to expand the lumen size and prevent acute closure or restenosis

▶ Coronary atherectomy—excision and removal of plaque through cutting, shaving, or grinding

▶ Coronary artery bypass grafting—saphenous vein grafts on internal mammary artery grafting to bypass the occluded area of the vessel

Cardiac procedures

Procedure	Indications	Key assessments	Complications	Nursing management
Coronary artery bypass graft	• Severe angina from atherosclerosis • Coronary artery disease (CAD) with high risk of myocardial infarction (MI)	• Vital signs • Hemodynamics • Electrocardiogram (ECG) • Electrolytes • Complete blood count • Intake and output • Pain • Neurologic status • Incision	• Cerebral or myocardial infarct • Hemorrhage • Cardiac tamponade • Arrhythmias • Hemodynamic instability	• Control pain • Monitor hemodynamics • Administer medications to increase cardiac output and decrease myocardial oxygen consumption (dopamine, dobutamine, nitroglycerin) • Monitor for hemorrhage (chest tube drainage, perfusion); administer I.V. fluids and blood products if needed • Monitor ECG for onset of arrhythmias and blocks • Monitor and replace electrolytes
Valve replacement (mitral, pulmonic, or aortic)	• Stenosis, insufficiency, or regurgitation of one of the cardiac valves	• Same as above	• Same as above	• Same as above with increased monitoring for development of arrhythmias and blocks
Percutaneous coronary interventions (includes coronary angioplasty and coronary artery stent placement)	• Angina • Acute MI • Nonoperative CAD	• Vital signs • ECG • Catheter insertion site • Affected limb for perfusion	• Coronary artery dissection • Arrhythmias • Hematoma formation at catheter insertion site • Pseudoaneurysm formation • Retroperitoneal bleeding • Acute reocclusion	• Monitor catheter insertion site for bleeding or hematoma • Monitor ECG • Keep affected limb immobile per practitioner instructions (usually 2 to 8 hours) • Administer antiplatelet drugs as ordered • Control pain • Monitor affected limb for perfusion • Administer I.V. fluids to flush out dye

◆ Administer oxygen for 24 to 48 hours to prevent or treat hypoxia
◆ Maintain continuous cardiac monitoring to detect ventricular arrhythmias
◆ Maintain the patient on bed rest with bedside commode privileges
◆ Administer stool softeners and antiplatelet agents
◆ Administer nitroglycerin to dilate coronary arteries and to reduce afterload, workload of the heart, and chest pain
■ Nursing management
◆ Assess the patient's chest pain on a scale of 1 to 10; note its type, location, and duration as well as precipitating events and relieving factors
◆ Administer medication, as prescribed, and assess the patient's response to pain medication

◆ Be prepared to initiate thrombolytic therapy; because 85% of coronary artery occlusions are caused by a blood clot, initiating thrombolytic treatment (to reestablish perfusion) within 4 to 6 hours after onset of chest pain can significantly reduce mortality

◆ Maintain a patent I.V. line to ensure access if emergency medications need to be given

◆ Monitor the patient's use of oxygen for the first 24 to 48 hours, as prescribed; oxygen therapy is used to prevent and treat hypoxia; the nasal cannula commonly isn't worn properly by the patient

◆ Maintain continuous cardiac monitoring, especially in the leads showing ST-segment elevation and depression, to detect ventricular arrhythmias and to monitor ST-segment status in the leads that reflect the affected area of heart

◆ Explain to the patient that bed rest decreases the heart's workload and myocardial oxygen consumption

◆ Make the patient as comfortable as possible; tell him to avoid using the knee gatch on the bed and crossing his legs in bed (these actions slow venous return and increase the risk of thrombus formation)

◆ Assess for normal bowel habits, and administer stool softeners, as prescribed, to decrease the risk of constipation and straining; if possible, maintain the patient's normal bowel regimen

◆ Administer anticoagulants, as prescribed, to decrease the incidence of embolic complications; monitor the patient, as needed, to assess the effectiveness of therapy

◆ Monitor prothrombin time (PT); normal PT is 11 to 12.5 seconds, and the therapeutic range is 1.5 to 2 times the normal range

  ▶ Monitor partial thromboplastin time (PTT); notify the practitioner if it isn't within the normal range (35 to 45 seconds)

  ▶ Monitor the International Normalized Ratio (INR); the recommended INR target range for a patient on warfarin is 2.5 to 3.5

◆ Unless contraindicated, administer antiplatelet agents, as prescribed, to decrease platelet aggregation

◆ Assess the patient's anxiety level, and initiate measures to decrease anxiety, including maintaining a quiet environment, maintaining a calm demeanor, offering reassurance, permitting family members to visit, and providing explanations for all procedures; high anxiety levels contribute to increased myocardial oxygen demands

◆ Educate the patient about the atherosclerotic disease process, modification of risk factors, diet and exercise programs, medication regimen, cardiac rehabilitation, and available support groups; increasing the patient's knowledge level can help him make informed health care decisions

◆ Monitor for complications, such as ventricular aneurysm, ventricular septal defect, papillary muscle rupture, and pericarditis

❖ **Acute heart failure**
  ■ Description
    ◆ Acute heart failure has a sudden onset; it occurs secondary to a precipitating factor that causes a decrease in cardiac output

◆ Left-sided heart failure is caused by failure of the left ventricle to pump, resulting in pulmonary congestion and edema or decreased cardiac output; it usually is secondary to left ventricular infarction, hypertension, or aortic or mitral valve disease

◆ Right-sided heart failure is usually caused by failure of the right ventricle to pump, secondary to left-sided heart failure; it may also be caused by a pulmonary embolus or right ventricular infarction

◆ In patients with nonacute heart failure, three compensatory mechanisms that enhance cardiac output (by manipulating heart rate, preload, contractility, and afterload) are activated

▶ Increased sympathetic activity in the adrenergic system stimulates the release of epinephrine, resulting in peripheral vasoconstriction, increased venous return, and increased preload

▶ The renin-angiotensin-aldosterone system constricts the renal arterioles, which decreases the glomerular filtration rate, increases the reabsorption of sodium, and promotes fluid retention

▶ The development of ventricular hypertrophy increases the force of each contraction, which helps the ventricles overcome an increase in afterload

■ Clinical signs and symptoms

◆ Left-sided heart failure: dyspnea, orthopnea, wheezing, tachypnea, S_3 gallop, nocturnal angina, paroxysmal nocturnal dyspnea, PAWP greater than 20 mm Hg, and moist crackles

◆ Right-sided heart failure: systemic venous congestion, jugular venous pressure greater than 8 cm, elevated CVP, hepatomegaly, dependent pitting edema, and peripheral edema

■ Medical management

◆ Remove the precipitating cause, and correct the underlying cause

◆ Reduce cardiac workload by prescribing bed rest, small meals, weight reduction if the patient is overweight, and small doses of sedatives if the patient is anxious

◆ Enhance myocardial contractility by administering cardiac glycosides (such as digoxin), sympathomimetic agents (such as dopamine or dobutamine), or other drugs that have a positive inotropic effect (such as amrinone)

◆ Biventricular pacemaker (or cardiac resynchronization therapy) may be placed if patient has systolic heart failure and ventricular dyssynchrony (By causing both ventricles to contract simultaneously, cardiac output is improved)

◆ Control excess fluid retention with a low-sodium diet, diuretic therapy, and vasodilating therapy with nitrates

◆ Administer morphine sulfate to effect vasodilation and to decrease the patient's anxiety

◆ Administer oxygen therapy

◆ Insert a pulmonary artery catheter to monitor left ventricular function

◆ Raise the head of the bed, or let the patient dangle his legs over the bed with feet dependent; this helps improve the patient's pulmonary status

■ Nursing management

◆ Monitor blood pressure, heart rate, respirations, heart and lung sounds, LOC, and hemodynamic parameters every 1 to 2 hours (or as needed) to detect signs and symptoms of decreased cardiac output or disease progression or improvement

◆ Maintain the patient on bed rest with the head of the bed elevated 30 to 60 degrees, administer oxygen as prescribed, and promote rest by spacing treatments; these interventions can decrease myocardial oxygen demand and facilitate ventilation

◆ Administer drugs, as prescribed, and monitor for signs and symptoms of toxicity; vasodilators decrease preload and afterload, inotropic agents improve contractility and renal blood flow, and diuretics decrease circulating volume

◆ To detect fluid retention, weigh the patient daily, keep an accurate record of intake and output, and auscultate heart and lung sounds

◆ Maintain a patent I.V. line to ensure access if emergency medications need to be given

◆ Restrict dietary sodium and fluid intake to control sodium reabsorption and fluid retention

◆Monitor electrolyte results and report abnormalities to the practitioner; loop diuretics typically cause hypokalemia

◆ Provide frequent, small meals; patients with heart failure often have a feeling of fullness, experience nausea and vomiting, and have difficulty eating and breathing simultaneously

◆ Assess skin integrity and initiate measures to prevent skin breakdown and enhance circulation, including turning the patient every 2 hours with a turning sheet and keeping linens clean and wrinkle-free

◆ Educate the patient about the disease process, the drug regimen and possible adverse effects, and the need for a sodium-restricted diet

◆ Tell the patient to weigh himself every morning, reporting a weight gain of more than 2 lb (0.9 kg) in a 24-hour period

◆ Instruct the patient to pace all activities for adequate rest periods

❖ Angina

■ Description

◆Angina is a severe, constricting pain that's classified as stable, variant, or unstable

◆ Stable angina begins gradually, reaching maximal intensity in a few minutes before dissipating

▶ It's precipitated by activity, tachycardia, systemic hypertension, thyrotoxicosis, sympathomimetic drugs, systemic illness, or anemia

▶ Correction of the precipitating event or the administration of I.V. nitroglycerin usually terminates the episode

◆ Variant (Prinzmetal's) angina is a reversible reduction in the diameter of the coronary artery that's caused by coronary artery spasms and results in severe myocardial ischemia

▶ Variant angina often occurs when the patient isn't active and has no precipitating factors

▶ Treatment aims at decreasing the incidence of spasm with vasodilators or calcium channel blockers

◆ Unstable angina is a change in previously stable angina or new onset of severe angina

  ▶ Makes up a spectrum of diseases in acute coronary syndrome, along with acute myocardial infarction

  ▶ There's a progressive increase in the frequency and severity of anginal pain, and the pain is induced by less exertion than previously; the pain may last up to 30 minutes and may be only partially relieved by rest or nitrates; pain isn't accompanied by cardiac enzyme level changes or ECG changes characteristic of infarction

  ▶ Precipitating factors include worsening of atherosclerosis in multiple vessels, left main coronary artery disease, increases in localized platelet agglutination, acute or chronic thrombosis, plaque hemorrhage or fissure, acute vasoconstriction, and mechanical problems after acute MI (such as left ventricular aneurysm, a ruptured papillary muscle, ventricular septal defect, or left-sided heart failure)

■ Clinical signs and symptoms

  ◆ Chest pain lasting up to 30 minutes
  ◆ Transient ECG changes with chest pain
  ◆ No changes in cardiac enzyme levels

■ Medical management

  ◆ Administer beta-blocking agents to reduce heart rate, contractility, and blood pressure
  ◆ Administer nitrates to decrease blood flow to the heart, thereby reducing left ventricular filling pressure; nitrates also dilate coronary arteries and decrease peripheral resistance, reducing myocardial oxygen consumption
  ◆ Administer calcium channel blockers to relax the vascular smooth muscle
  ◆ Consider cardiovascular revascularization procedures (as discussed under acute MI)
  ◆ Control hypertension and heart failure to help relieve angina
  ◆ Maintain bed rest until the anginal episode is controlled
  ◆ Administer sedatives to reduce the patient's anxiety
  ◆ Administer I.V. heparin to prevent thromboembolism formation during bed rest
  ◆ Administer oxygen to reduce ischemia

■ Nursing management

  ◆ Assess the patient's anginal pain and his activity before the onset of pain to determine precipitating factors
  ◆ Administer medications, as prescribed, to control pain
    ▶ Nitrates relieve pain through venous and arterial dilation
    ▶ Morphine sulfate relieves pain by reducing the autonomic response
  ◆ Request an immediate ECG while the patient is experiencing chest pain to document if ischemia or infarction exists
  ◆ To reduce myocardial oxygen demand, restrict the patient's activity until the angina is controlled
  ◆ Administer nitrates and beta-blocking agents, as prescribed
    ▶ Nitrates reduce afterload
    ▶ Beta-blocking agents decrease myocardial ischemia by decreasing contractility and reducing the workload of the heart

◆ Educate the patient about the atherosclerotic disease process, modification of risk factors, diet and exercise programs, the drug regimen, cardiac rehabilitation, and available support groups; increasing the patient's knowledge level can help him make informed health care decisions

■ Cardiac assist devices
  ◆ Intra-aortic balloon counterpulsation
    ▶ Description
      • 34-, 40-, or 50-cc balloon-tipped catheter placed in the descending aorta between the left subclavian artery and the renal artery, connected to a console that synchronously inflates and deflates the balloon timed according to the cardiac cycle
      • Balloon inflation occurs during ventricular diastole, augmenting the patient's baseline diastolic arterial pressure
      • Primary benefit is enhancement of coronary artery perfusion; secondary benefits are enhanced cerebral and renal arterial flow
      • Balloon deflation occurs just before ventricular ejection, lowering intra-arterial resistance and left ventricular afterload
      • Primary benefit is reduction of left ventricular workload; secondary benefit is enhancement of cardiac output
    ▶ Medical management
      • Balloon catheters are typically inserted percutaneously through the femoral artery or may be placed transthoracically during surgery
    ▶ Nursing management
      • Concerns include optimizing and ensuring correct timing of the balloon inflation and deflation cycles, ECG monitoring and prevention or management of dysrhythmias, hemodynamic monitoring and maintenance of cardiac output, monitoring for peripheral ischemia, monitoring insertion site for hematoma formation, maintenance of the balloon lumen, monitoring for evidence of balloon rupture, monitoring for evidence of balloon malposition, prevention of skin impairment, anxiety management, and patient or family education
  ◆ Ventricular assist devices
    ▶ Description
      • Diversion of varying amounts of blood flow around a failing ventricle through use of an extracorporeal pump
      • Ventricular assist devices (VADs) can be centrifugal, rotary, pneumatic, or electric
      • VADs can provide right ventricular support, left ventricular support, or biventricular support
      • Temporary adjunctive therapy for persistent cardiac failure with hope of recovery, or as a bridge to cardiac transplantation
    ▶ Medical management
      • Device selection depends on the physician's preference and patient need
      • Implantation occurs by surgical procedure
    ▶ Nursing management

Junctional rhythm

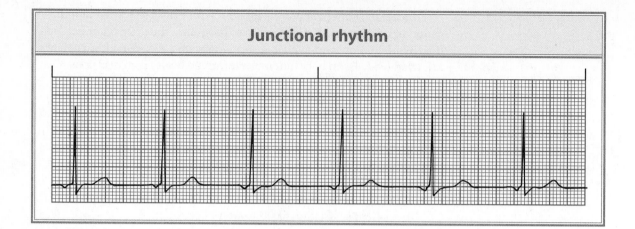

● Concerns include monitoring for hemodynamic changes, optimization of cardiac output, monitoring for device failure, maintenance of anticoagulation, monitoring for bleeding, managing and minimizing infection risk, prevention of skin impairment, anxiety management, and patient or family education

❖ **Myocardial conduction system defects**
  ■ Junctional rhythm
    ◆ Description
      ▶ Rhythm initiating in the AV junction
    ◆ ECG recognition
      ▶ P waves may be before the QRS, but with a PR of less than 0.12 second; P waves may be buried in the QRS (absent); P waves may be retrograde to the QRS; P waves may be inverted in lead II, regular rhythm, rate 40 to 60 beats/minute, QRS normal (for a sample ECG rhythm strip, see *Junctional rhythm*); if the rate is 60 to 100 beats/minute, it's called accelerated junctional rhythm; if it's 100 to 200 beats/minute, it's junctional tachycardia
    ◆ Clinical signs and symptoms of low cardiac output may be present
    ◆ Medical management
      ▶ Correct the underlying cause, such as drug toxicity, excess vagal tone, SA or AV node ischemia, or sinus node suppression
      ▶ Administer oxygen and I.V. atropine if symptomatic
      ▶ Anticipate the potential need for temporary or permanent pacing
    ◆ Nursing management
      ▶ Assess the patient for signs of low cardiac output and ECG changes
      ▶ Administer medications, as prescribed
      ▶ If the patient is hypotensive, lower the head of the bed as tolerated, and keep atropine at the bedside
  ■ Premature junctional complexes
    ◆ Description
      ▶ A premature complex that's initiated by irritable junctional tissue, frequently asymptomatic and considered normal in some individuals
    ◆ ECG recognition
      ▶ Underlying sinus rhythm interrupted by a premature complex in which the P waves may be before the QRS, but with a PR of less than

Premature junctional complex

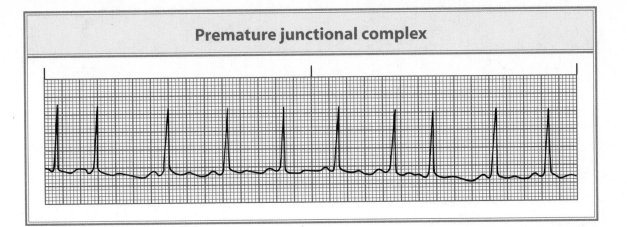

0.12 second; P waves may be buried in the QRS (absent), retrograde to the QRS; and inverted in lead II, with a normal QRS (for a sample ECG rhythm strip, see *Premature junctional complex*)

◆ Medical management
  ❭ Correct the underlying cause of irritable junctional tissue
  ❭ Prophylactic treatment with digoxin may be ordered
◆ Nursing management
  ❭ Assess the patient for signs of low cardiac output and ECG changes
  ❭ Administer medications, as prescribed
■ First-degree atrioventricular block
  ◆ Description
    ❭ First-degree AV block results when conduction is delayed at the AV node or the His-Purkinje system, causing a prolonged PR interval on the ECG
    ❭ A first-degree AV block may occur in healthy people, secondary to treatment with antiarrhythmic medications, or in association with rheumatic fever, chronic degenerative disease of the conduction system, hypokalemia, hyperkalemia, hypothyroidism, or inferior wall MI
  ◆ Defining characteristics
    ❭ Atrial and ventricular rhythm: regular (for a sample ECG rhythm strip, see *First-degree atrioventricular block*, page 52)
    ❭ Atrial and ventricular rates are usually 60 to 100 beats/minute
    ❭ P wave: normal
    ❭ PR interval: prolonged, but constant
    ❭ A PR interval of 0.21 to 0.24 second indicates slight block; 0.25 to 0.29 second indicates moderate block; 0.30 second or more indicates severe block
    ❭ QRS complex: usually within normal limits
    ❭ T wave: normal
  ◆ Clinical signs and symptoms
    ❭ Usually asymptomatic
    ❭ Pulse rate slow to normal
  ◆ Medical management
    ❭ Treat the underlying cause
    ❭ Monitor ECG for worsening of AV block
    ❭ Administer I.V. atropine if symptomatic bradycardia occurs

First-degree atrioventricular block

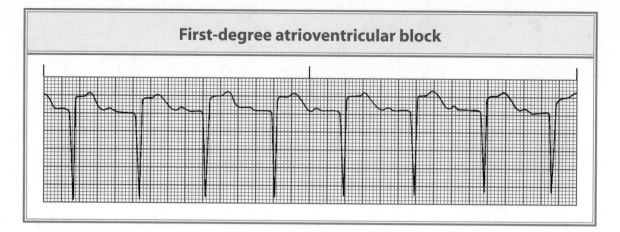

◆ Nursing management

▶ Maintain continuous ECG monitoring to observe for worsening of AV block

▶ Be prepared to administer I.V. atropine if symptomatic bradycardia develops; atropine is a cholinergic blocker that blocks the action of acetylcholine in the SA and AV nodes

■ Second-degree atrioventricular block, Mobitz type I

◆ Description

▶ Second-degree AV block, Mobitz type I, results when diseased AV nodal tissue conducts impulses increasingly earlier in the refractory period until an impulse arrives during the absolute refractory period, when it can't be conducted

▶ Second-degree AV block, Mobitz type I, may be caused by inferior wall MI, cardiac surgery, acute rheumatic fever, vagal stimulation, cardiac glycoside toxicity, or use of propranolol, quinidine, or procainamide

▶ The ECG shows a constant P-P interval, a progressively longer PR interval, and a progressively shorter R-R interval; after several cycles, there's a missing QRS complex; the PR interval shortens after the missed beat, then progressively lengthens again; this pattern has the visual effect of "group beating"

◆ Defining characteristics

▶ Atrial rhythm: regular (for a sample ECG rhythm strip, see *Second-degree atrioventricular block, Mobitz type I*)

▶ Ventricular rhythm: irregular, with the R-R interval shortening until a P wave appears without a QRS complex

▶ Atrial rate: greater than the ventricular rate but usually within normal limits

▶ Ventricular rate: slower than the atrial rate but usually within normal limits

▶ P wave: normal

▶ PR interval: progressively lengthens until a P wave appears without a QRS complex; the PR interval after the nonconducted beat is shorter than the previous beat's PR interval

▶ QRS complex: periodically absent but within normal limits

▶ T wave: usually normal

Second-degree atrioventricular block, Mobitz type I

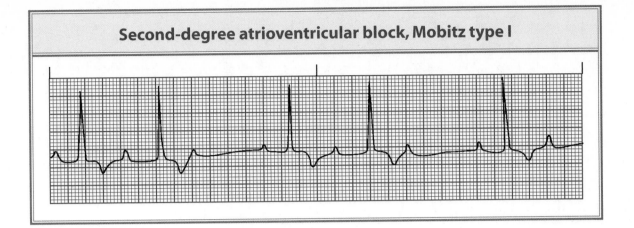

- ◆ Clinical signs and symptoms
  - ▶ Usually asymptomatic
  - ▶ Pulse rate usually normal, with occasional irregularity
  - ▶ Symptoms of decreased cardiac output if ventricular rate is too slow
- ◆ Medical management
  - ▶ Treat the underlying cause
  - ▶ Monitor ECG for worsening of AV block
  - ▶ If symptomatic bradycardia occurs, administer I.V. atropine and consider a temporary pacemaker
- ◆ Nursing management
  - ▶ Maintain continuous ECG monitoring to observe for worsening of AV block
  - ▶ Be prepared to administer I.V. atropine if symptomatic bradycardia develops; atropine is a cholinergic blocker that blocks the action of acetylcholine in the SA and AV nodes
- ■ Second-degree atrioventricular block, Mobitz type II
  - ◆ Description
    - ▶ Second-degree AV block, Mobitz type II (also called classic second-degree AV block) results when a conduction disturbance in the His-Purkinje system causes an intermittent block
    - ▶ Second-degree AV block, Mobitz type II, is caused by organic heart disease, acute anterior wall MI, severe coronary artery disease, and acute myocarditis
    - ▶ There's no warning on the ECG before a beat is blocked, and there can be any number of dropped beats before a beat is conducted; the block is referred to by the number of beats dropped, that is, 2:1, 3:1, or 4:1 block
  - ◆ Defining characteristics
    - ▶ Atrial rhythm: regular (for a sample ECG rhythm strip, see *Second-degree atrioventricular block, Mobitz type II*, page 54)
    - ▶ Ventricular rhythm: regular (even if block is constant) or irregular
    - ▶ Atrial rate: usually within normal limits
    - ▶ Ventricular rate: normal to slow; may be slower than the atrial rate
    - ▶ P wave: normal, with regular P-P interval

Second-degree atrioventricular block, Mobitz type II

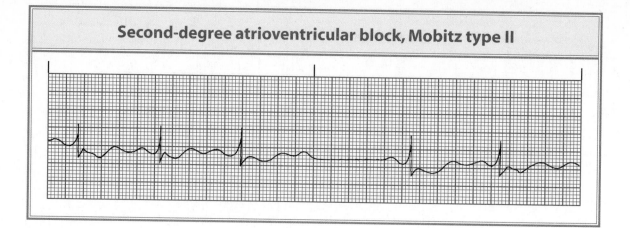

 ▶ PR interval: usually within normal limits; always constant when followed by a QRS complex (the PR interval after a nonconducted beat may be slightly shortened)
 ▶ QRS complex: within normal limits but absent with nonconducted beat or may be slightly widened
 ▶ T wave: normal
 ◆ Clinical signs and symptoms
 ▶ Pulse rate slow to normal
 ▶ Pulse regular or irregular
 ▶ Symptoms of decreased cardiac output if pulse rate is too slow
 ◆ Medical management
 ▶ Monitor ECG continuously for worsening of AV block
 ▶ If symptoms of decreased cardiac output develop, apply an external pacemaker to increase the heart rate
 ▶ Consider inserting a permanent pacemaker, if indicated (see *Programmable pacemaker codes*)
 ◆ Nursing management
 ▶ Monitor ECG continuously for worsening of AV block
 ▶ Be prepared for insertion of external, temporary or permanent pacemaker if symptomatic bradycardia develops
 ▶ Transcutaneous (external) pacemakers are used in an emergency situation; two-layer skin electrodes are applied to the patient to depolarize the heart
 ● Transvenous pacemakers are temporary or permanent; the pacing electrode is inserted and advanced through the brachial, subclavian, or femoral vein to the right atrium, right ventricle, or both to pace the heart
 ● Epicardial pacing electrodes are attached to the epicardium during cardiac surgery to pace the heart
 ▶ Assess the patient's LOC, heart rate, and blood pressure every 2 hours, or as needed, to evaluate changes in clinical status that may indicate decreased cardiac output
 ▶ If symptoms of decreased cardiac output occur, apply an external pacemaker; symptoms of decreased cardiac output can usually be alle-

Programmable pacemaker codes

Programmable pacemakers use a five-letter coding system to help identify chambers paced and sensed.

First letter	Second letter	Third letter	Fourth letter	Fifth letter
Chamber paced	Chamber sensed	Response to sensing	Programmability	Anti-tachyarrhythmia functions
A = Atria	A = Atria	I = Inhibited	P = Simple program-mability	P = Pacing (anti-tachyarrhythmia)
V = Ventricle	V = Ventricle	T = Triggered	M = Multiprogram-mability	S = Shock
D = Dual	D = Dual	D = Dual	C = Communicating	D = Dual
O = None	O = None	O = None	R = Rate modulation	O = None
			O = None	

viated by increasing the heart rate to within normal limits; the external pacemaker is the treatment of choice if personnel are trained in its use

- Pacing delivers an electronic stimulus to the myocardium, producing a pacemaker spike on the ECG
- Capture is evidenced when the appropriate wave of depolarization (P wave for atrial pacemakers, QRS for ventricular pacemakers) immediately follows the spike
- Sensing (if programmed) is evidenced when the pacemaker pauses pacing due to the presence of intrinsic cardiac activity

▶ Assess the patient's level of anxiety and degree of understanding of the problem; remain with him when he's frightened

▶ Explain all procedures and protocols; information usually alleviates anxiety and gives the patient a sense of control

▶ If applicable, educate the patient about permanent pacemaker implantation

■ Third-degree atrioventricular block

◆ Description

▶ Third-degree AV block, or complete heart block, results when no impulses are conducted from the atria to the ventricles

- The ventricular rhythm is either junctional escape or ventricular escape, depending on whether it originates in the bundle of His or the Purkinje system, respectively
- Ventricular escape rhythms are slower and less stable; they place the patient at risk for ventricular standstill and decreased cardiac output

▶ Acute third-degree AV block may be caused by severe cardiac glycoside toxicity or inferior wall MI; it may also occur transiently during cardiac catheterization or angioplasty

▶ Chronic third-degree AV block may be caused by bilateral bundle branch block, congenital abnormalities, rheumatic fever, hypoxia, postoperative complications of mitral valve replacement, Lev's disease, or Lenègre's disease

Third-degree atrioventricular block

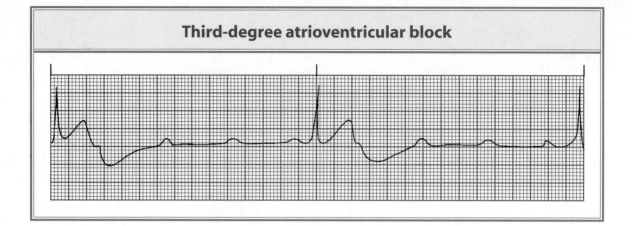

◆ Defining characteristics
  ▶ Atrial and ventricular rhythms: regular (for a sample ECG rhythm strip, see *Third-degree atrioventricular block*)
  ▶ Atrial rate: usually within normal limits but faster than the ventricular rate
  ▶ Ventricular rate: usually 25 to 40 beats/minute
  ▶ P wave: normal
  ▶ PR interval: varies
  ▶ QRS complex: wide, bizarre complex if it originates in the ventricles; normal if it originates in the junction
  ▶ T wave: normal
  ▶ QT interval: may be normal
◆ Clinical signs and symptoms
  ▶ Slow, regular pulse
  ▶ May be asymptomatic
  ▶ Signs and symptoms of decreased cardiac output if pulse rate is too slow
◆ Medical management
  ▶ Monitor ECG continuously for worsening of AV block
  ▶ Administer I.V. atropine if symptomatic bradycardia occurs
  ▶ Insert a temporary pacemaker; consider a permanent pacemaker if indicated
◆ Nursing management
  ▶ Monitor ECG continuously for worsening of AV block
  ▶ Be prepared to administer an infusion of I.V. atropine if symptomatic bradycardia develops
  ▶ Assess the patient's LOC, heart rate, and blood pressure every 2 hours, or as needed, to evaluate changes in clinical status that may indicate decreased cardiac output
  ▶ If symptoms of decreased cardiac output occur, apply an external pacemaker; symptoms of decreased cardiac output can usually be alleviated by increasing the heart rate to within normal limits; the external pacemaker is the treatment of choice, if personnel are trained in its use
  ▶ Assess the patient's level of anxiety and degree of understanding of the problem; remain with him when he's frightened

▶ Explain all procedures and protocols; information usually alleviates anxiety and gives the patient a sense of control

▶ If applicable, educate the patient about permanent pacemaker implantation

❖ **Pulmonary edema**
  ■ Description
    ◆ In pulmonary edema, increased left atrial and left ventricular pressures cause an excessive accumulation of serous or serosanguineous fluid in the interstitial spaces and alveoli of the lungs
      ▶ In stage I disease, interstitial edema and increased lymphatic flow occur
      ▶ In stage II disease, the fluid moves from the interstitium into the alveoli
    ◆ Fluid in the alveoli interferes with the diffusion of oxygen and leads to tissue hypoxia; the resulting feeling of suffocation increases the patient's fear and elevates the heart rate, decreasing ventricular filling and further depressing cardiac function
  ■ Clinical signs and symptoms
    ◆ Coughing, extreme shortness of breath, wheezing, intense anxiety, crackles, and tachypnea
    ◆ Frothy sputum that may be blood-tinged
    ◆ Sensation of drowning, fear of impending death
    ◆ Pallid complexion with cold, clammy, cyanotic skin
    ◆ Pulmonary artery diastolic pressure and PAWP greater than 30 mm Hg
    ◆ Respiratory alkalosis secondary to hyperventilation in initial stages; respiratory acidosis and hypoxemia as pulmonary edema progresses
    ◆ Decreased urine output
    ◆ X-ray shows pulmonary venous congestion and interstitial edema
  ■ Medical management
    ◆ Same as for acute heart failure (see page 46)
    ◆ Short-term intubation and mechanical ventilation may be required
  ■ Nursing management
    ◆ Same as for acute heart failure (see pages 46 and 47)
    ◆ Closely monitor the patient for progression to cardiogenic shock

❖ **Hypertensive crisis**
  ■ Description
    ◆ A hypertensive crisis is defined as a diastolic blood pressure of 120 mm Hg or higher
    ◆ It occurs in less than 1% of hypertensive patients, and usually in those whose hypertension is poorly controlled or untreated
    ◆ Although the cause is unknown, hypertensive crisis commonly is associated with preeclampsia, acute or chronic renal disease, acute central nervous system (CNS) events, and ingestion of foods that contain tyramine by patients taking monoamine oxidase inhibitors
    ◆ Hypertensive crisis is a life-threatening event that can cause irreversible damage to vital organs

◆ Pathologic changes associated with hypertensive crisis include arterial dilation and contraction resulting in encephalopathy, microangiopathic hemolytic anemia contributing to deterioration of renal function, and arteriolar fibrinoid necrosis

◆ Activation of the renin-angiotensin-aldosterone system, in response to decreased renal blood supply caused by hypertensive changes, can raise blood pressure even higher

■ Clinical signs and symptoms
  ◆ Rapid increase in blood pressure, usually above 120 mm Hg diastolic
  ◆ Grade III or IV retinopathy with or without papilledema
  ◆ Restlessness, confusion, somnolence, blurred vision, headache, nausea, and vomiting
  ◆ Proteinuria, hematuria, red blood cell casts, azotemia, oliguria, hemolytic anemia, and epistaxis
  ◆ Hypertensive encephalopathy with severe headache, vomiting, vision disturbances, seizures, stupor, and coma

■ Medical management
  ◆ Administer antihypertensives, vasodilators, beta-blocking agents, and diuretics to reduce blood pressure
  ◆ Recommend a sodium-restricted diet, exercise program, weight reduction in overweight patients, stress reduction, and smoking cessation

■ Nursing management
  ◆ Continuously monitor blood pressure, heart rate, and ECG to assess the effects of antihypertensive medications
  ◆ Maintain a patent I.V. line for administration of antihypertensive medications; assess the line every 4 hours for infiltration or extravasation, which may cause localized tissue damage
  ◆ Titrate antihypertensive medications carefully because hypertensive patients can rapidly become hypotensive
  ◆ Monitor for toxic effects of medications; nitroprusside sodium infusions are associated with bleeding tendencies and may cause agitation and disorientation at toxic doses
  ◆ Assess urine output, monitor CVP or PAWP if available; check neurologic function; report trends or changes in the patient's condition to the practitioner
  ◆ Check for symptoms of hypovolemia or hypervolemia
  ◆ Because uncompensated sensory losses place the patient at risk for physical injury, implement safety precautions, including monitoring the patient's LOC every hour, implementing seizure precautions, reorienting the patient as needed, decreasing sensory stimulation, and applying adequate pressure to puncture sites
  ◆ Assess the patient's level of pain (patients in hypertensive crisis typically complain of severe headache), and administer analgesics, as prescribed; when dressing and immobilizing cannulated areas, be sure to maximize patient movement and comfort
  ◆ Help the patient change position gradually to reduce the likelihood of orthostatic hypotension
  ◆ Provide the patient with hard candy, ice chips, and good oral care to alleviate dry oral mucosa (an adverse effect of antihypertensive therapy)

◆ Assess the patient's level of anxiety, and administer sedatives, as prescribed; he may be anxious due to an unfamiliar environment, perceived lack of control, and fear of death or unknown consequences of the crisis

◆ Allow family members to visit, and ensure the patient's privacy

❖ **Cardiogenic shock**

■ Description

◆ Cardiogenic shock results from loss of more than 40% of the functional myocardium

◆ It may be caused by left ventricular dysfunction (secondary to acute MI), ischemia, inflammatory diseases, papillary muscle rupture, left ventricular free wall rupture, acute ventricular septal defect, end-stage cardiomyopathy, severe valvular dysfunction, myocardial contusion, cardiac tamponade, or left atrial myxoma

◆ It may also result from thrombus formation or massive pulmonary embolus formation, which causes hypoperfusion of vital organs; this lack of perfusion results in inadequate cellular oxygen delivery and local accumulation of toxic cellular waste

■ Stages of cardiogenic shock

◆ Stage I (initial stage): asymptomatic decreased cardiac output

◆ Stage II (compensatory stage): decreased cardiac output with early clinical signs and symptoms

▶ Sympathetic compensatory mechanisms are activated, resulting in increased heart rate and ventricular contractility

▶ Hormonal compensatory mechanisms trigger secretion of renin, angiotensin, and aldosterone, resulting in increased reabsorption of sodium and water

◆ Stage III (progressive stage): compensatory mechanisms become ineffective as cardiac workload and oxygen demands increase

▶ Acidosis allows blood to leak out of the capillary bed, causing fluid to shift into the interstitial space

▶ Sustained vasoconstriction results in cold and pulseless fingers, toes, tip of the nose, and earlobes

◆ Stage IV (refractory stage): shock state is irreversible

■ Clinical signs and symptoms

◆ Systolic blood pressure less than 90 mm Hg, or a 30- to 60-mm Hg decrease in systolic pressure in a previously hypertensive patient

◆ Tachycardia with jugular vein distention

◆ Increased CVP, pulmonary artery pressures, PAWP, and systemic vascular resistance (SVR)

◆ Decreased cardiac output

◆ Oliguria (less than 20 ml/hour) secondary to decreased renal perfusion

◆ Rapid, thready pulse

◆ Rapid, shallow respirations with crackles and rhonchi; may progress to pulmonary edema

◆ Decreased heart sounds; S_3, S_4 may be present; rhythm may be irregular

◆ Decreased peristalsis, resulting in absent bowel sounds

◆ Restlessness, agitation, confusion, or obtundation

◆ Cool, pale, diaphoretic skin becoming mottled and cyanotic as cardiogenic shock progresses

■ Medical management

◆ Insert an arterial line and a pulmonary artery catheter to monitor arterial pressure, left ventricular filling pressure, and cardiac output

◆ Administer oxygen therapy based on the patient's oxygen saturation level

◆ Use intra-aortic balloon counterpulsation (IABP) to decrease afterload or ventricular assist devices, as needed

◆ Administer analgesics to control pain, vasopressors to raise the arterial pressure, crystalloids or diuretics to keep PAWP at less than 20 mm Hg, positive inotropic agents to increase contractility, and venous vasodilators to decrease preload

■ Nursing management

◆ Continuously monitor PAP, PAWP, cardiac output, urine output, skin color and temperature, peripheral pulses, LOC, respiratory status, and bowel sounds; these evaluations are needed to assess tissue and organ perfusion

◆ Administer medications as prescribed; use the smallest amount of solution possible when mixing I.V. infusions; use infusion pumps; keep precise records of intake and output

▶ I.V. drugs are potent medications that must be carefully administered

▶ Fluids are commonly restricted in cardiogenic shock to decrease circulating volume

◆ Implement safety precautions (including monitoring the patient's LOC, reorienting the patient as needed, and decreasing sensory stimulation); administer oxygen therapy, as prescribed; changes in mentation occur secondary to decreased cerebral perfusion or tissue hypoxia

◆ Maintain skin integrity by using heel and elbow protectors, special mattresses, frequent turning, and passive range-of-motion exercises; skin breakdown may result from hypoperfusion

❖ **Structural heart defects**

■ Aortic insufficiency

◆ Description

▶ Aortic insufficiency results from incompetency of the aortic valve, which may be caused by rheumatic fever, syphilis, infectious endocarditis, or connective tissue disorders (such as Marfan syndrome)

▶ Aortic insufficiency causes the left ventricle to become overloaded and hypertrophied

▶ Left ventricular end-diastolic pressure and left atrial pressure increase over time while myocardial contractility diminishes, resulting in heart failure

◆ Clinical signs and symptoms

▶ Dyspnea on exertion, palpitations, orthopnea, chest pain on exertion, bounding pulse, and widened pulse pressure

▶ Decrescendo diastolic murmur (blowing) and high-pitched heart sounds (best heard at the base of the heart)

◗ Systolic ejection murmur (best heard at the base of the heart)
◆ Medical management
   ◗ Intervene surgically at the onset of left ventricular dysfunction, before severe symptoms develop
   ◗ Differentiate between aortic insufficiency and aortic stenosis
◆ Nursing management
   ◗ Prepare the patient for surgical intervention
   ◗ Differentiate between aortic insufficiency and aortic stenosis

■ Aortic stenosis
   ◆ Description
      ◗ Aortic stenosis most often is associated with congenital bicuspid or unicuspid valve formation and degenerative changes associated with aging; sometimes it's associated with rheumatic heart disease
      ◗ Degenerative aortic stenosis is caused by thickening and calcification of the aortic cusps in people older than age 65
      ◗ In patients with aortic stenosis, increased left ventricular pressure develops; this propels blood across the valve into the aorta and leads to left ventricular hypertrophy
   ◆ Clinical signs and symptoms
      ◗ Fatigue, dyspnea, orthopnea, angina pectoris, dizziness, and syncope
      ◗ Narrowed pulse pressure
      ◗ Crescendo-decrescendo, harsh systolic murmur (best heard at the base of the heart)
   ◆ Medical management
      ◗ Restrict strenuous physical activity
      ◗ Intervene surgically, including commissural incision into the valve under direct visualization to release the valve flaps and improve blood flow, or valve replacement
   ◆ Nursing management
      ◗ Instruct the patient to avoid strenuous physical activity
      ◗ Prepare the patient for surgical intervention

■ Mitral stenosis
   ◆ Description
      ◗ In mitral stenosis, the mitral valve orifice is less than one-half the normal size
      ◗ As a result, increased left atrial pressure is needed to propel blood from the left atrium through the stenotic valve to the left ventricle
      ◗ The elevated left atrial pressure raises the pulmonary venous and arterial pressures, reducing pulmonary compliance and causing dyspnea on exertion
      ◗ Usually a result of rheumatic fever, mitral stenosis causes the valve leaflets to thicken with fibrous tissue or calcific deposits; the mitral commissures fuse, the chordae tendineae fuse and shorten, and the valvular cusps become rigid, leading to a narrowing of the valve
      ◗ The physiologic changes resulting from mitral stenosis cause a low-pitched, rumbling, diastolic murmur that's best heard at the apex of the heart

◆ Clinical signs and symptoms
  ❱ Mild disease: dyspnea and cough on exertion and when blood flow is increased secondary to stressors
  ❱ Severe disease: orthopnea, paroxysmal nocturnal dyspnea, pulmonary edema, atrial arrhythmias, hemoptysis, increased incidence of pulmonary infarction and bronchitis, chest pain, and reduced pulmonary compliance
◆ Medical management
  ❱ Administer penicillin prophylaxis for beta-hemolytic streptococcal infections and endocarditis
  ❱ Restrict the patient's sodium intake, and prescribe maintenance doses of oral diuretics
  ❱ Administer cardiac glycosides for atrial fibrillation and right-sided heart failure
  ❱ Administer anticoagulants for embolization or intermittent atrial fibrillation
  ❱ Recommend that the patient avoid physically strenuous occupations
  ❱ Consider valvulotomy and valve replacement for symptomatic patients
◆ Nursing management
  ❱ Monitor vital signs, heart sounds, and arrhythmias to assess the development of right- or left-sided heart failure
  ❱ Be prepared to assist with cardioversion of atrial fibrillation; loss of atrial kick can decrease cardiac output by 25% to 30%
  ❱ Restrict the patient's dietary intake of sodium to minimize water retention
  ❱ Assess the patient's LOC and neurologic status, and administer anticoagulants as prescribed; mitral valve disease, an enlarged left atrium, and atrial fibrillation place the patient at increased risk for embolus formation
  ❱ Limit the patient's level of activity during the acute phase to conserve energy and decrease myocardial oxygen demand
  ❱ Educate the patient about the disease process, drug regimen, activity restrictions, diet and fluid restrictions; include appropriate choice of contraception for women, as pregnancy severely strains the cardiovascular system and may result in heart failure, valve rupture, or death
  ❱ Discuss the need for antibiotic prophylaxis to prevent endocarditis; the need to notify the dentist, urologist, and gynecologist of the patient's valvular heart disease; and the need to maintain good oral hygiene with regular visits to the dentist
■ Mitral insufficiency
  ◆ Description
    ❱ Mitral insufficiency results from rheumatic fever, which causes thickening, scarring, rigidity, and calcification of the valve leaflets; the commissures become fused with the chordae tendineae, causing shortening and retraction of the leaflets and preventing them from completely closing during systole
    ❱ Mitral insufficiency may also result from malposition of the papillary muscles

◗ Floppy valve syndrome is a loss of the fibrous and elastic tissue of the chordae tendineae, which keep the valve from opening backward; if the chordae tendineae rupture or break, blood flows backward, causing a murmur

◗ Papillary muscle rupture occurs secondary to acute MI, acute myocardial ischemia, or dilation of the left ventricle and displacement of the papillary muscles; these muscles are attached to the chordae tendineae

◆ Clinical signs and symptoms

◗ Dyspnea, fatigue, orthopnea, exercise intolerance, and palpitations

◗ Wide splitting of the S_2 heart sound and holosystolic murmur (best heard at the apex of the heart)

◗ Atrial dilation and enlargement

◗ Hypertrophied left ventricle

◆ Medical management

◗ Restrict the patient's level of physical activity

◗ Reduce the patient's sodium intake and prescribe diuretic therapy

◗ Administer cardiac glycosides and anticoagulants

◗ Consider surgical valve replacement

◗ Differentiate between mitral insufficiency and mitral stenosis

◆ Nursing management

◗ Restrict the patient's level of physical activity to reduce the heart's workload

◗ Reduce sodium intake and administer diuretic therapy, as prescribed, to reduce fluid retention

◗ Administer cardiac glycosides and anticoagulants, as prescribed, to increase cardiac output

◗ Prepare the patient for surgical valve replacement, if indicated

◗ Differentiate between mitral insufficiency and mitral stenosis

❖ **Aortic aneurysms (ruptured or dissecting)**

■ Description

◆ There are two types of aortic aneurysm: saccular and fusiform

◗ A saccular aortic aneurysm is a balloonlike dilation produced by a weakened area in the aorta and involves only a portion of the circumference of the aorta

◗ A fusiform aortic aneurysm is a diffuse area of weakness that produces a spindle-shaped, balloonlike dilation that affects the total circumference of the aorta

◆ The aneurysm expands at an unpredictable rate; incidence of aortic rupture increases dramatically when the aneurysm reaches 6 cm in diameter

◆ Risk factors for aortic aneurysm include atherosclerosis, increasing age, smoking, hypertension, increased triglyceride and low-density lipoprotein levels, decreased high-density lipoprotein levels, aortic necrosis, and trauma

◗ Atherosclerosis, the most common underlying disease, initially affects the intima of the vessel; hemorrhage into the plaque formation may invade the medial layer, causing weakness and generalized dilation of the aorta; the abdominal aorta is most commonly affected by this atherosclerotic process

▶ Increasing age is linked to a reduction in the elastin content within the media aorta, contributing to weakness of the aortic wall

▶ Smoking causes an increase in atherosclerotic plaques, ulceration, and calcification within the aorta

▶ Hypertension increases injury to the endothelium and may accelerate medial degeneration

■ Clinical signs and symptoms

◆ Usually asymptomatic until the aneurysm begins to leak or reaches a size that impinges on other organs

◆ Ascending aortic aneurysm: commonly asymptomatic or associated with dyspnea and chest pain, widened pulse pressure, bounding pulse, aortic murmur, pulsating abdominal mass, and abdominal bruits

◆ Aortic arch aneurysm: dyspnea, stridor, cough, chest pain, distended jugular and arm veins, left vocal cord paralysis, abnormal pulsation of the upper anterior chest, absent breath sounds or dullness on percussion, crackles, and an S_3 heart sound

◆ Descending thoracic aortic aneurysm: intermittent or constant dull pain between the shoulders and in the lower back, abdomen, shoulders, arms, or neck; occasionally, hoarseness caused by pressure on the laryngeal nerve; seldom detected by physical examination

◆ Abdominal aneurysm: dull and constant back pain caused by pressure on the lumbar nerves, abdominal pain and bloating caused by stretching of the duodenum over an enlarged aorta

■ Medical management

◆ Check the size of the aneurysm every 6 months, and repair surgically when it reaches 6 cm in diameter, or before

◆ Repair of thoracic aneurysm may necessitate use of cardiopulmonary bypass or concurrent aortic valve replacement

◆ Control risk factors (hypertension, hypercholesterolemia, hyperlipidemia, and smoking) through changes in diet, exercise, medications, and smoking-cessation support

■ Nursing management

◆ Assess the patient's level of anxiety, and administer sedatives, as prescribed; explain procedures and protocols; remain with the patient and offer realistic assurance, as needed; remember that the sympathetic response to anxiety can have detrimental hemodynamic effects in the perioperative period

◆ Monitor vital signs, hemodynamic parameters, and LOC every 15 minutes to 1 hour, as needed; early recognition of deteriorating hemodynamic status increases the patient's chances of survival

◆ Keep in mind that symptoms of hypovolemia will be present if the aneurysm ruptures

◆ Maintain the patient on bed rest in the supine position to prevent further decreases in blood pressure

◆ Maintain a patent I.V. line to ensure venous access if emergency drugs and fluids need to be given

◆ Administer fluids, as prescribed, to restore circulating blood volume

◆ Record intake and output every hour to assess kidney function and circulating fluid volume

◆ Educate the patient about the disease process and the importance of controlling blood pressure and adhering to a low-sodium diet; hypertension places added stress on the aneurysm, and sodium retention increases blood pressure

◆ Teach the patient about signs and symptoms, including back and chest pain (which indicate leakage of the aneurysm), that should be reported to the practitioner

■ Ruptured aortic aneurysm
  ◆ Description
    ❯ When a weakened aorta ruptures, blood flows freely into the thoracic or abdominal cavity
    ❯ Extreme tenderness of the mass in the abdominal aorta is symptomatic of imminent rupture
  ◆ Clinical signs and symptoms
    ❯ Unremitting back or abdominal pain
    ❯ Hypovolemia: weakness, light-headedness, nausea, vomiting, low blood pressure, tachycardia, and unconsciousness
  ◆ Medical management
    ❯ Control hypovolemia
    ❯ Apply an external counterpulsation device (such as a pneumatic antishock garment) to minimize leakage
    ❯ Surgically repair the ruptured area by using a synthetic graft to replace the section containing the aneurysm
  ◆ Nursing management
    ❯ Control hypovolemia by administering I.V. fluids, blood, or plasma as ordered
    ❯ Apply an external counterpulsation device (such as a pneumatic antishock garment) to minimize leakage

■ Aortic dissection
  ◆ Description
    ❯ Aortic dissection primarily results from a longitudinal tearing of the aortic media caused by a dissecting hematoma; blood is propelled through the torn intima into the media
    ❯ Aortic dissection occurs most frequently in the thoracic aorta
    ❯ It's more common in men than in women, and typically occurs in people in their 60s and 70s; mortality is 90% for those who don't receive treatment
    ❯ The underlying pathophysiologic causes of aortic dissection include intimal damage as seen with atherosclerosis, syphilis, infection, or trauma; medial degeneration secondary to Marfan syndrome, aging, or hypertension; and shearing stress related to the hemodynamic forces of the pulse wave
  ◆ Clinical signs and symptoms
    ❯ Acute chest pain spreading down into the back and abdomen; pain may be intense, sharp, tearing, or stabbing
    ❯ Symptoms indicating compromised circulation to a major artery
      • Coronary arteries: MI

- Aortic valve: systolic or diastolic murmur
- Carotid artery: strokelike symptoms
- Aortic bifurcation: loss or decrease of femoral pulses
- Subclavian artery: blood pressure between the two arms differs significantly
- Erosion into esophagus: nausea and vomiting with hematemesis
  ◗ Signs of shock, but normal to high blood pressure
◆ Medical management
  ◗ Administer nitrates and beta-blocking agents to decrease blood pressure and contractility of the heart
  ◗ Maintain the patient on bed rest
  ◗ Administer morphine sulfate to relieve pain
  ◗ Repair dissected area surgically, if indicated
◆ Nursing management
  ◗ Monitor blood pressure, cardiac rhythm, CVP, PAP, urine output, and peripheral pulses; changes in hemodynamic pressures may indicate progression of the dissection or aortic rupture; oliguria may indicate renal artery dissection
  ◗ Assess the location, quality, and radiation of the patient's pain; location of pain can help pinpoint the location of the dissection, and pain that increases or subsides and returns may indicate the initiation of a dissection
  ◗ Administer medications as prescribed; opioid analgesics relieve pain; nitrates and beta-blocking agents decrease blood pressure and myocardial contractility, which reduces the shearing effect that causes dissection
  ◗ Auscultate bowel sounds and palpate the abdomen every 2 hours to detect signs of acute abdominal process, which may indicate involvement of the mesenteric artery
  ◗ Maintain the patient on bed rest in a quiet environment
  ◗ Assess the patient's anxiety level; institute measures to decrease anxiety (to reduce stimulation and sympathetic response)
  ◗ Educate the patient about the disease process and the importance of controlling blood pressure and abstaining from tobacco product use; hypertension and smoking increase the risk of aortic dissection
  ◗ Discuss the drug regimen, activity restrictions, and the need to avoid isometric exercises
  ◗ Teach the patient about signs and symptoms, including pain, pallor, paresthesia, paralysis, and pulselessness, that should be reported to the practitioner

❖ **Hypovolemic shock**
  ■ Description
    ◆ Hypovolemic shock results when 30% to 40% of blood volume is lost
    ◆ Hemorrhage and dehydration are the principal causes
      ◗ Fluid loss may result from diarrhea, diabetes insipidus, vomiting, or overuse of diuretics
      ◗ Fluid loss into the extravascular compartment is a nonhemorrhagic cause of hypovolemic shock

◆ If the vascular volume isn't replaced within 90 minutes, the state of shock may be irreversible
- Clinical signs and symptoms
  ◆ Cool, clammy, mottled skin
  ◆ Systolic blood pressure less than 90 mm Hg or a 30- to 60-mm Hg decrease in systolic pressure in a previously hypertensive patient
  ◆ Agitation, confusion, or obtundation
  ◆ Urine output less than 30 ml/hour
- Medical management
  ◆ Initiate rapid corrective fluid therapy—including blood, blood products, and plasma expanders—to replace blood loss and crystalloid solutions to replace plasma or fluid losses
  ◆ Use oxygen therapy to maintain partial pressure of arterial oxygen at 80 mm Hg or above
  ◆ Monitor hemodynamic parameters to assess fluid status
  ◆ Monitor ABG values to assess acid-base balance
  ◆ Monitor urine output
  ◆ Give nothing by mouth if the patient is unconscious; give ice chips and liquid if he can swallow
  ◆ Maintain the patient on complete bed rest with the head of the bed flat
  ◆ Treat the underlying cause after the immediate crisis has passed
- Nursing management
  ◆ To facilitate circulation and increase venous return, maintain the patient on complete bed rest with the head of the bed flat and legs elevated 6″ to 8″ (15 to 20 cm), or place the patient in mild Trendelenburg's position, if tolerated
  ◆ Monitor vital signs, neurologic function, intake and output, and peripheral pulses every 15 minutes to 1 hour, as indicated; if the state of shock progresses, vital functions deteriorate rapidly
  ◆ Monitor for symptoms of decreased cardiac output and report changes to the practitioner
  ◆ Administer fluids, as prescribed, to restore blood volume
  ◆ Maintain an accurate record of intake and output to assess kidney function
  ◆ Administer oxygen therapy and monitor ABG values, as prescribed, to ensure optimal oxygen delivery and gas exchange
  ◆ Weigh the patient daily to assess overall fluid status
  ◆ Assess skin integrity and initiate measures to prevent skin breakdown and enhance circulation, including turning the patient every 2 hours using a turning sheet and keeping linens clean and wrinkle-free
  ◆ Assess the patient's level of anxiety, and administer sedatives, as prescribed; the patient may be anxious due to an unfamiliar environment, perceived lack of control, and fear of death or the unknown consequences of the crisis
  ◆ Allow family members to visit, and ensure the patient's privacy

❖ **Acute inflammatory cardiac diseases**
- Myocarditis
  ◆ Description

◗ Myocarditis is an inflammation of the myocardium caused by bacterial, viral, or autoimmune disease

- It may result from exposure to radiation or chemotherapy or from chronic cocaine use
- It may also occur as a complication of rheumatic fever, infectious mononucleosis, polio, mumps, or typhoid fever

◗ Myocardial damage results from invasion by the causative agent, myocardial toxin production, or autoimmunity

◗ Myocarditis may have no residual effects or may lead to acute dilated cardiomyopathy and death

◗ Viral myocarditis may be difficult to treat and requires an extended recovery period

◆ Clinical signs and symptoms

◗ Fatigue, dyspnea, and fever

◗ Palpitations, pericardial discomfort and chest pain, tachycardia, nonspecific ECG abnormalities, and pericardial friction rub

◆ Medical management

◗ Administer antibiotics for bacterial myocarditis, and treat the symptoms of viral infection

◗ Prescribe bed rest with restricted activity during periods of fever, fatigue, and pain

◗ Administer oxygen therapy and antipyretic agents

◗ Make sure that the patient receives adequate nutrition

◗ Restrict fluid and sodium intake, and prescribe digoxin therapy if the patient has symptoms of heart failure

◗ Consider immunosuppressant therapy with corticosteroids or cyclosporine

◆ Nursing management

◗ Maintain the patient on bed rest with restricted activity, and plan the patient's care to include periods of rest; bed rest reduces the workload of the heart, decreases residual myocardial damage, and promotes healing

◗ Administer oxygen, as prescribed, and verify that the patient is wearing the oxygen delivery device correctly

◗ Administer antipyretic agents, as prescribed; fever increases the heart's workload

◗ Maintain continuous ECG monitoring to detect and treat arrhythmias

◗ Monitor the patient for signs and symptoms of decreased cardiac output, heart failure, heart block, and pulmonary or systemic emboli; these conditions are the most common complications of myocarditis

◗ Educate the patient about the disease process and signs and symptoms that should be reported to the practitioner; tell him to consult with the practitioner before resuming physical activities

■ Infectious endocarditis

◆ Description

◗ Endocarditis is caused by a microbial infection of the endothelial tissue of the heart valves; pathogens are typically bacteria (often *Rickettsia*), fungi, or *Chlamydia*

- Acute infectious endocarditis ordinarily involves the normal heart and is common in I.V. drug abusers
- Subacute infectious endocarditis usually involves the abnormal heart
- Right-sided endocarditis is most common in I.V. drug abusers but may occur as a result of an infected peripheral or CVP catheter or transvenous pacing wire; it manifests as acute endocarditis with pulmonary infarction and abscess formation

▶ Patients at greatest risk for infectious endocarditis are those with preexisting heart disease, including congenital disease involving bicuspid aortic valves, mitral and aortic valves damaged by rheumatic fever, calcified mitral and aortic valves, mitral valve prolapse, prosthetic heart valves, Marfan syndrome, hypertrophic cardiomyopathy, coarctation of the aorta, arteriovenous shunt, ventricular septal defect, and patent ductus arteriosus

▶ Bacteria can seed and proliferate on an abnormal valve
- As a result, sterile platelet-fibrin thrombi, called vegetations, form on the injured valve leaflets
  - These vegetations may cause valvular destruction and ulceration associated with valvular insufficiency, obstruct the valve, or become dislodged (producing emboli)
  - Embolism causes infarctions and abscesses in the heart, brain, lungs, kidneys, spleen, and extremities

▶ The infection can extend to surrounding structures, causing a mycotic aneurysm, myocardial abscess, or cardiac conduction defect; acute valvular insufficiency may occur if the chordae tendineae rupture

◆ Clinical signs and symptoms
  ▶ Acute infective endocarditis: high fever, chills, petechiae, prominent embolic phenomena, Roth's spots, Janeway lesions, and headache
  ▶ Subacute infective endocarditis: low-grade fever with afternoon and evening peaks; night sweats; headache; anorexia and weight loss; malaise; fatigue; weakness; arthralgia; petechiae in the mucosa of the mouth, pharynx, conjunctiva, and upper anterior trunk; Osler's nodes; and symptoms of embolism
  ▶ Right-sided endocarditis: high fever, pleuritic chest pain, hemoptysis and sputum production, dyspnea on exertion, malaise, anorexia, and fatigability

◆ Medical management
  ▶ Obtain blood samples to determine the causative organism
  ▶ Administer bactericidal antibiotics for 2 to 6 weeks; prescribe antipyretic agents for fever, and anticoagulants if a large thrombus or atrial fibrillation develops
  ▶ Supplement the patient's regular diet with high-calorie feedings if he can't eat well
  ▶ Consider surgical intervention, if indicated

◆ Nursing management
  ▶ Monitor the patient's temperature every 1 to 4 hours; elevated temperature is a sign of infection

▶ Monitor intake and output every shift, assess for dehydration, weigh the patient daily, and encourage oral fluid intake, as tolerated; fever causes a water loss in the tissues, and oral fluids help maintain the fluid balance; daily weigh-ins provide a good indication of fluid balance (1 L of fluid weighs about 2.2 lb [1 kg])

▶ During every shift, assess for symptoms of embolization, including neurologic changes, splenomegaly, decreased urine output, hematuria, and symptoms of pulmonary embolus

  • CNS emboli occur in one-third to one-half of all patients with infectious endocarditis; splenic emboli occur in 44% of cases

    • Renal and pulmonary emboli or pulmonary infarction may also occur

▶ Administer antibiotics, as prescribed and according to the dosing schedule, to maintain therapeutic blood levels

▶ To prevent parenteral I.V. line sepsis, monitor the I.V. site for redness and signs of infection; change the site according to facility protocol, or as needed

▶ Check for signs of malnutrition: weigh the patient daily; monitor the patient's daily food intake; offer small, frequent feedings or supplemental feedings high in calories and protein; consult a dietitian; and allow family members to bring food from home, if the practitioner approves

▶ The infectious process increases metabolic needs, and chronic illness leads to anorexia; malnourishment also decreases the body's resistance to infection

▶ Provide diversionary activities, as needed; as the patient's condition improves, he may complain of boredom, depression, or a feeling of being trapped

▶ Educate the patient about the disease process and its treatment; discuss precipitating factors for reinfection (such as poor oral hygiene, dental work, GI or genitourinary procedures, vaginal deliveries, furuncles [boils], staphylococcal infections, and surgical procedures); the need to notify practitioners and dentists before undergoing procedures; and the importance of antibiotic prophylaxis

■ Pericarditis

◆ Description

▶ Pericarditis is an inflammation of the pericardium commonly caused by bacterial or viral infections, cardiac injury, uremia, or trauma

▶ Pericarditis is categorized as acute (lasting less than 6 weeks), subacute (lasting 6 weeks to 6 months), or chronic (lasting more than 6 months)

▶ In constrictive pericarditis, thick scar tissue fuses the visceral and parietal layers of the pericardium, resulting in a stiff pericardium that prevents adequate diastolic filling and leads to heart failure

▶ In postmyocardial infarction pericarditis, fibrin is deposited between the pericardial layers at the site of necrosis after a transmural MI

▶ Dressler's syndrome (postmyocardial infarction syndrome) usually occurs weeks to months after the MI and causes fever, pleuritis, and pericardial inflammation; this syndrome may have an autoimmune cause

▶ Postcardiotomy syndrome usually occurs 2 to 3 weeks after open-heart surgery; it's similar to Dressler's syndrome, but the irritation to the pericardium is caused by the surgical procedure

◆ Clinical signs and symptoms

▶ Sharp, stabbing precordial or substernal chest pain exacerbated by deep inspiration, coughing, or swallowing and usually relieved by sitting upright and leaning forward

▶ Pericardial friction rub and atrial fibrillation

▶ Dyspnea, chills, fever, diaphoresis, and pericardial effusion

▶ Elevated erythrocyte sedimentation rate

◆ Medical management

▶ Maintain the patient on bed rest until fever and pain subside

▶ Administer nonsteroidal anti-inflammatory drugs to relieve pain

▶ Administer short-term corticosteroid therapy

▶ Administer antibiotics for bacterial pericarditis

▶ Treat constrictive pericarditis surgically

▶ Consider pericardiocentesis, if indicated

◆ Nursing management

▶ Assess the characteristics of the patient's pain to distinguish pericardial pain from myocardial ischemia

▶ Administer medications, as prescribed, and evaluate the effectiveness of pain-relief measures

▶ Encourage bed rest, elevate the head of the bed, and make sure that the patient is comfortable; bed rest can reduce the workload of the heart, alleviate pain, and promote healing

▶ Check for paradoxical pulse, narrowing pulse pressure, and tachycardia—early signs of cardiac tamponade

▶ Maintain continuous ECG monitoring to detect ECG changes (diffuse ST segment elevation in all leads except aV_L and V_1) and tachycardia

▶ Check for muffled heart sounds, paradoxical pulse, decreased cardiac output, and distended jugular veins—signs of pericardial effusion and cardiac tamponade

▶ Provide emotional support to decrease the patient's anxiety

▶ Educate the patient about the disease process and the signs and symptoms of recurring inflammation

▶ Instruct the patient to avoid overexertion and heavy lifting for 2 weeks or longer (based on the practitioner's preference) and to notify the practitioner if symptoms continue or worsen

❖ **Cardiomyopathies**

■ General information

◆ Cardiomyopathies are classified as primary (if the heart is the only organ affected with no involvement of valves or other cardiac structures) or

Morphologic and hemodynamic characteristics of cardiomyopathies

	Dilated	Hypertrophic	Restrictive
Morphologic characteristics	Biventricular dilation	Marked hypertrophy of left ventricle and, occasionally, of right ventricle; usually, but not always, disproportionate hypertrophy of septum	Reduced ventricular compliance; usually caused by infiltration of myocardium (for example, by amyloid or glycogen deposits)
Hemodynamic characteristics			
Cardiac output	Decreased	Normal	Normal to decreased
Stroke volume	Decreased	Normal or increased	Normal or decreased
Ventricular filling pressure	Increased	Normal or increased	Increased
Chamber size	Increased	Normal or decreased	Normal or increased
Ejection fraction	Decreased	Increased	Normal to decreased
Diastolic compliance	Normal or decreased	Decreased	Decreased
Other findings	• May have associated functional mitral or tricuspid insufficiency	• Obstruction may develop between interventricular septum and septal leaflet of mitral valve • Mitral insufficiency may be present	• Characteristic ventricular pressure tracings that resemble those recorded in constrictive pericarditis

secondary (if the myocardial abnormality is related to another abnormality or condition and if other organs are affected)

◆ Cardiomyopathies are further classified by pathophysiologic changes as dilated, hypertrophic, or restrictive (see *Morphologic and hemodynamic characteristics of cardiomyopathies*)

■ Dilated cardiomyopathy

◆ Description

▶ Dilated cardiomyopathy results from damage to the myofibrils

◗ All four heart chambers are dilated, and contractile function of the ventricles is impaired; thrombus formation occurs most commonly in the ventricles

◗ Cardiomegaly and impairment of systolic pump function leads to heart failure

◗ Cardiac output declines as the disease progresses, with the final result being biventricular pump failure

◆ Clinical signs and symptoms

◗ Dyspnea on exertion that progresses to orthopnea, paroxysmal nocturnal dyspnea, and dyspnea at rest

◗ Fatigue and weakness, symptoms of biventricular failure

◗ Chest pain

◗ Narrowed pulse pressure

◗ Laterally displaced apical pulse

◗ Decreased cardiac output

◗ Increased RAP, PAP, PAWP, and SVR

◆ Medical management

◗ Restrict the patient's activity, sodium intake, and fluid intake

◗ Maintain continuous ECG monitoring

◗ Administer oxygen, as needed

◗ Monitor hemodynamic parameters to assess left ventricular function and cardiac output

◗ Use IABP or a ventricular assist device, as needed

◗ Administer cardiac glycosides, diuretics, vasodilators, and antiarrhythmic medications

◗ Consider heart transplantation, if indicated

◆ Nursing management

◗ Monitor blood pressure, hemodynamic parameters, and intake and output to detect early or progressive signs of low cardiac output

◗ Monitor for excessive fluid volume and increased congestion by weighing the patient daily, recording intake and output, auscultating breath sounds and heart sounds, and checking RAP, PAP, and PAWP; weighing the patient daily can help to determine the response to therapy and the amount of fluid retention

◗ Restrict sodium and fluid intake, as prescribed, to decrease fluid retention

◗ Coordinate care to provide the patient with frequent rest periods; uninterrupted rest can help restore the patient's physical and psychological well-being

◗ Increase the patient's level of activity gradually, and help the patient with activities, as needed

◗ Assess the patient's level of knowledge about the disease process, and educate him about the disease and its treatment

◗ Help the patient develop coping strategies that give him a sense of control over the situation

◗ Refer the patient to support groups for people with heart disease; support groups can alleviate feelings of isolation and are a source of information about the disease

▶ Encourage family members to learn CPR; ventricular arrhythmias associated with dilated cardiomyopathy are a common cause of sudden cardiac death; performing CPR can increase the patient's chances of survival

■ Hypertrophic cardiomyopathy
  ◆ Description
    ▶ Hypertrophic cardiomyopathy is a disproportionate thickening of the interventricular septum; this overgrowth of muscle makes the ventricular walls rigid, obstructing left ventricular outflow and impeding left ventricular ejection during systole
    ▶ The atria become hypertrophied and dilated as a result of the high resistance to ventricular filling
    ▶ Hypertrophic cardiomyopathy may be genetically transmitted, occurs equally in men and women, and is seen in young adults
  ◆ Clinical signs and symptoms
    ▶ Dyspnea, shortness of breath, angina, fatigue, palpitations, and syncope
    ▶ Normal cardiac output with elevated RAP, PAP, PAWP, and SVR
  ◆ Medical management
    ▶ Restrict the patient's activity and sodium and fluid intake
    ▶ Maintain continuous ECG monitoring
    ▶ Administer oxygen, as needed
    ▶ Monitor hemodynamic parameters to assess left ventricular function and cardiac output
    ▶ Use intra-aortic balloon counterpulsation, as needed
    ▶ Administer beta-adrenergic blocking agents, calcium channel blockers, and antiarrhythmic medications
    ▶ Consider myotomy or myectomy, if indicated
  ◆ Nursing management
    ▶ Same as for dilated cardiomyopathy
    ▶ Educate the patient about a low-sodium, fluid-restricted diet

■ Restrictive cardiomyopathy
  ◆ Description
    ▶ Restrictive cardiomyopathy results in abnormal diastolic filling secondary to excessively rigid ventricular walls
    ▶ Fibroelastic tissue infiltrates the endocardium or myocardium; contractility is mostly unimpaired, with normal systolic emptying of the ventricles
    ▶ Hemodynamically, restrictive cardiomyopathy resembles constrictive pericarditis
  ◆ Clinical signs and symptoms
    ▶ Fatigue, exercise intolerance, and symptoms of right-sided heart failure
    ▶ Narrowed pulse pressure
    ▶ Low cardiac output with increased RAP, PAP, PAWP, and SVR
  ◆ Medical management
    ▶ Restrict the patient's activity and sodium and fluid intake
    ▶ Maintain continuous ECG monitoring
    ▶ Administer oxygen, as needed

▶ Monitor hemodynamic parameters to assess left ventricular function and cardiac output

▶ Use IABP, as needed

▶ Administer cardiac glycosides and diuretics

▶ Consider excision of fibrotic endocardium, if indicated

◆ Nursing management

▶ Same as for dilated cardiomyopathy

▶ Educate the patient about dietary restrictions and the proper use of medications and their adverse effects

❖ **Cardiac trauma**

■ Penetrating cardiac trauma

◆ Description

▶ Fatal in 90% of cases, penetrating cardiac trauma is caused by stabbing or bullet wounds

▶ Penetrating trauma can lacerate any anatomic part of the heart, causing shunts, fistulas, and valve disruptions that result in murmurs

▶ Pericardial laceration resulting in cardiac tamponade or exsanguination is the most common consequence of penetrating cardiac trauma

▶ If the penetrating wound is small, cardiac tamponade can help reduce the severity of bleeding, thus improving the patient's chances of survival

◆ Clinical signs and symptoms

▶ Hypotension secondary to cardiac tamponade or hemorrhage

▶ Penetrating mediastinal wound

▶ X-ray showing object in or near cardiac silhouette

◆ Medical management

▶ Immediately transport patient from the scene to a health care facility

▶ Initiate pericardiocentesis to stabilize cardiac tamponade until an emergency thoracotomy can be performed

▶ Perform immediate emergency thoracotomy to control bleeding (once bleeding is controlled, the recovery rate is about 80%)

◆ Nursing management

▶ Maintain continuous ECG monitoring; damage to the heart muscle can cause ventricular arrhythmias and AV block

▶ Assess for symptoms of chest pain, and have the patient rate the pain on a scale of 1 to 10; obtain an immediate ECG to determine nature of chest pain

• Chest pain caused by penetrating trauma is similar to that caused by an acute MI

• An ECG is needed to differentiate among acute MI, myocardial contusion, and pericardial chest pain

▶ Monitor blood pressure, heart rate, and urine output

• Hypotension may signal cardiac injury

• Hypotension with tachycardia may indicate cardiac tamponade or hypovolemia

• Urine output provides an indication of kidney function

▶ Auscultate breath sounds and heart sounds to assess for new murmurs and the onset of heart failure

■ Nonpenetrating cardiac trauma

◆ Description
  ▮ In nonpenetrating cardiac trauma, or blunt trauma, there may be no evidence of trauma to the chest wall; the severity of the chest wall trauma doesn't correlate with the likelihood or extent of cardiac injury
  ▮ Blunt trauma commonly is caused by impact (such as with the steering wheel in a car accident), resulting in an injury to the sternum; tearing of the aorta or other great vessels results from the shearing forces associated with sudden deceleration
  ▮ Other causes of blunt trauma include a hard blow to the chest from sports activities, industrial crush injuries, falls or accidents, and personal assaults
  ▮ Blunt trauma may result in myocardial contusion, rupture of the ventricle or interventricular septum, pericardial laceration, valve disruption, coronary artery thrombosis, or great vessel rupture
  ▮ Myocardial contusion (usually in the right ventricle) is the most common blunt injury; chest pain may be masked by musculoskeletal pain, and myocardial necrosis can range from petechiae to transmural necrosis
  ▮ Myocardial contusion has several consequences:
    • Arrhythmias may occur, and ventricular tachycardia should be vigorously suppressed; high-grade AV block usually is transient, but may require temporary pacing
    • Right-sided heart failure may be caused by severe right ventricular injury; it's usually treated with digitalization, maintenance of high right-sided filling pressures, and reduction of elevated PAP
    • Rupture of the myocardium and tearing of the interventricular septum, papillary muscles and chordae tendineae, valve cusps, or aortic annulus are usually treated surgically
    • Cardiac tamponade typically is treated by pericardiocentesis until the cause can be determined
◆ Clinical signs and symptoms
  ▮ Chest pain (the most common symptom) and hypotension
  ▮ Ventricular arrhythmia or AV block
  ▮ ECG changes indicating acute MI or pericarditis
  ▮ Pericardial rub, murmur, or muffled heart sounds
  ▮ Symptoms of heart failure
◆ Medical management
  ▮ Perform cardiac catheterization with coronary angiography if cardiac enzyme levels are elevated
  ▮ Control pain and arrhythmias; don't administer anticoagulants
  ▮ Perform thoracotomy with surgical intervention, if indicated
◆ Nursing management
  ▮ Prepare the patient for cardiac catheterization
  ▮ Control pain and arrhythmias; don't administer anticoagulants, as internal bleeding may occur
  ▮ Prepare the patient for thoracotomy and surgical intervention, if indicated

❖ Cardiac tamponade

- ■ Description
  - ◆ Accumulation of fluid in the pericardial space leading to compression of the heart chambers
  - ◆ As the right ventricle volume increases during inspiration, the right ventricle is unable to properly expand due to the maximally stretched pericardium; the intraventricular septum displaces to the left, decreasing the left ventricle's end diastolic volume, which decreases the cardiac output
  - ◆ Fluid accumulation can be gradual, leading to an accumulation of 1 to 2 L before symptoms are seen, or acute, where as much as 50 to 100 ml will cause symptoms to appear
  - ◆ Causes include idiopathic (Dressler's syndrome), effusion, hemorrhage due to traumatic or nontraumatic causes, viral or postirradiation pericarditis, chronic or acute renal failure, drug reactions, connective tissue disorders, acute MI with ventricular rupture
- ■ Clinical signs and symptoms
  - ◆ The three classic features of cardiac tamponade are known as Beck's triad
    - ▶ Elevated CVP with jugular vein distention
    - ▶ Decreased heart sounds
    - ▶ Pulsus paradoxus—inspiratory drop in systemic blood pressure greater than 15 mm Hg
  - ◆ Diaphoresis and cool, clammy skin from decreased cardiac output
  - ◆ Anxiety, restlessness, and syncope
  - ◆ Weak, rapid pulse
  - ◆ Chest pain
  - ◆ ECG changes may include low-amplitude QRS complex and a generalized ST-segment elevation
  - ◆ Hemodynamic changes include increased right atrial pressure, right ventricular diastolic pressure, and CVP
- ■ Medical management
  - ◆ Trial volume loading with crystalloids to maintain systolic blood pressure
  - ◆ Inotropic drugs (isoproterenol or dopamine) to improve myocardial contractility and cardiac output
  - ◆ Surgical interventions to remove the fluid and relieve the compression on the heart
    - ▶ Pericardiocentesis—needle aspiration of the fluid in the pericardial cavity
      - • Pericardiectomy may be performed to allow communication with wpleura in cases of repeated tamponade that doesn't respond to pericardiocentesis
    - ▶ Pericardial window or drain—creating an opening in the pericardium to remove fluid
    - ▶ Repair of bleeding sites in cases of trauma
  - ◆ Administration of protamine or vitamin K to stop bleeding if heparin or warfarin induced
- ■ Nursing management

- ◆ Monitor ECG and hemodynamics continuously
- ◆ Assess ECG for changes indicative of cardiac tamponade
- ◆ Assess hemodynamic status for changes in CVP, right atrial pressure, pulmonary artery pressures, and decreased cardiac output
- ◆ Administer drugs as prescribed
    - ▶ I.V. solutions and blood products to maintain blood pressure
    - ▶ Inotropic agents to increase contractility and cardiac output
    - ▶ Protamine or vitamin K if indicated for anticoagulant-induced bleeding
    - ▶ Administer supplemental oxygen and be prepared for emergency intubation if cardiac respiratory function collapses
- ◆ Prepare patient for surgical procedures
- ◆ Monitor for signs of increasing tamponade—increased dyspnea and arrhythmia
- ◆ Assess renal function and notify practitioner if urine output less than 30 ml/hour
- ◆ Monitor capillary refill time, LOC, peripheral pulses, and skin temperature for decreasing tissue perfusion

❖ Acute peripheral vascular insufficiency

- ■ Description
    - ◆ The incidence of acute peripheral vascular insufficiency increases with age; the chief contributing factors are atherosclerosis, hypertension, and certain cardiac disorders (including mitral valve disease, rheumatic heart disease, atrial fibrillation, left atrial myxoma, and prosthetic valves)
    - ◆ Acute peripheral vascular insufficiency is primarily caused by thrombi resulting from cardiac disorders; in 95% of cases, the lower extremities are involved
        - ▶ Venous thrombosis can be precipitated by injury to the vessel, hypercoagulability, or prolonged immobility
        - ▶ Acute arterial insufficiency can result from thrombosis, embolism, or trauma
    - ◆ An embolus can travel through the systemic circulation and lodge in an arterial branch, occluding blood flow
        - ▶ This blockage causes a secondary thrombus to form along the arterial wall, which compromises collateral circulation
        - ▶ The distal tissues are deprived of oxygen, leading to ischemia, pain, and paresthesia in the affected area
        - ▶ If ischemia is prolonged, cellular damage leads to muscle necrosis
    - ◆ Complications of acute peripheral vascular insufficiency include gangrene and muscle necrosis, with the possible need for limb amputation
- ■ Medical management
    - ◆ Perform arteriography with percutaneous transluminal coronary angioplasty, if indicated
    - ◆ Administer anticoagulants to maintain the PTT at twice the normal value
    - ◆ Administer fibrinolytic agents
    - ◆ If possible, perform an embolectomy or insert a peripheral stent before advanced ischemia occurs

◆ Amputate the limb if advanced ischemia has occurred
■ Nursing management
◆ Assess arterial pulses distal to the occlusion every 1 to 2 hours to check arterial blood flow to the extremity; use Doppler ultrasonography to evaluate the presence of hard-to-palpate pulses
◆ Check skin color and temperature of the affected extremity, and assess for absence of sensation and level of motor deficit
◆ Monitor vital signs and cardiac rhythm; an arterial embolus commonly is associated with myocardial disease
◆ Maintain the patient on bed rest during the acute phase to reduce the oxygen demand of the extremity
◆ To maintain optimal gravitational blood flow, don't raise the affected extremity above the level of the heart
◆ To prevent further embolization, administer anticoagulants, as prescribed; monitor PTT results and notify the practitioner if they aren't within the therapeutic range (that is, twice the normal value)
◆ Assess the patient's level of pain, and administer analgesics, as prescribed; pain is usually alleviated when the obstruction and ischemia are relieved
◆ Use a bed cradle, cotton blankets, or sheepskin, as needed, to protect the extremity from injury
◆ Educate the patient about the disease process, its possible causes, and treatment; tell the patient to avoid crossing his legs and sitting or standing for prolonged periods (which can cause pooling or obstruction of blood flow); teach the patient about the importance of anticoagulant therapy and follow-up clotting studies to monitor the effectiveness of anticoagulant therapy; and advise the patient to avoid extreme temperatures and to always wear shoes

❖ Carotid artery stenosis
■ Description
◆ Carotid artery stenosis is caused by a buildup of plaque in the internal carotid arteries
◆ Blockage of the internal carotid arteries blocks the flow of blood to the brain and can lead to transient ischemic attacks (TIA) and strokes
◆ The incidence of carotid artery stenosis increases with age and contributing factors; the chief contributing factors are hypertension, hyperlipidemia, high stress levels, diabetes mellitus, smoking, obesity, and lack of exercise
■ Clinical signs and symptoms
◆ Typically asymptomatic
◆ Temporary symptoms may include difficulty speaking, loss or blurred vision in one eye, numbness or weakness in one extremity
◆ Bruit heard in affected artery when stethoscope placed over artery
■ Medical management
◆ Evaluate degree of blockage using cerebral angiography, carotid ultrasound, or magnetic resonance angiography
◆ Blockage of 70% or greater, or blockage between 50% and 69% with recent symptoms of stroke, surgical treatment is indicated

> ▶ Carotid endarterectomy excises plaque from inner lining of artery
> ▶ Carotid angioplasty and stenting involve dilating artery with a catheter-tipped balloon and flattening the plaque; a mesh stent is then placed in the artery to help prevent the artery from collapsing
> ◆ Antiplatelet therapy with aspirin and antiplatelet agents
> ◆ Reduction of risk factors
> ■ Nursing management
> ◆ Monitor neurological status frequently for signs of a TIA or stroke
> ◆ Administer aspirin and antiplatelet agents as prescribed
> ◆ Educate the patient about the disease process, possible causes, and treatments
> ◆ Encourage patient to modify risk factors
> ◆ Closely monitor patient after endarterectomy or stenting
> ◆ Neurologic checks every 1 to 2 hours
> ◆ Monitor operative site for drainage, pain, and hematoma formation
> ◆ Monitor airway for signs of swelling; stridor, difficulty breathing, pain
> ◆ Monitor vital signs as ordered

Review questions

1. To optimize patient outcomes for a patient with complete heart block, the nurse would prepare for which one of the following?

○ **A.** Administration of adenosine

○ **B.** Administration of lidocaine

○ **C.** Defibrillation

○ **D.** Temporary pacemaker insertion

Correct answer: D Temporary pacemaker insertion may enhance heart rate and alleviate low cardiac output produced by complete heart block. Adenosine is used for tachycardic arrhythmias, lidocaine is used to suppress ventricular arrhythmias, and defibrillation is used to convert ventricular fibrillation.

2. You're caring for a patient recently admitted with an inferior wall MI. Which of the following combinations of 12-lead ECG findings would you anticipate seeing?

○ **A.** T-wave inversion in leads I, aV_L, V_5, and V_6

○ **B.** Q-wave formation and ST elevation in leads II, III, and aV_F

○ **C.** QRS duration > 0.10 second in all 12 leads

○ **D.** R wave taller in lead V_6 than V_5

Correct answer: B Leads II, III, and aV_F are used to view the heart's inferior wall. Q-wave formation and ST elevation indicate myocardial injury and infarction. T-wave inversion indicates myocardial ischemia. A QRS duration greater than 0.10 second may indicate bundle branch block. An R wave taller in lead V_6 than V_5 may indicate left ventricular hypertrophy.

3. Management of a patient experiencing heart failure includes all of the following EXCEPT:

    ○ **A.** enhancement of cardiac workload.

    ○ **B.** monitoring of fluid balance and retention.

    ○ **C.** prevention of skin breakdown.

    ○ **D.** patient education about lifestyle changes.

Correct answer: A Enhancing cardiac workload would produce negative effects on cardiac pumping ability. Monitoring for fluid retention is paramount, as is prevention of skin breakdown due to the potential for decreased circulation; patient education to prevent recurrence and management is also important.

4. The best definition of hypertrophic cardiomyopathy is:

    ○ **A.** abnormal diastolic filling secondary to excessively rigid ventricular walls.

    ○ **B.** damage to the myofibrils.

    ○ **C.** disproportionate thickening of the interventricular septum.

    ○ **D.** death of myocardial muscle cells.

Correct answer: C Thickening of the interventricular septum, the primary pathologic process in hypertrophic cardiomyopathy, frequently leads to restriction of the outflow tract. Option A defines restrictive cardiomyopathy, option B defines dilated cardiomyopathy, and option D defines MI.

5. Primary patient care management of pericarditis includes all of the following EXCEPT:

    ○ **A.** monitoring for signs of cardiac tamponade.

    ○ **B.** evaluating the effectiveness of pain relief strategies.

    ○ **C.** maintaining the patient's bowel regimen.

    ○ **D.** providing emotional support.

Correct answer: C Maintaining the patient's bowel regimen isn't a primary concern when caring for a patient with pericarditis. For an acute MI patient, it's a significant concern because of the potential for vagal stimulation and straining. Pericarditis patients must be monitored for cardiac tamponade and pain relief, and they require emotional support throughout the course of their illness.

CHAPTER 3

Pulmonary disorders

❖ **Anatomy**
- ◼ Nose
  - ◆ The area from the nose to the terminal bronchioles where the gas flows but isn't exchanged is called the anatomic dead space; it's calculated as 2 ml per kg of body weight
  - ◆ Ciliated mucous membrane lines the nose and the respiratory tract; it warms the air to 2% to 3% of body temperature, humidifies air, and filters particles larger than 6 μm in diameter
- ◼ Pharynx
  - ◆ Posterior to the nasal cavities and mouth
  - ◆ Separates food from air through local nerve reflexes; contains lymphatic tissue to control infection
  - ◆ Opens to eustachian tube to regulate middle ear pressure
- ◼ Larynx
  - ◆ Located at the upper end of the trachea, the larynx is constructed of incomplete rings of cartilage; contains the vocal cords for speech function
  - ◆ The epiglottis helps prevent aspiration
  - ◆ The cricoid cartilage is the only complete rigid ring and sets the inner diameter limit for endotracheal tube size
- ◼ Trachea
  - ◆ The trachea is composed of smooth muscle embedded with C-shaped cartilage rings
  - ◆ The trachea helps warm and humidify air, while mucosal cells trap foreign material
  - ◆ At the carina tracheae, the tracheal bifurcation, the cough reflex is present
- ◼ Primary and secondary bronchi
  - ◆ The right bronchus is slightly larger and more vertical than the left bronchus; the left bronchus is smaller and more horizontal than the right bronchus
  - ◆ Before the bronchi enter the lungs, the bronchial walls are composed of incomplete cartilaginous rings; after the bronchi enter the lungs, the rings are complete
  - ◆ Just after entering the lungs, the primary bronchi are divided into secondary bronchi, which are divided into small bronchioles, and further divided into smaller alveolar ducts
- ◼ Terminal bronchioles

       ◆ The terminal bronchioles are composed of only smooth muscle; bronchospasms narrow the lumen and increase airway resistance

       ◆ They are sensitive to carbon dioxide (CO_2) levels; increased levels cause bronchiolar dilation; decreased levels cause bronchiolar constriction

    ■ Alveoli

       ◆ The alveoli are small, grapelike sacs surrounded by a network of capillaries

       ◆ Type I alveolar cells are composed of squamous epithelium and adapted for gas exchange; they're sensitive to injury by inhaled agents and prevent fluid transudation into the alveoli

       ◆ Type II cells are secretory and the origin of surfactant; this phospholipid decreases surface tension, lessens the work of breathing, keeps alveoli inflated at low pressures, detoxifies gases, and traps inhaled and deposited particles

    ■ Lungs

       ◆ The lungs are cone-shaped organs that fill the pleural portion of the thoracic cavity

       ◆ The bronchi enter the lungs through the hilum, a slit on the medial surface of the lungs

       ◆ At their base, the lungs are broad and rest on the diaphragm; at the apex in the upper part of the chest cavity, the lungs are pointed

       ◆ The left lung has two lobes (upper and lower); the right lung has three lobes (superior, middle, and inferior) (These divide into bronchopulmonary segments that subdivide into secondary lobules, the primary functional units of the lung; the terminal bronchioles, alveolar ducts and sacs, and pulmonary circulation compose the secondary lobules)

    ■ Thorax

       ◆ The thorax, or chest, is encased by the ribs

       ◆ Parietal pleura lines the entire thoracic cavity; visceral pleura covers and adheres to the outer surface of the lungs; a small amount of pleural fluid is contained between these layers to reduce friction and maintain negative pressure

       ◆ The diaphragm, the principal muscle of ventilation, lies outside the pleura

       ◆ The intercostal muscles, which aid in ventilation, lie between the ribs

❖ **Physiology**

    ■ Upper airways

       ◆ Air reaches the lungs through the upper airways; air passing through the upper airways also produces the voice

       ◆ The upper airways heat, filter, and humidify the air before it enters the lungs

       ◆ They also protect the lungs from foreign objects and liquids

    ■ Lower airways

       ◆ The bronchioles and alveoli compose the lower airways

       ◆ Diffusion of gases between the air and the blood takes place in the lower airways; oxygen (O_2) and CO_2 move easily across the thin membranes of the alveoli and capillaries

- ◆ The exchange of gases is called respiration
  - ▶ External respiration is the exchange of gases in the lungs
  - ▶ Internal respiration is the exchange of gases at the cellular level between the blood and cells of the organs and muscles
- ◆ The movement of air into and out of the lungs is called ventilation; the normal adult respiratory rate is 12 to 20 breaths/minute
  - ▶ Air moves into and out of the lungs because of a pressure gradient
  - ▶ Inhalation (inspiration) creates a negative pressure in the chest cavity compared with the atmosphere, and air moves into the lungs; inhalation is an active process and requires the use of the respiratory muscles (The diaphragm, innervated from the C3 to C5 level, is the primary muscle of inspiration; it also facilitates vomiting, coughing, sneezing, defecation, and parturition)
  - ▶ Exhalation (expiration) creates a positive pressure in the chest cavity compared with the atmosphere, and air moves out of the lungs; exhalation is a passive process and occurs when the muscles of respiration relax
- ■ Principles that affect gas exchange
  - ◆ Air flows into the lungs when the intrapulmonary air pressure falls below atmospheric pressure; when intrapulmonary air pressure exceeds atmospheric pressure, air flows out
  - ◆ Intrapleural pressures are normally negative, with respect to atmospheric air, due to elastic recoil of the lungs; this negative pressure prevents lung collapse
  - ◆ The pleural space is a potential space (or vacuum) due to a constant negative pressure
  - ◆ Compliance of the lung is an expression of its elastic property; if compliance is high, the lung is more easily distended; if compliance is low, the lung is stiff and difficult to distend
  - ◆ Airway resistance must be overcome to generate airflow through the passages (If airway caliber is decreased, resistance is then increased; airflow is also dependent upon differences between atmospheric and alveolar pressures)
- ■ Control of respirations
  - ◆ The CO_2 level in the blood is the primary and most powerful stimulant of respiration; when CO_2 levels increase above normal (45 mm Hg), the respiratory center in the brain stem is stimulated, and the respiratory muscles contract; chemoreceptors located centrally (in the medulla) and peripherally (in the carotid body and aortic arch) are sensitive to changes in CO_2 levels, initiating a feedback loop if blood gases aren't maintained within the normal range
  - ◆ The O_2 level in the blood is a backup control for respiration; it doesn't stimulate respiration, as long as the CO_2 level remains normal; when the O_2 level falls below normal (70 mm Hg), combined with a high CO_2 level, respirations are stimulated
  - ■ Arterial blood pressure helps to control respirations through a pressure-reflex mechanism
    - ▶ A sudden rise in blood pressure slows respirations
    - ▶ A sudden drop in blood pressure increases the rate and depth of respirations

◆ Hering-Breuer reflexes control the depth and regularity of normal respirations at rest

◆ The pneumotaxic center in the pons regulates the rhythmicity of respirations by ending inspirations

◆ The cerebral cortex can override automatic respiratory functions, allowing the rate and depth of respirations to be voluntarily increased or decreased within limits

◆ The buildup of certain substances in the body, particularly those that affect blood pH, can affect respirations by stimulating irritant receptors

■ Diffusion of gases

◆ Diffusion is the process by which air gases move across the alveolar-capillary membrane to the capillary bed and back again

▶ Diffusion occurs from higher to lower areas of concentration; CO_2 is 20 times more diffusible than O_2

▶ O_2 concentration is greater in the alveoli than in the capillaries; O_2 diffuses from the alveoli into the blood

▶ The CO_2 concentration in the blood is greater than that in the alveoli; CO_2 diffuses from the blood into the alveoli

◆ The amount of surface area for gas exchange, integrity of the alveolar-capillary membrane, amount of hemoglobin (Hb), alveolar gas tensions, and diffusion coefficient of gas as well as contact time determine diffusion

◆ The A-a gradient (PAO_2-PaO_2) is the difference between the partial pressure of O_2 in the alveolar gas spaces and the pressure in the systemic arterial blood; it indicates the gas transfer gradient between the pulmonary capillary and alveolar capillary; the normal gradient in young adults is less than 10 mm Hg on room air; this rate increases with age and can be as high as 20 mm Hg in those over age 60

■ Transport of gases

◆ The oxyhemoglobin (O_2-Hb) dissociation curve expresses the relationship between O_2 saturation (and content) and the partial pressure of arterial oxygen (PaO_2) as an S-shaped curve; it describes the ability of Hb to bind with O_2 at normal arterial O_2 tension levels and release it at lower PaO_2 levels (see *Oxyhemoglobin dissociation curve*, page 86)

◆ The upper part of the O_2-Hb dissociation curve represents arteriolar association, while the lower steep portion shows venous dissociation

▶ When PaO_2 is increased (as in the pulmonary capillaries), O_2 binds readily with Hb; when PaO_2 is decreased (as in the tissues), O_2 unloads from Hb

◆ Shift of the O_2-Hb curve to the right (meaning O_2 delivery to tissues increased) is caused by pH decrease (acidosis), partial pressure of arterial carbon dioxide ($PaCO_2$) increase, increased body temperature, and increased levels of 2,3-diphosphoglycerate (2,3-DPG)

◆ Shift of the O_2-Hb curve to the left (meaning O_2 delivery to tissues decreased) is caused by pH increase (alkalosis); $PaCO_2$ decrease; temperature decrease; lowered levels of 2,3-DPG; and carbon monoxide poisoning

◆ The amount of O_2 transported per minute is a factor of both the O_2 content (CaO_2) and the cardiac output; it depends on the circulatory system (arterial blood delivery), erythropoietic system (Hb amount),

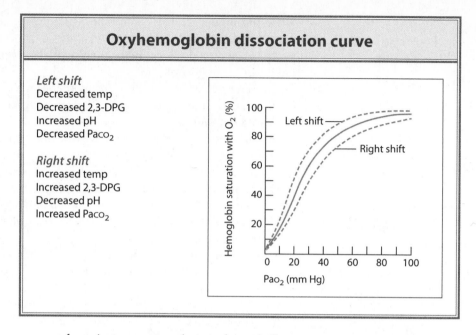

Oxyhemoglobin dissociation curve

Left shift
Decreased temp
Decreased 2,3-DPG
Increased pH
Decreased Pa_{CO_2}

Right shift
Increased temp
Increased 2,3-DPG
Decreased pH
Increased Pa_{CO_2}

and respiratory system (gas exchange); O_2 transport range is 1,000 to 1,200 ml/minute

◆ An arterial-mixed venous difference in O_2 content (Ca_{O_2}-Cv_{O_2}) is the difference between the arterial O_2 content and mixed venous O_2 content; this reflects the amount of O_2 extracted from the blood during passage through the tissues; normal Ca_{O_2}-Cv_{O_2} is 4.5 to 6 ml/dl

◆ In the lung, the measurement of flow resistance is termed pulmonary vascular resistance

❖ **Pulmonary assessment**

■ Noninvasive assessment techniques

◆ Patient history

▶ The patient's presenting symptoms or complaints provide the starting point for obtaining the patient history; common symptoms include dyspnea, cough, sputum, hemoptysis, and pain

▶ The patient history should include the medical history; family history; social history and habits (tobacco, alcohol and drug use, and home conditions); current medications; and past diagnostic studies

◆ Physical examination

▶ Inspection includes observation of the patient's general appearance, condition, and musculoskeletal development

• During the physical examination, note the patient's weight, state of debilitation, and evidence of chronic disease

• Observe the shape and diameter of the thorax, slope of the ribs, and evidence of asymmetry, retractions, or bulging of interspaces

• Observe the ventilatory pattern for dyspnea, stridor, paradoxical breathing, and evidence of splinting

• Note the position in which the patient breathes most comfortably

— Assess for presence of pursed lip breathing, nasal flaring, or paradoxical movement of the diaphragm

Abnormal respiratory patterns

Tachypnea
Shallow breathing with increased respiratory rate

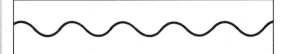

Bradypnea
Decreased rate but regular breathing

Apnea
Absence of breathing; may be periodic

Hyperpnea
Deep breathing at a normal rate

Kussmaul's respirations
Rapid, deep breathing without pauses; in adults, more than 20 breaths/minute; breathing that usually sounds labored with deep breaths that resemble sighs

Cheyne-Stokes respirations
Breaths that gradually become faster and deeper than normal, then slower, during a 30- to 170-second period; alternates with 20- to 60-second periods of apnea

Biot's respirations
Rapid, deep breathing with abrupt pauses between each breath; equal depth to each breath

─ Observe and assess the breathing rate and depth (see *Abnormal respiratory patterns*)
● Note general state, such as restlessness, pain, mental status, fear, or distress
● If O_2 is being administered, note amount and delivery method
● Inspect extremities for clubbing, cigarette stains, and edema; assess for cyanosis
● Assess for jugular vein distention, masses, enlarged lymph nodes, and superior vena cava syndrome (distended jugular veins with edema of neck, eyelids, and hands)
❱ Palpate the thoracic muscles and skeleton for pulsations, fremitus, tenderness, bulges, depressions, crepitus, or subcutaneous emphysema
● Assess expansion by placing hands over the lower aspect of the chest with the thumbs meeting in the midline along the costal mar-

gins, anteriorly or posteriorly; note symmetry on inspiration and expiration as well as reduced chest wall movement
- Assess position and mobility of the trachea
- Locate point of maximal impulse (apical pulse)
- Examine the patient for vocal fremitus, noting any areas of diminished intensity or increased fremitus

▶ Percuss the chest, comparing bilaterally; note areas of resonance, hyperresonance, tympany, or dullness
- Percuss for diaphragmatic excursion

▶ Auscultate the patient's lungs, comparing bilaterally, while the patient breathes through his mouth
- Breath sounds vary according to the site of auscultation and may be vesicular, bronchial, or bronchovesicular
  - Vesicular sounds are soft and normally heard over the anterior, lateral, and posterior chest on inspiration
  - Bronchial sounds are high-pitched, loud expirations normally heard over the trachea; if heard over lung fields, they may indicate consolidation or increased density
  - Bronchovesicular sounds are harsh and normally heard over the large bronchi; if heard over lung fields, they may indicate consolidation
- Listen for absent or diminished breath sounds that may indicate decreased airflow
- Listen for adventitious sounds, such as crackles (rales), wheezes, gurgles (rhonchi), pleural friction rub, mediastinal crunch, and pericardial friction rub; note the location and the influence of patient position and coughing on sounds
  - Crackles may be fine or coarse popping sounds on inspiration, which signify opening of collapsed alveoli and small airways
  - Wheezes are high-pitched sounds occurring on expiration and may also occur on inspiration as air passes through constricted airways
  - Gurgles are low-pitched, continuous sounds due to air passing through secretions; they often disappear with coughing
  - Inflammation and loss of pleural fluid may result in pleural friction rub, which sounds like a harsh grating sound on inspiration and expiration
  - A mediastinal crunch can be heard during systole and indicates air in the pericardium or mediastinum
  - Pericardial friction rub is heard most clearly at the left lower sternal border during atrial and ventricular systole; it persists during held breath
- Assess for voice sounds by having the patient say "ninety-nine" while auscultating the lung fields
  - Increased sounds occur when normal tissue is replaced with solid tissue; decreased sounds occur when bronchi are obscured, with pneumothorax, or with collection of fluid or tissue between the lung and chest wall

- Noninvasive diagnostic testing
    - ◆ Sputum examination shows color, consistency, volume, and odor of secretions; samples are obtained by having the patient cough, by suctioning, or by bronchoscopy
        - ❭ Microscopic cytological examination can detect malignant cells; Gram stain may detect bacteria; infections or drug resistance may also be identified
        - ❭ Special stains for cultures may detect mycobacteria, fungi, and other pathogens
    - ◆ Pleural fluid obtained from thoracentesis or pleural biopsy may be examined to determine protein, lactate dehydrogenase levels, bleeding, cell counts, glucose, amylase, pH, microorganisms, and malignant cells
    - ◆ Skin tests may be done for type I hypersensitivity (those mediated by immunoglobulin E, such as pollen, mold, dust, or grasses) and type II hypersensitivity (mediated by T lymphocytes such as purified protein derivative for tuberculosis)
    - ◆ Serologic tests may be used to determine bacterial, viral, parasitic, and mycotic pathogens
    - ◆ Radiologic studies, including chest X-ray, may be used to confirm findings
        - ❭ Posteroanterior and lateral views are most common
        - ❭ Lateral decubitus films help determine fluid levels of pleural effusions or abscesses
        - ❭ Oblique views help localize lesions and infiltrates
        - ❭ Lordotic views show the apical lung area and middle lobe or lingula and are helpful in determining a lesion's anterior or posterior position
        - ❭ Expiratory films help visualize pneumothorax or air trapping
    - ◆ Fluoroscopy shows structural movement and diaphragmatic motion, localizes lesions, and helps monitor special procedures, such as catheter insertion, thoracentesis, and chest tube placement
    - ◆ Tomography provides a plane view of the lungs, showing better definition and location of lesions
    - ◆ Computed tomography (CT) scan provides axial cross-sections of the body and helps detect subtle tissue density differences
    - ◆ Magnetic resonance imaging (MRI) can distinguish tumors from other structures
    - ◆ Pulmonary angiography visualizes the pulmonary arterial system using radiopaque dye; it's useful in thromboembolic disease, congenital circulatory abnormalities, and definition of masses
    - ◆ Ventilation-perfusion lung scans use radioisotopes to describe blood flow and ventilation, pulmonary emboli, and lung function
    - ◆ Ultrasonography helps evaluate pleural disease, fluid location, thickening, and status of the diaphragm and inferior areas such as subphrenic abscesses
    - ◆ Pulmonary function studies assess pulmonary status, detect early disease, and quantify lung function; volumes, capacities, ventilatory mechanics, lung compliance, and gas transfer and exchange studies provide information about the patient's pulmonary status

▶ Tidal volume (V_T) is the amount of gas inspired and expired during each respiratory cycle; normal is 7 ml/kg

▶ Inspiratory reserve volume (IRV) is the maximal volume that can be inspired after a tidal breath is taken; normal 3,000 ml

▶ Expiratory reserve volume (ERV) is the maximal volume that can be expired from end-expiratory breath; normal 1,000 ml

▶ Residual volume (RV) is the volume of gas remaining in the lungs after maximal expiration; normal 1,000 ml

▶ Total lung capacity (TLC) is the volume of gas in the lung at the end of a maximal inspiration (TLC = V_T + IRV + ERV + RV); normal 5,500 to 6,000 ml

▶ Vital capacity (VC) is the maximal volume of gas expelled from the lungs by forceful effort after maximal inspiration (VC = V_T + IRV + ERV); normal 4,500 ml

▶ Inspiratory capacity (IC) is the maximal volume that can be inspired from a resting expiratory level (IC = V_T + IRV); normal 3,500 ml

▶ Functional residual capacity (FRC) is the volume remaining in the lungs at resting end expiration (FRC = ERV + RV); normal 2,000 ml

  • Ventilatory mechanics are forced breathing maneuvers by the patient that can provide information about dynamic lung function (forced expiratory spirograms, flow-volume loop studies, and maximum voluntary ventilation)

  • Lung compliance studies assess the ability of the lung to distend (lung elasticity)

  • Gas transfer and exchange studies (blood gas and acid-base analysis) help diagnose and manage pulmonary problems; diffusing capacity measures the amount of functioning alveolar-capillary surface area for gas exchange

■ Invasive assessment techniques

  ◆ Lung biopsy may be performed through needle biopsy or open lung technique (thoracotomy) to diagnose malignancy or infection

  ◆ Bronchoscopy through insertion of a fiber-optic scope into the airways is performed to directly visualize the airways and obtain specimens

    ▶ It's useful in diagnosing lung malignancy, evaluating hemoptysis, and removing secretions or foreign bodies

    ▶ Washings, brushings, or biopsy of specimens may be obtained for testing

  ◆ Mediastinoscopy may be performed for diagnostic exploration of the mediastinum and to obtain biopsy specimens

  ◆ Arterial blood gases (ABGs) are used to evaluate ventilation and acid-base status (see *ABG analysis*)

    ▶ pH—normal value is 7.35 to 7.45

    ▶ $Paco_2$—normal value is 35 to 45 mm Hg

    ▶ HCO_3^-—normal value is 22 to 26 mm Hg

    ▶ Pao_2—normal value is 80 to 100 mm Hg

      • greater than 100 indicates hyperoxemia

      • less than 80 indicates mild hypoxemia

      • less than 60 indicates moderate hypoxemia

      • less than 40 indicates severe hypoxemia

ABG analysis

Imbalance	Causes	Signs and symptoms	Nursing management
Respiratory acidosis pH < 7.35 ↑ $PaCO_2$ (primary) ↑ HCO_3^- (compensatory)	Hypoventilation • Atelectasis • Central nervous system (CNS) depression • Neuromuscular abnormality • Obstructed airway • Obstructive lung disease • Pneumonia • Pulmonary edema • Respiratory arrest • Restrictive lung disease	Early • Tachycardia • Increased respiratory rate Late • Arrhythmias • Confusion • Decreased respiratory rate • Headache • Hypotension • Lethargy	• Treat cause of hypoventilation • Improve ventilation • Administer medication therapy • Maintain patent airway • Use mechanical ventilation • If mechanical ventilation being used, increase rate or tidal volume
Respiratory alkalosis pH > 7.45 ↓ $PaCO_2$ (primary) ↓ HCO_3^- (compensatory)	Hyperventilation • Anxiety • CNS infection • CNS injury • Excessive mechanical ventilation • Fever • Hepatic failure • Hyperthyroidism • Pain • Pneumothorax • Pulmonary embolism	• Anxiety • Coma • Diaphoresis • Dizziness • Increased respiratory rate • Palpitations • Seizures • Syncope • Tingling around mouth	• Treat cause of hyperventilation • Decrease ventilation • Administer sedatives or pain medication • Decrease anxiety • Use a nonrebreather mask • If mechanical ventilation being used, decrease rate or tidal volume
Metabolic acidosis pH < 7.35 ↓ HCO_3^- (primary) ↓ $PaCO_2$ (compensatory)	Acid gain • Drugs and toxins • Ketoacidosis • Renal failure • Tissue hypoxia Bicarbonate loss • Diarrhea • Excessive bile drainage • Pancreatic fistula	• Arrhythmias • Coma • Confusion • Headache • Hypotension • Increased respiratory rate • Lethargy • Nausea, vomiting • Weakness • Tremors	• Treat cause • Administer antidiarrheals • Administer I.V. bicarbonate • Dialysis • If diabetic ketoacidosis, give insulin • Improve oxygenation • Improve tissue perfusion
Metabolic alkalosis pH > 7.45 ↑ HCO_3^- (primary) ↑ $PaCO_2$ (compensatory)	Acid loss • Cushing's disease • Hepatic disease • Nasogastric suctioning • Potassium-wasting diuretics • Steroid therapy • Vomiting Bicarbonate gain • Bicarbonate administration • Excessive lactated Ringer's infusion	• Coma • Confusion • Decreased respiratory rate • Diarrhea • Dizziness • Nausea, vomiting • Seizures • Tingling around mouth • Tetany	• Treat cause • Replace electrolytes as needed • Administer buffer

❖ **Mechanical ventilation**
- Indications
  - ◆ Hypoxemia in the presence of maximum oxygen therapy
  - ◆ Increased CO_2 retention caused by relief of hypoxemia
  - ◆ Apnea
  - ◆ Respiratory rate sustained greater than 30 to 35 breaths/minute
  - ◆ Acute ventilatory failure
  - ◆ Any other condition where the patient is not able to adequately oxygenate or ventilate
- Modes of ventilation
  - ◆ Assist-control (AC) ventilation delivers a preset tidal volume for each patient respiratory effort, whether the patient initiates the respiratory effort or the respiration is delivered by the ventilator
    - ◗ AC ventilation lessens the work of breathing for the patient
    - ◗ Patient may be overventilated due to set amount of tidal volume delivered with all breaths
    - ◗ Overventilation may result in respiratory alkalosis
    - ◗ Patient may need to be sedated to control respiratory rate
    - ◗ AC ventilation may decrease cardiac output due to changes in intrathoracic pressure
  - ◆ Synchronized intermittent mandatory ventilation (SIMV) delivers a preset tidal volume at a preset rate; any spontaneous breaths by the patient aren't augmented by the ventilator
    - ◗ Breaths initiated by ventilator are synchronized with patient to not interrupt patient's breathing effort
    - ◗ Helps the patient regain muscle conditioning
    - ◗ Less potential for overventilation than with AC mode
    - ◗ Increases work of patient breathing compared with AC mode
    - ◗ Less effect on hemodynamics
  - ◆ Controlled mandatory ventilation (CMV) or pressure control ventilation (PCV) delivers a preset volume to the patient at a preset rate; there's no spontaneous ventilation allowed by the patient
    - ◗ Patient must be heavily sedated or paralyzed to tolerate this mode
    - ◗ Ensures complete control of patient ventilation
    - ◗ Generally used if patient doesn't tolerate or respond to other modes of ventilation
  - ◆ Positive end-expiratory pressure (PEEP) delivers a constant preset amount of pressure at the end of expiration; this pressure helps prevent alveolar collapse and improves ventilatory function and eases the work of breathing
    - ◗ Does not help improve lung function
    - ◗ Helps improve atelectasis due to underventilation
    - ◗ May compromise hemodynamic status due to increased intrathoracic pressure
    - ◗ High levels of PEEP (greater than 20 cm H_2O) may cause pneumothorax
  - ◆ Continuous positive airway pressure (CPAP) maintains positive airway pressure throughout the respiratory cycle
    - ◗ May be delivered via an endotracheal tube or a tight-fitting face mask

> ▶ Often used to wean patients from ventilator
> ▶ Used to try to treat respiratory distress without intubating patient
> ▶ Used to treat sleep apnea

◆ Bilevel positive airway pressure (Bi-PAP) alternates inspiratory positive pressure and expiratory positive pressure to reach a desired tidal volume

> ▶ May be used with a ventilator or as a stand-alone machine
> ▶ May be used with endotracheal tube or face mask
> ▶ Used to treat respiratory distress without intubation
> ▶ Used as at-home nocturnal treatment for restrictive and obstructive airway diseases

■ Nursing management

◆ Assessment

> ▶ Note airway size, type, and position
> > • Change position of airway daily to prevent necrosis of tongue and oral mucosa
> > • Check cuff pressure
> > • Overinflation can cause necrosis of the trachea
> > • Underinflation allows air to escape around the cuff and underventilation of the patient and also increases risk for aspiration
> ▶ Provide frequent oral care to prevent formation of bacteria
> ▶ Patient respiratory status including use of accessory muscles and independent respiratory effort (if present)
> ▶ Note ventilator settings including mode, tidal volume, rate, forced inspiratory oxygen (FIO_2), PEEP, and alarms
> ▶ Monitor patient vital signs and hemodynamic status
> > • Cardiac output may decrease if patient placed on AC mode or if PEEP used
> ▶ Assess for pain or anxiety and administer medication as needed
> ▶ Monitor breath sounds; breath sounds should be equal on both sides
> > • If breath sounds are absent or diminished on left side, obtain chest X-ray to check placement of endotracheal tube
> ▶ Draw ABGs and make ventilator changes as ordered

◆ Complications

> ▶ Barotrauma and pneumothorax from increased intrathoracic pressures
> > • May necessitate insertion of chest tube to remove air from pleural cavity
> ▶ If patient develops increased respiratory rate, decreased SaO_2, increased peak pressures, or decreased breath sounds, obtain chest X-ray to evaluate for pneumothorax
> ▶ Atelectasis may result from underventilation
> ▶ Respiratory alkalosis may result from hyperventilation
> > • Monitor ABGs and make ventilator changes as needed
> ▶ Aspiration of stomach contents, oral secretion, and tube feeding due to delayed gastric emptying or gastroesophageal reflux
> > • Ensure proper cuff inflation
> > • Keep head of bed elevated at least 30 degrees (if possible)

- Check nasogastric (NG) tube placement and residual at least every 4 hours
▶ Gastric ulcer formation due to physiological pressure and stress
  - Initiate enteral feedings as soon as possible
  - Administer H_2 receptor agonist as prescribed
▶ Infection from bypassing normal upper airway defenses and compromised immune system
  - Ventilator-associated pneumonia most common infection for patients being mechanically ventilated
  - Administer antibiotics as prescribed
  - Make sure that bronchial suctioning is sterile
  - Use proper hand-washing and infection-control techniques
▶ Anxiety from loss of control of breathing, inability to communicate and discomfort
    - Explain procedures to patient and provide reassurance
    - Sedation may be necessary to optimize ventilation (see *American Association of Critical-Care Nurses sedation assessment scale*)
    - Minimize interruptions in sleep pattern when possible
    - Place call bell by patient and explain use

❖ **Acute respiratory failure**
  ■ Description
    ◆ Acute respiratory failure is characterized by the inability of the lungs to maintain Pao_2 and removal of CO_2 ($Paco_2$)
    ◆ Abnormalities in ABGs for hypoxemic respiratory failure (abnormality in Pao_2) is Pao_2 less than 60 mm Hg or Sao_2 less than 90%; acute hypercapnic respiratory failure (abnormality in $Paco_2$) is a value of $Paco_2$ above 50 to 55 mm Hg with a pH less than 7.30
    ◆ In diagnosing respiratory failure, the patient's preexisting ABG values are considered as well as the rapidness of onset of signs and symptoms (minutes to days)
    ◆ The primary conditions associated with acute respiratory failure are hypoventilation, ventilation-perfusion mismatching, right-to-left pulmonary shunting, and impaired diffusion; these result in extravascular lung fluid and impaired ventilation
      ▶ *Alveolar hypoventilation* is indicated by an increased $Paco_2$
        - It's caused by a decrease in total minute ventilation or an increase in dead-space ventilation
        - C4 or higher spinal cord injuries impair movement of the diaphragm and intercostal nerves; T4 to C4 spinal cord injuries cause paralysis of the abdominal wall and lower intercostal muscles, resulting in paradoxical chest and abdominal wall movements and reduction in the patient's ability to breathe
        - Neck and cardiac surgery can cause paralysis of the phrenic nerve, which enervates the diaphragm and reduces the patient's ability to breathe
      ▶ *Ventilation-perfusion mismatching* occurs when the lungs are adequately ventilated but inadequately perfused (or vice versa)
        - In a high-ventilation–low-perfusion condition, the lungs compensate for a low $Paco_2$ by contracting the airway's smooth mus-

American Association of Critical-Care Nurses Sedation Assessment Scale

Domain or obstacle	Indicator	Best 1	2	3	4	Worst 5
				Score		
Consciousness	Awake and aware of self and environment	Spontaneously opens eyes and initiates interaction with others	Wakens and responds after light verbal or tactile stimuli May return to sleep when stimuli stop	Wakens and responds after strong or noxious verbal or tactile stimuli Returns to sleep when stimuli stop	Displays localization or withdrawal behaviors to noxious stimuli	Displays posturing or no response to strong or noxious stimuli
Agitation	Body movement, patient/staff safety*	Calm body movements and tolerance of treatments and restrictions Movements don't pose a significant risk for safety of patient or staff		Body movements or noncompliance with treatments or restrictions don't pose a significant risk for safety of patient or staff		Body movements or noncompliance with treatments or restrictions pose a significant risk for safety of patient or staff
	Noises of patient	No noises		Frequent moaning or calling out		Shouting, screaming, or other disruptive vocalizations
	Patients' statements†	Very calm				Very restless
Anxiety	Patient's perceived anxiety † (Faces Anxiety Scale)‡	No anxiety				Extreme anxiety
Sleep	Observed sleep	Looks asleep, calm, resting (eyes closed, calm face and body)	Looks asleep, periodically awakens and returns to sleep easily	Awake, naps occasionally for brief periods		Unable to sleep or nap
	Patient's preceived quality of sleep†	I slept well		I slept fair		I slept poorly
Patient-ventilator synchrony	Breathing pattern relative to ventilator cycle	Synchrony of patient and ventilator at all times, patient cooperative and accepting ventilation Coordinated, relaxed chest movement		Occasional resistance to ventilation, or spontaneous breathing is out of synchrony with the ventilator Chest movement occasionally not coordinated with ventilator		Frequent resistance to ventilation, or spontaneous breathing isn't synchronous with the ventilator Uncoordinated chest and ventilator movements

*This component is assessed in all patients, regardless of the goal of sedation.

† Assumes the patient has the ability to understand directions and communicate his or her perceptions verbally, in writing, or by pointing to words or pictures. If score is greater than 2 for this subscale, ask the patient if he or she needs something to help him or her relax.

‡ Faces Anxiety Scale reprinted from McKinley et al. with permission of Blackwell Publishing.

De Jong, M.M., et al. "Development of the American association of critical-care nurses' sedation assessment scale for critically ill patients," *American Journal of Critical Care* 14(6):531-44, November 2005. Used with permission.

cles, which increases airway resistance and decreases ventilation to an area

- In a low-ventilation–high-perfusion condition, the lungs respond to a high Pa_{CO_2} by relaxing the airway smooth muscles, which decreases airway resistance and increases ventilation to an area
- Ventilation-perfusion mismatching can be caused by pulmonary emboli, left-sided heart failure, pulmonary infection, atelectasis, or chronic obstructive pulmonary disease (COPD)

▶ *Right-to-left pulmonary shunting* is a common cause of hypoxemic pulmonary disease

- It occurs when blood passes by nonventilated alveoli; the subsequent return of unoxygenated blood to the left atrium results in a decreased Pa_{O_2}
- Conditions that cause right-to-left pulmonary shunting include acute respiratory distress syndrome (ARDS), pneumonia, atelectasis, and O_2 toxicity

▶ *Impaired diffusion* is caused by a physical alteration in the alveolocapillary membrane

- Because O_2 diffuses about 20 times more slowly than CO_2, impaired diffusion is most commonly indicated by a decreased Pa_{O_2} and O_2 saturation level, rather than an elevated Pa_{CO_2}
- The signs and symptoms of impaired diffusion are those of hypoxemia, hypercapnia, and the underlying disorder; they include anxiety, restlessness, tachycardia, central cyanosis, cool and dry skin, weakness, fatigue, disorientation, somnolence, coma, decreased blood pressure, and an increased rate and depth of respiration

■ Clinical signs and symptoms

◆ The patient most often complains of increased work of breathing and dyspnea; may appear confused, restless, irritable, or somnolent; and may need to sit upright to breathe more comfortably

◆ Inspection may reveal retractions, barrel chest, accessory muscle use, increased breath rate, stridor, cyanosis, and diaphoresis

◆ Signs of right-sided heart failure may be present (pitting edema of lower extremities, jugular venous distention, cardiac gallop)

◆ Signs of hypercapnia with acidemia may be present (muscle twitching, asterixis, miosis, papilledema, engorged fundal veins, diaphoresis, hypertension)

◆ Increased fremitus may be found in consolidated lung tissue; decreased fremitus indicates obstructed major bronchus, fluid in the pleural space, or severe COPD

◆ Decreased breath sounds are heard in COPD; adventitious sounds such as crackles (rales), rhonchi (gurgles), wheezes, or pleural friction rub may also be heard

■ Diagnostic tests

◆ ABG analysis

▶ Respiratory failure is defined by ABG as hypoxemia (decreased Pa_{O_2}), hypercapnia (decreased Pa_{O_2} and increased Pa_{CO_2}), or both

▶ Pao_2 below 60 mm Hg, $Paco_2$ above 50 mm Hg, or both are the criteria
  • Acute processes show acidosis with normal or mildly increasing bicarbonate (HCO_3^-)
  • Chronic processes show relatively normal pH with elevated HCO_3^-
◆ Radiologic findings may indicate primary disease process
◆ Intrapulmonary shunt is greater than 15%
■ Medical management
◆ Maintain or enhance O_2 delivery and CO_2 removal
  ▶ Adequate oxygenation is Pao_2 greater than 60 mm Hg
  ▶ Adequate oxygen saturation is Sao_2 greater than 90 mm Hg
  ▶ Adequate red blood cell counts are Hb levels greater than 12 g/dl or hematocrit greater than 36%
  ▶ Adequate cardiac index is 2.5 to 4 L/minute
  ▶ Adequate CO_2 elimination is a pH of 7.35 to 7.45
◆ Manage hypoxemia with supplemental O_2 therapy; administer O_2 cautiously to patients with underlying pulmonary disease, as it can suppress the hypoxic respiratory drive
◆ In conditions characterized by right-to-left shunting, determine whether mechanical ventilation with PEEP is needed to maintain adequate tissue oxygenation
◆ If hypoventilation is related to drug use, administer an antidote or treat the patient's symptoms until the effects of the drug wear off
◆ Encourage coughing, deep breathing, and turning; prescribe chest physiotherapy to help the patient expectorate retained pulmonary secretions
◆ Keep in mind that ventilation of patients with hypercapnic respiratory failure can result in metabolic alkalosis
  ▶ Metabolic alkalosis increases minute ventilation, Pao_2, and mixed venous O_2 tension and decreases O_2 consumption
  ▶ Metabolic alkalosis can be reversed by correcting fluid and electrolyte abnormalities and administering acetazolamide, ammonium chloride, hydrochloric acid, or arginine hydrochloride
■ Nursing management
◆ Assess breath sounds every 1 to 4 hours, and note wheezes, crackles, and rhonchi; acute respiratory failure always causes some degree of pulmonary congestion and bronchospasm; frequent auscultation helps determine if the patient's condition is worsening
◆ Monitor the patient's respiratory rate; tachypnea with rapid, shallow, ineffective respirations is often present
◆ Encourage and assist with abdominal respirations, pursed-lip breathing, and respiratory therapy; these measures help control dyspnea, reduce air trapping, and open blocked or constricted bronchi
◆ Increase the patient's fluid intake to 2,000 ml/day, if appropriate, and provide warm liquids; hydration helps to decrease the viscosity of secretions and facilitates expectoration; warm fluids decrease bronchospasms; mucolytic agents may also be used

Conditions leading to acute respiratory distress syndrome

A common form of respiratory failure, acute respiratory distress syndrome occurs in response to a direct or indirect systemic insult, such as those listed below.

Direct pulmonary injury	Indirect pulmonary injury
Aspiration of gastric contents or other toxic substances	Sepsis—especially gram-negative
Near-drowning	Multiple emergency blood transfusions
Inhalation of toxic substances	Multiple trauma
Some infections	Disseminated intravascular coagulation
Radiation	Shock or prolonged hypotension
Pulmonary contusion, secondary trauma	Head trauma
Drugs: heroin, bleomycin, salicylates	Drug overdose
Embolism: fat, air, amniotic fluid	Pancreatitis
Postlung transplant	Diabetic coma
	Cardiopulmonary bypass
	Burns
	Hypo/hyperthermia

◆ Encourage expectoration of sputum and use suction, as necessary; secretions in the respiratory tract are a prime source of impaired gas exchange

◆ Monitor serial ABG values; changes in ABG values provide an indication of treatment effectiveness

❖ Acute respiratory distress syndrome
 ■ Description
  ◆ ARDS is a group of occurrences spiraling to severe diffuse lung injury; high mortality occurs when ARDS is accompanied by sepsis, especially from an abdominal source
  ◆ Various conditions can lead to ARDS (see *Conditions leading to acute respiratory distress syndrome*)
  ◆ No single common mechanism that causes ARDS has been found (see *Pathogenesis of acute respiratory distress syndrome*)
  ◆ In the acute phase, pulmonary mechanisms associated with ARDS include defects of the alveolar epithelium, interstitial lung edema, and microthrombosis
   ▶ Defects of the type I alveolar epithelium cause loss of vascular proteins from the capillaries to the pulmonary interstitial spaces
    • As a result, large amounts of fluid enter the pulmonary interstitial spaces, overwhelming the pulmonary lymphatic drainage system
    • The increased hydrostatic pressure eventually collapses the terminal bronchioles, causing hypoxemia
    • Fluids subsequently enter the alveoli, decreasing surfactant activity, promoting alveolar collapse and increasing pulmonary

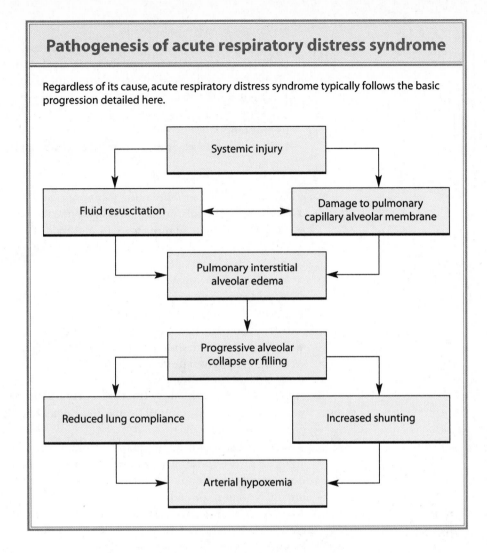

Pathogenesis of acute respiratory distress syndrome

Regardless of its cause, acute respiratory distress syndrome typically follows the basic progression detailed here.

Systemic injury

Fluid resuscitation

Damage to pulmonary capillary alveolar membrane

Pulmonary interstitial alveolar edema

Progressive alveolar collapse or filling

Reduced lung compliance

Increased shunting

Arterial hypoxemia

shunting; this results in marked reduction of gas exchange and pronounced hypoxemia
- This chain of events increases pulmonary shunting, which results in significant reduction of gas exchange and marked hypoxemia
- Physiologic dead space is increased and large minute ventilation may be required
- Compliance of areas of lung parenchyma is reduced; increased stiffness occurs, requiring high peak inspiratory pressures
- Narrowing or obstruction of blood vessels occurs, resulting in increased pulmonary arterial pressures, even though the pulmonary artery wedge pressure (PAWP) remains normal or low
◆ The chronic phase of ARDS is characterized by thickening of the endothelium, epithelium, and interstitial spaces
  ❱ Type I cells are destroyed and replaced by type II cells (neutrophils)
  ❱ Interstitial spaces are increased by edema, fibers, and cell proliferation

> ◗ Fibrosis occurs after 1 week

> ◗ Within the alveoli, protein-rich fluid that enters the pulmonary interstitial spaces forms hyaline membranes that further decrease compliance, widen the A-a gradient, and result in refractory hypoxemia

> ◗ Alveolar structure is destroyed, resulting in increased vascular resistance, hypoxemia from ventilation-perfusion mismatch, and decreased tissue compliance

> ◗ Microthrombosis often accompanies ARDS and can be a complicating factor

■ Clinical signs and symptoms

◆ Hypoxemia, hyperventilation, tachypnea, and tachycardia

◆ Shortness of breath, anxiety, and orthopnea

◆ PaO_2 greater than 60 mm Hg; SaO_2 less than 90 mm Hg

◆ PAWP less than 18 mm Hg; high wedge pressures are seen in patients with left-sided heart failure

◆ Respiratory rate greater than 30 breaths/minute, intercostal retractions, and use of accessory muscles

◆ Diffuse crackles and rhonchi on auscultation and bronchovesicular breath sounds due to increased lung density

◆ Dullness on percussion and increased vocal fremitus, related to increased density from pulmonary edema

◆ Production of frothy, pink sputum

■ Diagnostic tests

◆ Chest X-ray findings vary from diffuse patchy infiltrates to "white out" of the lung

◆ ABGs show hypoxemia due to intrapulmonary shunting (hallmark sign), and the hypoxemia is refractory to O_2 therapy; respiratory alkalosis due to hyperventilation occurs in the early phase; hypercapnia isn't seen initially and is an ominous sign

◆ Pulmonary function tests may indicate large right-to-left shunting, increased A-a gradient, reduced compliance, reduced functional residual capacity secondary to microatelectasis and edema, and increased dead space ventilation

◆ Pulmonary artery pressure is often elevated, but pulmonary artery occlusive pressure may be normal or low

■ Medical management

◆ Administer supplemental O_2 therapy; the lung can tolerate O_2 concentrations of 40% to 50% indefinitely, but higher concentrations can cause increasing alveolar collapse, type II granular pneumocyte dysfunction, and impaired mucociliary clearance within 3 to 4 days

◆ Use mechanical ventilation to maintain or restore an adequate PaO_2

> ◗ The tidal volume usually is set at 6 mg/kg

> ◗ FIO_2 is set to maintain a PaO_2 greater than 70 mm Hg

> ◗ Rate of ventilation is set to maintain a $PaCO_2$ of 35 to 45 mm Hg

◆ Use PEEP, if indicated, to maintain adequate oxygenation; PEEP is often useful for maintaining alveolar airflow during expiration

> ◗ Closely monitor the patient's cardiovascular status as PEEP is increased

▶ The increased intrathoracic pressure caused by PEEP can decrease cardiac output; high levels of PEEP also predispose the patient to pneumothorax

▶ PEEP greater than 15 cm H_2O is generally not recommended

◆ Use pressure-controlled inverse ratio ventilation (PC-IRV), a mode of ventilation that reverses the conventional inspiratory-expiratory ratio (I:E ratio), if indicated

▶ PC-IRV delivers each breath at a set pressure, rather than a set tidal volume, and at an I:E ratio of 1:1, 2:1, or higher

▶ The effects of PC-IRV include reduced peak inspiratory pressure, decreased mean airway pressure, increased compliance, reduced minute ventilation, and improved oxygenation with a lower delivered FIO_2

■ Nursing management

◆ Use a closed suction system when suctioning the patient

▶ Hypoxemia can rapidly develop when patients are disconnected from the ventilator; a closed system maintains oxygenation

▶ A closed system also prevents the loss of PEEP, which may result when the ventilator is disconnected

◆ Reposition the patient at regular intervals and note changes in oxygenation; the prone position may improve oxygenation, possibly by increasing perfusion of the anterior apical regions; if the prone position isn't feasible, use a semiprone position; continuous rotational beds are also useful

◆ Implement measures to decrease O_2 consumption, which is necessary for adequate perfusion of vital organs; methods of decreasing O_2 consumption range from anxiety reduction and pain control to pharmacologic paralysis of a restless patient

◆ Keep in mind that inotropic support may be required to maintain adequate cardiac output; because dobutamine decreases the PAWP, this inotropic agent is more useful than dopamine in ARDS treatment

◆ Administer fluid therapy to maintain the PAWP between 10 and 12 mm Hg, as indicated

▶ PEEP greater than 10 cm H_2O can interfere with cardiac output, lowering blood pressure and causing increased antidiuretic hormone secretion and fluid retention

◆ Use venoarterial or venovenous extracorporeal membrane oxygenation (ECMO); ECMO facilitates gas exchange and rests the lungs of patients with severe reversible respiratory failure

❖ **Acute respiratory infections**

■ Description

◆ The principal acute respiratory tract infection is pneumonia, which is caused when infectious organisms enter the sterile lower respiratory tract, overcome host defenses, and multiply

◆ Pneumonia can be bacterial, viral, or fungal

▶ Bacterial pathogens include *Legionella pneumophila, Moraxella* (formerly *Branhamella*) *catarrhalis, Staphylococcus, Haemophilus* influenzae, *Streptococcus pneumoniae* (*Pneumococcus*), *Enterobacter, Escherichia coli, Proteus,* and *Pseudomonas*

▶ Viral pathogens include influenza virus, adenovirus, cytomegalovirus, and herpes virus

▶ Fungal pathogens include *Aspergillus, Candida, Cryptococcus, Nocardia, Mycoplasma* (a common cause in young, healthy people), and *Pneumocystis carinii* (commonly seen in acquired immune deficiency syndrome)

◆ Bacterial pneumonia is much more common than viral pneumonia; hospital-acquired (nosocomial) respiratory tract infections are typically caused by gram-negative enteric bacteria

◆ Upper airway defenses (nasopharyngeal filtration, mucosal adherence, saliva, secretory immunoglobulin A) may be altered by nasotracheal intubation, endotracheal intubation, tracheostomy suction catheters, and NG tubes

◆ Lower airway defenses (cough reflex, mucociliary clearance, humoral and cellular factors) can be affected by advanced age, underlying disease (diabetes or chronic bronchitis), hypoxia, pulmonary edema, malnutrition, decreased level of consciousness (LOC), and drug and O_2 therapy

◆ Infectious organisms can enter the respiratory tract through inhalation or aspiration, inoculation, direct spread from contiguous sites, hematogenous spread, or colonization in chronic lung disease (COPD, cystic fibrosis)

◆ Infection occurrence depends on the nature of the infecting organism, the immediate environment, and the host's defense status

◆ Respiratory tract infection produces inflammation with or without exudate

▶ Inflammation of the lung parenchyma is characterized by the influx of polymorphonuclear leukocytes, fluid, and fibrin into alveolar spaces

▶ Inflammation leads to a ventilation-perfusion abnormality and hypoxemia; right-to-left shunting can also occur

■ Clinical signs and symptoms

◆ Dyspnea, fever, hyperpnea, and tachycardia

◆ Bacterial pneumonia: productive cough with yellow-green or rust-colored sputum

◆ Viral pneumonia: nonproductive cough and low-grade or absent fever

◆ *P. carinii* pneumonia: nonproductive cough

◆ Pleuritic pain caused by pleural surface inflammation

◆ Crackles and wheezes over the affected area on auscultation; an increase in vocal fremitus may occur with frank consolidation; egophony, bronchophony, or whispered pectoriloquy is usually present over areas of consolidation

◆ Dullness on percussion of the affected area

■ Diagnostic tests

◆ Chest X-ray findings vary with the areas of involvement and may show segmental or lobar consolidation, multiple infiltrates, pleural effusions, abscesses, or cavities

◆ Sputum cultures may identify the organism or assist in differential diagnosis

◆ Blood cultures help determine bacteremia (poor prognosis)

◆ Elevated white blood cell (WBC) count, with a shift to the left (characterized by an increased number of immature neutrophils) in bacterial pneumonia; normal or depressed WBC count may be present in immunocompromised patients, patients with viral pneumonia, or those with overwhelming infection

◆ ABGs may reveal hypoxemia and hypocapnia in lobar pneumonia

◆ Thoracentesis may be indicated if significant pleural effusion is present

■ Medical management

◆ Support the patient's respiratory function

◆ Culture sputum and blood specimens to guide the choice of antibiotic therapy; a saline mist treatment with an ultrasonic nebulizer may be helpful in obtaining the sputum specimen

◆ Prescribe empiric antibiotic therapy until Gram stain and culture results are available

■ Nursing management

◆ Institute chest physiotherapy, including postural drainage, percussion, and vibration

◆ To facilitate lung expansion and help expectorate sputum, encourage coughing and deep breathing

◆ When only one lung is involved, position the patient on the unaffected side to decrease the ventilation-perfusion imbalance

◆ Closely monitor fluids in patients with *P. carinii* pneumonia; increased alveolocapillary membrane permeability causes fluids to build up in the alveoli

◆ Control fever with tepid sponge baths and prescribed antipyretics

◆ Maintain head of bed at least 30 degrees or higher to help prevent aspiration

❖ **Status asthmaticus**

■ Description

◆ Asthma is a state of increased airway responsiveness (hyperreactivity) related to altered immune response

◆ Characterized by bronchoconstriction, mucosal edema, and excessive production of thick, tenacious mucus, which increases the work of breathing and impairs gas exchange

❯ Bronchoconstriction and mucus plugging cause trapping of air, resulting in hyperinflation of the lungs

❯ The bronchial walls hypertrophy, leading to bronchiolar obstruction, which reduces alveolar ventilation and causes hyperinflation of the alveoli and increased residual volume

◆ Pathologic airway changes associated with asthma include hypertrophy of smooth muscle, thickening of the respiratory epithelial basement membrane, hypertrophy and hyperplasia of mucous glands, and proliferation of goblet cells

◆ Status asthmaticus is a severe attack of asthma that doesn't respond to conventional therapy; hypoxemia and a widened A-a gradient are signs of status asthmaticus

❯ Peak expiratory flow rates are reduced

▶ Airway narrowing is due to smooth muscle spasm, inflammation of bronchial walls (causing increased mucosal permeability and basement membrane thickening), and mucus plugging

◆ The most common causes of an asthma attack are exposure to allergens; inappropriate bronchodilator use; respiratory tract infections; emotional stress; environmental exposure (air pollution, ingestion of food preservative metabisulfite); exercise; occupational exposure; reflux esophagitis; sinusitis; mechanical stimulation (coughing, laughing, cold air inhalation); and use of aspirin, nonsteroidal anti-inflammatory drugs, or nonselective beta-blocking medications such as propranolol (Inderal)

■ Clinical signs and symptoms

◆ Dyspnea, chest tightness, restlessness, and anxiety

◆ Pursed-lip breathing, nasal flaring, and intercostal bulging on expiration

◆ Minimal chest expansion on inspiration and decreased vocal fremitus caused by hyperinflation of the lungs

◆ Cough that may produce thick, tenacious mucus

◆ Inspiratory or expiratory wheezes caused by bronchoconstriction; decreased or absent breath sounds (silent chest) are ominous signs

◆ Prolonged expiratory phase of the respiratory cycle as the patient attempts to exhale trapped air

◆ Impaired diaphragmatic excursion caused by trapped air

◆ Tachypnea or hyperpnea

◆ Tachycardia

◆ Use of accessory muscles

■ Diagnostic tests

◆ Evidence of infection (positive sputum cultures), elevated WBC count

◆ ABG analysis may initially show low normal or reduced Pa_{CO_2}, high pH, and low Pa_{O_2} (less than 60 mm Hg); in a severe asthmatic attack, there may be a normal or increased Pa_{CO_2} level, which may be a sign of impending respiratory failure

◆ The chest X-ray may be normal or hyperlucent; X-ray may help rule out other conditions that mimic asthma

◆ Pulmonary function tests may show a peak expiratory flow less than 60 L/minute or one that doesn't improve to greater than 50% of predicted value after 1 hour of treatment; forced expiratory volume in 1 second (FEV_1) may be less than 30% of predicted value or doesn't improve to at least 40% of predicted value following 1 hour of aggressive therapy

■ Medical management

◆ Rehydrate the patient with oral or I.V. fluids to liquefy pulmonary secretions

◆ Initiate bronchodilator therapy to relieve bronchospasm; agents include epinephrine given subcutaneously or inhaled ipratropium bromide (by metered-dose inhaler or nebulizer)

▶ Epinephrine is used cautiously with coexisting cardiac disease; doses may be repeated every 20 minutes as needed

▶ Theophylline has been shown to have increased side effects, especially of cardiac origin

◆ Prescribe corticosteroids to reduce the lung's inflammatory response

◗ Inhaled steroids may be administered in an acute attack
◆ Administer sedatives with extreme caution, if at all
◆ Administer supplemental O_2, ranging from nasal cannula to mechanical ventilation, to prevent hypoxemia
◆ Prescribe antibiotics, as indicated by results of sputum cultures, to eradicate respiratory tract infection
■ Nursing management
◆ Position the patient for comfort, as tolerated; sitting up with the shoulder girdle elevated (for example, with the hands over the head or leaning on a bedside table) often helps lessen the feeling of air hunger
◆ Implement chest physiotherapy (postural drainage with percussion and vibration, coughing, and deep breathing) in conjunction with bronchodilator therapy to remove retained pulmonary secretions; monitor results of FEV comparisons with treatments
◆ Implement interventions similar to those for patients with acute respiratory failure (see pages 97 to 99)
◆ Intensive asthma education is necessary regarding peak flow monitoring, proper inhalation technique, spacer use, and medication therapy

❖ **Acute pulmonary embolus**
■ Description
◆ Acute pulmonary embolus is caused by the movement of a clot from its site of origin, through the right side of the heart, then lodging in a branch of the pulmonary circulation
◗ The degree of patient compromise caused by pulmonary embolus depends on the extent of the vascular occlusion and degree of preexisting cardiopulmonary disease
◗ Massive pulmonary embolus can result in a sudden shocklike state and may cause death
◆ Pulmonary embolism produces an area in the lung that's ventilated but underperfused, increasing physiologic dead-space ventilation; right or left shunting and low ventilation-perfusion ratios occur
◆ In some situations, the dual circulation (pulmonary and bronchial) in the lungs may provide adequate circulation distal to the occlusion; if the pulmonary vascular bed is sufficiently reduced by a large embolus or by recurrent multiple emboli, pulmonary hypertension can result (although two-thirds of the vascular bed must be obliterated before this occurs)
◆ Nearly 95% of all pulmonary emboli arise from thrombi in the deep veins of the legs; pulmonary emboli of nonthrombotic origin are uncommon and may be caused by air, fat, or amniotic fluid
◆ The principal contributing factors of venous thrombosis (Virchow's triad) are stasis of blood flow, endothelial injury or vessel wall abnormalities, and hypercoagulability
◗ Other risk factors for thrombosis include history of thrombosis, immobility, chronic heart failure, cancer, use of estrogen contraceptives, blood dyscrasias, advancing age, leg or pelvic trauma or surgery, obesity, and poor postoperative status
◗ Thrombus formation can also result from heart failure, atrial fibrillation, endocarditis, and myocardial infarction (MI)

◆ Deep vein thrombosis (DVT) is an insidious problem that can lead to pulmonary embolus; in some patients with DVT, secondary arterial compromise may occur with massive venous thrombosis due to vascular compression or spasm; diminished arterial pulses and pallor may result

■ Clinical signs and symptoms

◆ In a patient with signs of thrombophlebitis in leg veins: sudden onset of unexplained dyspnea, tachypnea, tachycardia, and restlessness

◆ In a patient on bed rest: sudden onset of tachypnea, tachycardia, and hypoxemia

◆ In a patient with massive pulmonary embolus: tachycardia, hypotension, cyanosis, stupor, syncope, cardiac arrest, and distended jugular veins

◆ In a patient with pulmonary infarction: pleuritic chest pain, dyspnea, hemoptysis, fever, rales, wheezes, and pleural friction rub

◆ Pleuritic pain, friction rub, hemoptysis, and fever, if pulmonary infarction occurs

◆ Fixed splitting of S_2 is an ominous sign related to marked right ventricular overload; murmurs and pleural friction rub may also be heard

◆ Inspiratory crackles on auscultation

■ Diagnostic tests

◆ Pulmonary angiography is the definitive diagnostic test for pulmonary embolus

◆ A lung ventilation or perfusion scan isn't definitive but is less risky than angiography

◆ A chest X-ray is nonspecific and frequently normal

◆ An electrocardiogram (ECG) is nonspecific but may show ventricular arrhythmias (in response to hypoxemia), sinus tachycardia, or transient ST-T wave changes

◆ABG levels indicating respiratory alkalosis (due to hyperventilation) and hypoxemia; possibly increased A-a gradient

■ Medical management

◆ Initiate cardiorespiratory support

◆ Treat hypoxemia with supplemental O_2 therapy; keep PaO_2 greater than 60 mm Hg

◆ Intubate and mechanically ventilate the patient, if indicated; a patient with massive pulmonary emboli may experience hypoxemia and hypercapnia, requiring mechanical ventilation

◆ Initiate intravascular volume expansion

▶ Pulmonary emboli reduce blood flow to the left side of the heart, consequently reducing cardiac output and arterial blood pressure

▶ The pulmonary vasculature triggers systemic arteriolar vasodilation, producing a relative volume depletion

◆ Administer anticoagulants to prevent further clot formation; anticoagulants are beneficial as prophylactic therapy to prevent thrombus formation and recurrent embolization in patients with emboli

◆ Administer heparin, which impedes clotting by interfering with fibrin formation, to maintain partial thromboplastin time at 1.5 times normal (generally 55 to 85 seconds)

▶ Although heparin doesn't dissolve emboli, it can prevent the formation of new thrombi and enhances fibrinolytic activity on fresh thrombi; heparin blocks platelet-thrombin interactions on the embolus that lead to the release of chemical mediators associated with bronchospasm and hypotension

▶ The effects of heparin can be reversed with protamine

◆ Administer oral anticoagulants, such as warfarin sodium (Coumadin)

▶ Before the patient is weaned from the heparin infusion, he may be started on oral anticoagulant therapy

▶ Warfarin is administered for 6 or more weeks to maintain prothrombin time at 1.5 times normal (generally 16 to 18 seconds)

▶ The effects of warfarin can be reversed with vitamin K

◆ Administer thrombolytic therapy; streptokinase, urokinase, and tissue plasminogen activator can be used to dissolve the clot

◆ In patients with recurrent emboli, consider surgical placement of a filter in the vena cava

◆ In patients with massive emboli, determine whether embolectomy is indicated

■ Nursing management

◆ Maintain the patient on bed rest to reduce the workload of the heart and lungs and to decrease the likelihood of embolus movement

◆ Administer stool softeners and mild cathartics, as needed; defecation increases the potential for pulmonary embolus in patients with DVT

◆ Monitor the patient for complications of pulmonary emboli, which include pulmonary infarction, pneumonia, pulmonary abscess, ARDS, MI, arrhythmias, and shock as well as complications of heparin therapy (bleeding overt or covert); signs of hemorrhage may include hematuria, hypotension, anemia, tachycardia, ecchymosis, and occult blood in the stool

❖ **Pulmonary contusion**

■ Description

◆ Approximately 75% of patients with blunt chest trauma, especially those with rib fractures, also have pulmonary contusion

◆ Signs and symptoms of pulmonary contusion may not develop until 4 to 24 hours after the injury

◆ Direct blunt trauma causes alveolar congestion and atelectasis

◆ The resulting decrease in intrathoracic pressure and expansion of the lung parenchyma under pressure rupture capillaries and produce localized edema and hemorrhage

◆ The localized edema and hemorrhage increase pulmonary vascular resistance, which decreases pulmonary blood flow

◆ Reduced chest wall motion caused by trauma can lead to an inability to cough, with resultant development of atelectasis; this in turn leads to shunting and alterations in ventilation and perfusion manifested as hypoxemia, hypercapnia, and metabolic acidosis and can lead to ARDS

■ Clinical signs and symptoms

◆ Ecchymosis on the chest wall at the site of impact

◆ Gradual onset of hypoxemia

◆ Coughing and expectoration of bloody sputum
◆ Tachycardia and tachypnea
◆ Diminished breath sounds or crackles on the affected side
◆ Dullness on percussion of the involved area
■ Diagnostic tests
◆ ABGs reveal decreased PaO_2 and $PaCO_2$
◆ Increased A-a gradient caused by decreasing pulmonary diffusion capacity
◆ Chest X-ray shows localized, patchy, poorly defined areas of increased parenchymal density reflecting intra-alveolar hemorrhage
■ Medical management
◆ Institute pulmonary care to mobilize secretions
◆ Maintain a patent airway and adequate oxygenation
◆ Use intubation and mechanical ventilation with PEEP, if indicated, to maintain oxygenation in severe cases
◆ Manage fluid intake carefully to minimize vascular fluid leakage into the lung tissue; PAWP should be kept at 10 to 12 mm Hg
■ Nursing management
◆ Position the patient with the uninjured side down to enhance ventilation and perfusion
◆ Place the patient with bilateral disease in the right lateral decubitus position, which places a larger surface area in the dependent position and may increase oxygenation; use a rotating bed to prevent pulmonary stasis
◆ Elevate the head of the bed to decrease the pressure of abdominal contents on the diaphragm
◆ Encourage deep breathing and coughing to keep lungs expanded and prevent complications

❖ **Rib fracture**
■ Description
◆ Simple rib fractures can cause a patient to avoid movement to prevent pain and to hypoventilate for prolonged periods; shallow breathing and ineffective cough can lead to atelectasis and pneumonia, which in turn may progress to respiratory failure
◆ Fracture of the first rib is uncommon; when it occurs, it may indicate severe underlying thoracic injuries, including brachial plexus injury, pneumothorax, aortic rupture, and thoracic outlet syndrome
◆ The most commonly fractured ribs are the third to eighth; in a single, simple rib fracture, the ribs above and below the fracture site stabilize the broken rib
◆ Any rib fracture below the seventh rib is also considered abdominal trauma; lower rib fractures, in particular, are associated with laceration or tear of the liver or spleen
■ Clinical signs and symptoms
◆ Chest pain, possible ecchymosis, splinting, or guarding of affected area
◆ Diminished breath sounds, shallow respirations, and signs of hypoxemia
■ Diagnostic tests

◆ Chest X-ray shows presence of fractured rib

◆ ABGs may show evidence of hypoxemia

■ Medical management

◆ Provide adequate analgesia, including an intercostal nerve block, if necessary; a patient who has a tidal volume less than 5 ml/kg despite adequate pain control should generally be admitted

◆ Don't use binders, which decrease chest excursion

■ Nursing management

◆ Encourage coughing and deep breathing, using bronchial hygiene and chest physiotherapy techniques; these actions keep the airways open and prevent secretion buildup

◆ Frequently monitor respiratory status, noting changes indicative of pneumothorax

◆ Institute pain management techniques (medication, splinting, relaxation techniques) before performing nursing procedures

❖ **Flail chest**

■ Description

◆ Flail chest is a chest injury in which three or more adjacent ribs are fractured in two or more places, causing a segment of the ribs and chest wall to work paradoxically with respiration

◆ The flail segment moves inward with inspiration and outward with expiration, causing diminished movement of air that leads to hypoxia; a decreased cough mechanism results in retained secretions

◆ The larger the flail, the less effective the gas exchange

◆ Interstitial and intra-alveolar edema and hemorrhage are caused by the underlying pulmonary contusion; sternal fractures are also frequently associated with myocardial injuries

◆ Flail chest is often associated with hemopneumothorax

■ Clinical signs and symptoms

◆ Hypoxia, according to the size of the flail

◆ Cyanosis, dyspnea, apprehension, and anxiety

◆ Diminished breath sounds, paradoxical chest wall movement, and crepitus over the flail segment

◆ Signs of decreased venous return to the heart: distended jugular veins, elevated central venous pressure, and decreasing blood pressure

■ Medical management

◆ Maintain airway, breathing, and circulation

◆ Use an intercostal nerve block to reduce pain and splint simple rib fractures

◆ Use mechanical ventilation with PEEP, if indicated; PEEP provides internal stabilization of the flail segment

■ Nursing management

◆ Monitor the patient's respiration status, vital signs, and capillary refill time

◆ Administer appropriate pain medication, as prescribed, to aid respiratory expansion

◆ Frequently assess the patient for complications of mechanical ventilation, PEEP, and bed rest

❖ **Hemothorax**
- ■ Description
  - ◆ Hemothorax refers to a condition in which blood is trapped in the pleural space, resulting in impaired respiration and hypovolemia
  - ◆ The chest cavity can hold up to 4 L of blood
  - ◆ The source of bleeding in hemothorax is generally the pulmonary parenchyma and vessels, the intercostal and internal mammary arteries, or the mediastinum (heart, aorta, and great vessels)
- ■ Clinical signs and symptoms
  - ◆ Hypovolemia (shock)
  - ◆ Diminished breath sounds on the affected side, and possible signs of hypoxemia
  - ◆ Marked dullness to percussion on the affected side
  - ◆ Mediastinal shift away from the affected side with an accumulation of more than 1,500 ml of blood
  - ◆ Pain that may radiate to the neck, shoulder, and upper abdomen
- ■ Medical management
  - ◆ Keep in mind that a small hemothorax may resolve spontaneously due to low pulmonary system pressures and thromboplastin in the lungs
  - ◆ Use thoracentesis or placement of a chest tube for a large hemothorax, if indicated
  - ◆ Replace blood volume with volume expanders and blood products, as indicated
- ■ Nursing management
  - ◆ Frequently assess respiratory status for changes in pleural drainage
  - ◆ Prepare the patient with a large hemothorax for thoracentesis or chest tube placement, if indicated
  - ◆ Administer blood products, as prescribed
  - ◆ Monitor chest tube drainage system for proper functioning (see *Management of a closed chest-drainage system*)
  - ◆ Encourage coughing and deep breathing to facilitate lung expansion
  - ◆ Institute pain relief measures (medication, splinting, relaxation techniques) before performing nursing management procedures, as indicated

❖ **Pulmonary aspiration**
- ■ Description
  - ◆ Aspiration is a situation in which solids or fluids from the oropharynx or GI tract enter the tracheobronchial tree
    - ▶ Vomiting is an active mechanism by which gastric contents are ejected out of the stomach
    - ▶ Regurgitation is a passive process by which gastric contents are expelled from the stomach; it can occur even in the presence of paralyzed muscles
  - ◆ Large particles, when aspirated, can obstruct the trachea or bronchi and cause asphyxia, leading to death
  - ◆ When the aspirated material has a pH less than 2.5, it causes a chemical burn to the lung, increasing the severity of the injury

Management of a closed chest-drainage system

One-piece, disposable plastic drainage systems, such as the Pleur-evac (shown right), contain three chambers. The drainage chamber is on the right and has three calibrated columns that display the amount of drainage collected. When the first column fills, drainage carries over into the second and, when that fills, into the third. The water-seal chamber is located in the center. The suction-control chamber on the left is filled with water to achieve various suction levels. Rubber diaphragms are provided at the rear of the device to change the water level or remove samples of drainage. A positive-pressure relief valve at the top of the water-seal chamber vents excess pressure into the atmosphere, preventing pressure buildup.

Nursing responsibilites
- assess drainage and record amounts
- medicate patient for pain as needed
- position patient in Semi-fowlers, if possible, to help facilitate drainage
- keep all tubes free from kinks and avoid dependant loops in the tubing
- there should be gentle bubbling in the suction-control chamber
- there should be gentle rise and fall of the water level in the water seal chamber
- if a patient has an air leak, there will be bubbling seen in the water seal chamber
- if chest tube becomes dislodged, place an occlusive dressing over site, and notify practitioner immediately

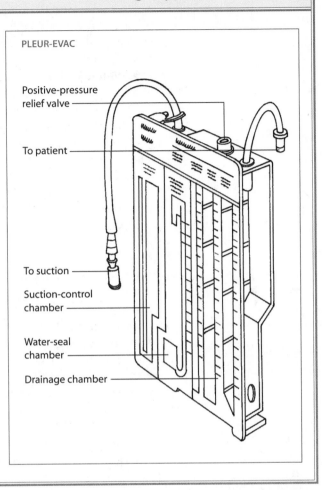

PLEUR-EVAC

Positive-pressure relief valve

To patient

To suction

Suction-control chamber

Water-seal chamber

Drainage chamber

▶ When acidic material is aspirated, type II alveolar cells are destroyed and alveolocapillary membrane permeability is increased, causing extravasation of fluid into the interstitium and alveoli
▶ Accumulation of blood and fluid diminishes functional residual capacity and compliance
▶ Alveolar ventilation decreases, leading to intrapulmonary shunting and hypoxia
▶ Bronchospasm results from irritation of the airways by the acidic aspirate; this irritation leads to epithelial injury and disruption of the alveolar membrane
▶ Peribronchial hemorrhage, pulmonary edema, and necrosis can also occur
◆ When the aspirated material is clear and nonacidic, the extent of the damage varies according to the volume of fluid aspirated; situations such as near-drowning, reflex airway closure, pulmonary edema, and alterations in surfactant lead to hypoxia

◆ Aspiration of small, solid particles can produce a severe, subacute, inflammatory reaction with extensive hemorrhage

◆ Aspiration of contaminated material (such as bacteria from a bowel obstruction) can be fatal

◆ The significant intrapulmonary shunting caused by pulmonary aspiration can lead to severe hypoxemia

   ▶ Within 6 hours after aspiration, hemorrhagic pneumonia occurs

   ▶ $Paco_2$ usually is much higher after aspiration of food

◆ The outcome of an aspiration event depends on the patient's preexisting physical state and the amount, type, and distribution of the aspirate in the lungs; silent aspiration is especially common in patients with altered LOC

  ◆ There are several risk factors for pulmonary aspiration

   ▶ Altered LOC caused by drugs, anesthesia, seizures, central nervous system disorders, or shock

   ▶ Altered anatomy through the presence of an endotracheal, tracheostomy, or NG tube; anomalies of the trachea or esophageal area; or trauma

   ▶ Decreased GI motility, intestinal obstruction, or protracted vomiting

   ▶ Improper patient positioning, especially if receiving hyperalimentation

■ Clinical signs and symptoms

  ◆ Dyspnea, cough, and wheezing, with aspiration of foreign bodies

  ◆ Respiratory distress with gastric acid aspiration

  ◆ Cough with pink, frothy exudate

  ◆ Fever and elevated WBC count if bacterial infection is present

■ Tachycardia and tachypnea

  ◆ Hypotension

  ◆ Inspiratory stridor if the airway is obstructed

   ▶ Decreased tactile fremitus if a foreign body obstructs a large bronchus; increased fremitus in an area of dependent lobe infiltrate or atelectasis

   ▶ If the airway is completely obstructed, breath sounds distal to the obstruction are absent

  ◆ Dullness on percussion of areas of atelectasis and infiltrate

  ◆ Audible wheezes if solids or liquids were aspirated; crackles or absent breath sounds can also occur, depending on the area of occlusion

  ◆ Aspiration of gastric contents in pulmonary secretions

■ Diagnostic tests

  ◆ A chest X-ray may show patchy alveolar infiltrates in portions of the lung

  ◆ The patient's position at the time of aspiration influences the pattern of lung involvement; superior segments of the lower lobes and posterior segments of upper and lower lobes are the most prone

  ◆ Pulmonary function studies may show decreased compliance or decreased diffusing capacity

  ◆ Sputum may help with cytology

  ◆ Fiber-optic bronchoscopy may be used for infectious processes

  ◆ ABGs may reveal hypoxemia

◆ Open lung biopsy may be done if the patient is unable to undergo transbronchial biopsy

■ Medical management

◆ Use an abdominal thrust when the airway is obstructed by large particles; bronchoscopy can be used to retrieve solid particles

◆ Prevent esophageal reflux; the presence of an NG tube prevents closure of the esophageal sphincter

◆ Prescribe appropriate antimicrobial therapy, as indicated by sputum culture

■ Nursing management

◆ If the patient is unconscious, avoid supine or any position that predisposes him to aspiration

◆ Elevate the head of the bed 30 to 45 degrees in patients receiving tube feedings to facilitate passage of gastric contents across the pylorus and to prevent reflux and aspiration; if elevation of the head of the bed is contraindicated, place the patient in a right lateral decubitus position

◆ Check NG tube placement at regular intervals to detect tube migration

◆ Monitor gastric residuals at regular intervals (every 2 to 4 hours); if the residual is greater than 20% of the hourly rate or greater than 100 ml in a patient receiving intermittent feedings, discontinue the tube feeding until the cause of the excess residuals is determined and corrected

◆ Maintain the patency and functioning of the gastric suctioning system; presence of an NG tube increases the risk of aspiration

◆ Treat nausea promptly to prevent vomiting and reduce the risk of aspiration

◆ Administer metoclopramide (Reglan), as prescribed; this medication increases upper GI motility and gastric sphincter tone

◆ Monitor gastric pH to ensure a pH greater than 2.5; an alkaline pH in the stomach promotes overgrowth of gram-negative organisms

◆ Administer histamine-2 receptor antagonists, as prescribed; these medications increase gastric pH, limiting chemical burn to pulmonary tissue if aspiration occurs

◆ Avoid using a syringe to introduce fluids into the patient's mouth as this increases the risk of aspiration by bypassing the tongue and interfering with the swallowing response

◆ Encourage patients with reasonable swallowing competence to eat semisolid foods, such as ice cream or pudding; semisolid foods are more easily swallowed than liquids or solids

◆ For patients with an endotracheal or a tracheostomy tube, monitor cuff pressures to maintain proper inflation; this reduces the possibility of aspiration of oropharyngeal secretions

◆ Suction the oropharynx at regular intervals to control the accumulation of oropharyngeal secretions above a cuffed endotracheal tube

◆ Administer supplemental O_2, ranging from nasal cannula to mechanical ventilation, to prevent hypoxemia

◆ Monitor the patient closely for signs of infection, a primary complication of pulmonary aspiration; prophylactic antibiotic therapy may be prescribed

❖ **Pneumothorax**
  ■ Description
    ◆ A pneumothorax is a defect in the visceral pleura that allows air to enter the pleural space
      ▶ A simple pneumothorax is one in which the defect doesn't continue to enlarge
      ▶ A tension pneumothorax is one in which the defect acts as a one-way valve, allowing air to enter the pleural space on inspiration but preventing it from exiting on expiration
      ▶ A spontaneous pneumothorax is one in which the defect occurs suddenly and without trauma; it may occur in lanky individuals with the rupture of a superficial bulla during a hearty cough or stretching exercises
      ▶ A traumatic pneumothorax is one in which chest wall penetration allows air to enter the pleural space; it may occur concurrently with a hemothorax
    ◆ A pneumothorax causes the lung to collapse to a varying extent, as the normal negative intrapleural pressure that counteracts elastic recoil is lost
    ◆ Air enters the pleural cavity through the chest wall or the parietal pleura
    ◆ Pleural causes of pneumothorax include rupture of a subpleural air pocket (bleb or bulla) and necrosis of adjacent lung parenchyma (necrotizing pneumonia or neoplasm); iatrogenic causes include accidental puncture during insertion of a subclavian catheter, tracheostomy, thoracentesis, and mechanical ventilation with PEEP
  ■ Clinical signs and symptoms
    ◆ Acute onset of dyspnea or chest pain
    ◆ Respiratory distress and hypoxemia (extent varies according to the size of the pneumothorax)
    ◆ Decreased breath sounds on the affected side
    ◆ Hyperresonance and diminished breath sounds on the affected side; decreased tactile fremitus and egophonies as the air-filled pleural space muffles sounds
    ◆ Tracheal deviation away from the affected side
    ◆ Chest wall asymmetry or crepitus (subcutaneous emphysema)
    ◆ Distended jugular veins
    ◆ Hypotension secondary to impaired venous return; venous return is impaired by the rising positive intrathoracic pressure
    ◆ Cyanosis (a late, ominous sign)
  ■ Diagnostic tests
    ◆ Chest X-ray shows a mediastinal shift to the contralateral side and loss of peripheral lung markings
    ◆ ABGs show a pH less than 7.35, a PaO_2 less than 80 mm Hg, and a $PaCO_2$ greater than 45 mm Hg
  ■ Medical management
    ◆ Perform emergency needle thoracentesis
    ◆ Insert a pleural chest tube at about the 4th, 5th, or 6th intercostal space
      ▶ If the pneumothorax is less than 20% of the total lung area, a chest tube may not be necessary, unless the patient is to undergo surgery

> ❭ The size of the air leak is determined at the time of the insult
>
> ❭ Recurrent pneumothorax may be treated with thoracotomy or pleurodesis (the intrapleural injection of doxycycline or talc)

- ■ Nursing management
  - ◆ Prepare the patient for emergency needle thoracentesis
  - ◆ Monitor respiratory status for worsening of condition
  - ◆ Monitor chest tube drainage system for proper functioning
  - ◆ Encourage coughing and deep breathing to facilitate lung expansion
  - ◆ Institute pain relief measures (medication, splinting, relaxation techniques) before performing nursing management procedures, as indicated

❖ **Penetrating chest trauma**
- ■ Description
  - ◆ Penetrating chest trauma is a situation where an object has penetrated chest wall and into the pleural cavity
  - ◆ Most common causes are motor vehicle accidents, falls, assault, bullets, knives, and industrial accidents
  - ◆ Injuries seen in conjunction with penetrating chest traumas include sucking chest wounds, hemothorax, pulmonary hemorrhage, esophageal injury, tracheal injury and perforation, cardiac or great vessel damage
  - ◆ Extent of injury and internal damage usually able to be predicted by cause of injury
  - ◆ Pneumothorax is common with penetrating chest trauma due to open chest cavity
- ■ Clinical signs and symptoms
  - ◆ Pain with chest wall movement
  - ◆ Tachypnea
  - ◆ Respiratory distress
  - ◆ Restlessness
  - ◆ Anxiety
  - ◆ If tracheal injury occurs, the trachea may be displaced
  - ◆ Crepitus
  - ◆ Cyanosis
  - ◆ Dullness of lung fields if hemothorax present; hyperresonance if pneumothorax present
  - ◆ Diminished breath sounds
  - ◆ Other signs and symptoms will vary based on type of penetrating trauma and injury
- ■ Diagnostic tests
  - ◆ Chest X-ray may show air or fluid in pleural space
  - ◆ Bronchoscopy may be performed to evaluate possible tracheal perforation or internal pulmonary hemorrhage
  - ◆ ABG analysis to determine extent of respiratory distress
  - ◆ ECG monitoring to evaluate cardiac function
  - ◆ Complete blood count to monitor extent of bleeding and clotting ability
  - ◆ CT or MRI scans may be used to determine extent of internal damage
- ■ Medical management
  - ◆ Chest tube may be used to remove air or fluid from chest cavity

Pulmonary procedures

Procedure	Key assessments	Complications	Nursing management
Thoracotomy—removal of part of a lung Lobectomy—removal of one or more lobes of the lungs Pneumonectomy—removal of an entire lung Wedge resection—removal of a small portion of the lung without regard to segments	• Breath sounds • Chest tube drainage • Pain • Vital signs • Incision • Oxygenation level	• Infection • Hemorrhage • Tension pneumo-thorax • Arrhythmias • Pneumonia	• Monitor chest tube for drainage • Monitor patient development of pneumothorax • Administer pain medication as needed • Position patient to increase lung expansion; encourage early ambulation • Monitor vital signs including respiratory rate and oxygen saturation • Monitor incision and chest tube site for signs of infection • Monitor for the onset of cardiac arrhythmias • Assess breath sounds • Administer oxygen therapy if needed
Tracheostomy—Airway for long-term mechanical ventilation and to facilitate removal of tracheo-bronchial secretions Tracheal resection—resection of a portion of the trachea	• Breath sounds • Oxygenation status • Secretions • Stoma condition	• Infection • Tracheoesophageal fistula • Hemorrhage • Tracheostomy tube dislodges • Aspiration • Obstruction of tube	• Explain procedure to patient and family • Assess cuff inflation • Monitor arterial blood gases and oxygen saturation for adequate oxygenation levels • Assess breath sounds • Suction patient as needed • Monitor for frank bleeding or constant oozing at site • Change ties and dressing per facility policy or as needed • Keep sterile tracheostomy tube at bedside for accidental dislodgement of tube • Provide oral care • Keep head of bed at 30 degrees if tolerated

♦ Intubation may be necessary depending on extent of damage and respiratory distress
♦ Use oxygen therapy to maintain adequate oxygenation
♦ Administer pain medication or anxiolytics as needed
♦ Thoracic surgery to repair internal damage if indicated (see *Pulmonary procedures*)
■ Nursing management
♦ Administer pain medications as ordered
♦ Position patient to improve ventilation
♦ Ensure proper functioning of chest tube and monitor drainage
♦ Assess respiratory status frequently

◆ Be prepared to assist with intubation or emergency procedures if respiratory status decreases
◆ Prepare patient for surgery if indicated
◆ Maintain patent airway
  ▶ Encourage patient to do frequent cough and deep-breathing exercises
  ▶ If patient mechanically ventilated, suction endotracheal tube as needed
  ▶ Monitor vital signs for hypotension, respiratory rate, and heart rate

Review questions

1. An unrestrained driver who suffered a blunt chest trauma in a motor vehicle accident is admitted to the critical care unit (CCU). Nursing management of this patient would include all of the following EXCEPT:

○ **A.** frequent monitoring of the patient's respiratory status for signs of pneumothorax, hemothorax, or acute respiratory failure.

○ **B.** placing a binder around the patient's chest to help stabilize the rib cage.

○ **C.** positioning the patient with the uninjured side down.

○ **D.** encouraging the patient to mobilize pulmonary secretions by coughing and deep breathing.

Correct answer: B Binding the chest decreases chest excursion, thereby leading to atelectasis and diminished gas exchange. Hemothorax, pneumothorax, and acute respiratory failure are frequent consequences of blunt chest trauma. Positioning the patient with the uninjured side down is appropriate in chest trauma because it enhances pulmonary ventilation and perfusion. Coughing and deep breathing help prevent atelectasis and pneumonia.

2. An elderly man with a history of stable angina is admitted to your unit for observation after receiving urgent treatent for status asthmaticus. The nurse notes that he's becoming increasingly anxious and dyspneic. The nurse's most appropriate initial response would be to:

○ **A.** administer a sedative to help him relax.

○ **B.** prepare to administer epinephrine 0.3 ml subcutaneously every 20 minutes for up to 3 doses to promote bronchodilation.

○ **C.** assist the patient into a sitting position and have him lean over the bedside table to lessen his feeling of air hunger.

○ **D.** ask a family member to stay with the patient for emotional support.

Correct answer: C Assisting the patient to assume a tripod position allows for greater chest expansion and promotes comfort. Sedatives are contraindicated because they may further depress the already compromised respiratory drive. Epinephrine is contraindicated in respiratory patients with cardiac disease because it may precipitate cardiac ischemia. Although the support of family members is comforting to the patient, maintaining airway patency is the primary concern at the moment.

3. The principal contributing factors to venous thrombosis include all of the following EXCEPT:

○ **A.** atrial fibrillation.

○ **B.** stasis of blood flow.

○ **C.** endothelial injury or vessel wall abnormalities.

○ **D.** hypercoagulability.

Correct answer: A Atrial fibrillation can precipitate pulmonary emboli, but it isn't a principal contributing factor. B, C, and D make up Virchow's triad, the three principal contributing factors for venous thrombosis.

4. A patient with ARDS is intubated and mechanically ventilated with PEEP. In caring for this patient, the critical care nurse must remember that PEEP may:

○ **A.** prevent pneumothorax.

○ **B.** significantly decrease intrathoracic pressure.

○ **C.** significantly increase cardiac output.

○ **D.** significantly decrease cardiac output.

Correct answer: D PEEP increases intrathoracic pressure, thereby decreasing cardiac output. PEEP can precipitate a pneumothorax.

5. The nurse assesses the respiratory status of a patient admitted to the CCU with bacterial pneumonia. The nurse can expect to find which of the following signs and symptoms?

○ **A.** Crackles and wheezes over the affected lobes

○ **B.** A decrease in vocal fremitus

○ **C.** Nonproductive cough

○ **D.** Low-grade or absent fever

Correct answer: A Crackles and wheezes are common findings in a patient with pneumonia, regardless of viral or bacterial origin. Vocal fremitus is increased over areas of consolidation. A nonproductive cough indicates viral pneumonia. Bacterial pneumonia is characterized by a cough that produces copious amounts of green-yellow or rust-colored sputum. Lack of fever or low-grade fever characterizes viral pneumonia.

CHAPTER 4

Endocrine disorders

❖ **Anatomy**
  ■ Pituitary gland
    ◆ The pituitary gland is located in the sella turcica of the sphenoid bone and connects to the hypothalamus by the pituitary stalk, which links the nervous and endocrine systems
    ◆ The two lobes of the pituitary gland are the anterior pituitary (adeno-hypophysis) and the posterior pituitary (neurohypophysis)
  ■ Thyroid gland
    ◆ The thyroid gland is located immediately below the larynx on either side of, and anterior to, the trachea
    ◆ The two lobes of the thyroid gland are connected by an isthmus
  ■ Parathyroid glands
    ◆ The parathyroid glands are four small glands located on the posterior surface of the thyroid gland at the upper and lower ends of each lobe
    ◆ They receive their blood supply from the thyroid gland and are often damaged by thyroid surgery
  ■ Adrenal glands
    ◆ The adrenal glands are located on the upper lobes of each kidney
    ◆ They are composed of two separate tissues: the adrenal cortex (outer layer or covering) and the adrenal medulla (inner layer)
  ■ Pancreas
    ◆ The pancreas is located transversely in the left upper abdominal quadrant, behind the peritoneum and stomach
    ◆ It contains specialized cells called alpha, beta, and delta cells

❖ **Physiology**
  ■ Pituitary gland
    ◆ The secretion of most pituitary hormones is controlled by the hypothalamus, which secretes releasing and inhibiting factors
    ◆ The term *hypothalamic-pituitary-adrenocortical axis* refers to the complex interrelationship among the central nervous system (CNS), the pituitary gland, and the adrenal gland
    ◆ Pituitary hormones regulate several other endocrine glands and affect many diverse body functions; most of the hormones produced by the anterior pituitary gland stimulate the secretion of other hormones

Principal hormones of the endocrine glands

Gland	Hormones
Anterior pituitary	Corticotropin (also known as adrenocorticotropic hormone or ACTH) Follicle-stimulating hormone (FSH) Growth hormone (GH) Luteinizing hormone (LH) Melanocyte-stimulating hormone (MSH) Prolactin Thyroid-stimulating hormone (TSH)
Posterior pituitary	Oxytocin Vasopressin (also known as antidiuretic hormone, or ADH)
Thyroid	Calcitonin Thyroxine Triiodothyronine
Parathyroid	Parathyroid hormone
Pancreas	Gastrin Glucagon Insulin
Adrenal	Adrenal androgens Aldosterone Catecholamines Cortisol
Ovary	Estrogen Progesterone
Testes	Testosterone

◆ The anterior pituitary gland produces several hormones (for a complete listing of the primary hormones, see *Principal hormones of the endocrine glands*)

▶ Thyroid-stimulating hormone (TSH) regulates the thyroid's production of hormones

▶ Corticotropin, also known as adrenocorticotropic hormone, regulates hormones produced in the adrenal cortex

▶ Luteinizing hormone and follicle-stimulating hormone stimulate ovulation, progesterone secretion, and spermatogenesis

▶ Prolactin regulates lactation

▶ Growth hormone (GH) regulates growth, metabolism, and secretion of growth-promoting peptides in the liver

▶ Melanocyte-stimulating hormone regulates skin pigmentation

◆ The posterior pituitary gland also produces hormones

▶ Antidiuretic hormone (ADH), also known as vasopressin, regulates homeostatic fluid balance by controlling plasma osmolality

- ADH acts to increase the permeability of the distal renal tubules
- The increased renal permeability leads to an increase in water reabsorption and the production of more concentrated urine

  ◗ Oxytocin regulates uterine contractions and lactation in pregnant women

■ Thyroid gland
  ◆ The thyroid gland produces three hormones: triiodothyronine (T_3), thyroxine (T_4), and calcitonin
  ◆ T_3 and T_4 regulate the body's metabolic rate and influence growth and development
  ◆ The exact role of calcitonin in humans is unknown but may be involved in bone preservation

■ Parathyroid glands
  ◆ The parathyroid glands produce parathyroid hormone (PTH)
  ◆ Also called parahormone, PTH regulates calcium and phosphorus metabolism

■ Adrenal glands
  ◆ The adrenal glands produce hormones specific to the adrenal cortex and adrenal medulla
  ◆ The adrenal cortex produces three hormones
    ◗ Aldosterone, the major mineralocorticoid, helps regulate electrolyte balance by promoting sodium retention and potassium loss
    ◗ Cortisol, the major glucocorticoid, influences carbohydrate storage, exerts anti-inflammatory effects, suppresses corticotropin secretion, and increases protein catabolism
    ◗ Adrenal androgens and estrogens play an important role in the development of secondary sex characteristics and in reproduction
  ◆ The adrenal medulla produces two catecholamines: epinephrine, a positive inotropic, and norepinephrine, a potent peripheral vasoconstrictor

■ Pancreas
  ◆ The pancreas produces insulin, glucagon, somatostatin, and gastrin
  ◆ Insulin is produced by the beta cells in the islets of Langerhans; the overall effect of insulin release is a decrease in the blood glucose level
    ◗ Insulin promotes the synthesis of proteins, carbohydrates, lipids, and nucleic acids
    ◗ It facilitates the transport of glucose across cell membranes sensitive to insulin
    ◗ It increases the liver's glucose uptake and stimulates glycogen and fatty acid synthesis in the liver
    ◗ It inhibits hepatic gluconeogenesis (glucose formation from nonglucose sources), glycogenolysis (splitting of glycogen to form glucose), and ketogenesis (formation of ketones from fats)
    ◗ It facilitates the intracellular transport of potassium
    ◗ In muscle, insulin increases glucose and amino acid uptake, increases glycogen synthesis, stimulates protein synthesis, and inhibits protein breakdown (proteolysis)

▶ In adipose tissue, insulin increases glucose uptake, stimulates fat synthesis, and inhibits fat breakdown (lipolysis); the net effect of insulin in these tissues is to stimulate cellular metabolism

◆ Glucagon, secreted by the alpha cells in the islets of Langerhans, stimulates glucose production in the liver and is an insulin antagonist

◆ Somatostatin, produced by the delta cells in the islets of Langerhans, inhibits the secretion of insulin, glucagon, GH, TSH, and GI hormones (gastrin and secretin)

◆ Gastrin, also secreted by the delta cells in the islets of Langerhans, regulates hydrochloric acid secretion

❖ **Endocrine assessment**
- ■ Noninvasive assessment techniques
  - ◆ Inspect the patient's general appearance, noting height, fat distribution, striae, neck scars or nodules, hair distribution and texture, and growth and developmental level; check for medical identification information
  - ◆ Palpate the skin for tissue turgor, diaphoresis, dryness, and texture and the neck for buffalo hump or enlarged or nodular goiter
  - ◆ Percuss for abnormal deep tendon reflexes
  - ◆ Auscultate the neck for bruits over the thyroid and the heart for remote or S_3 heart sounds
  - ◆ Check blood pressure for orthostatic hypotension or hypertension
  - ◆ Check heart rate and rhythm for presence of tachycardia, bradycardia, or arrhythmias
  - ◆ Assess the patient's respiratory pattern for tachypnea and Kussmaul's respirations
  - ◆ Check for hypoactive bowel sounds
- ■ Invasive assessment techniques
  - ◆ The water deprivation test measures a patient's ability to concentrate urine; it's used when diabetes insipidus (DI) is suspected
    - ▶ In a patient with neurogenic DI, a 9% increase in urine osmolality occurs after the administration of vasopressin
    - ▶ In a patient with nephrogenic DI, urine osmolality is unaffected after vasopressin administration
  - ◆ The water loading test measures a patient's ability to increase urine output in response to a large fluid challenge; this test is used to diagnose syndrome of inappropriate antidiuretic hormone secretion (SIADH)
- ■ Key laboratory values
  Normal reference values may vary by laboratory
  - ◆ Sodium (normal value: 135 to 145 mEq/L)
    - ▶ Sodium imbalance may result from a loss of sodium, a gain of sodium, or a change in water volume
    - ▶ Hypernatremia (serum sodium level greater than 145 mEq/L) may be caused by excessive sodium intake, insufficient water intake, water loss exceeding the sodium intake (which may result from DI, impaired renal function, or prolonged vomiting and diarrhea), or sodium retention secondary to aldosteronism

▶ Hypernatremia associated with hypovolemia manifests as increased serum sodium levels due to dehydration; this condition is seen in such disorders as diabetic ketoacidosis (DKA), hyperglycemic hyperosmolar nonketotic syndrome (HHNS), DI, heat stroke, and high fever

▶ Hyponatremia (serum sodium level less than 135 mEq/L) may result from inadequate sodium intake, excessive sodium loss secondary to gastric suctioning, diuretic therapy, diarrhea, vomiting, adrenal insufficiency, burns, or chronic renal insufficiency with acidosis; in SIADH, hyponatremia is caused by a dilutional sodium decrease

◆ Potassium (normal value: 3.5 to 5.5 mEq/L)

▶ A reciprocal relationship exists between sodium and potassium; a substantial increase in one substance usually causes a corresponding decrease in the other

▶ Because the kidneys have no efficient method for conserving potassium, potassium deficiency can develop rapidly and is quite common

▶ Hyperkalemia (potassium level greater than 5.5 mEq/L) is common in patients with renal failure, DKA, or HHNS; excessive cellular potassium enters the extracellular compartment in these conditions

▶ Hypokalemia (potassium level less than 3.5 mEq/L) may occur in the severe dehydration states associated with DKA as insulin is replaced; hypokalemia indicates severe, prolonged dehydration

◆ Serum calcium (normal value 8.5 to 10.5 mg/dl)

▶ Hypercalcemia (serum calcium level greater than 10.5 mg/dl) may result from hyperparathyroidism, bone metastases with calcium resorption, kidney stones, excess vitamin D intake

▶ Hypocalcemia (serum calcium level less than 8.5 mg/dl) may result from hypoparathyroidism, increased PTH, neoplastic bone metastases, blood administration, hypoalbuminemia

◆ Serum phosphate (normal value: 2.5 to 4.5 mEq/L)

▶ Hyperphosphatemia (serum phosphate level greater than 4.5 mEq/L) may result from hypoparathyroidism, chemotherapeutic agents, excess vitamin D intake, or renal failure

▶ Hypophosphatemia (serum phosphate level less than 2.5 mEq/L) may result from chronic alcoholism, malabsorption, total parenteral nutrition (TPN), hyperparathyroidism, renal tubular acidosis, or the treatment of DKA with glucose

◆ Anion gap (normal value: 8 to 14 mEq/L)

▶ The anion gap reflects the serum anion-cation balance and can be used to differentiate among types of metabolic acidosis

▶ An anion gap greater than 14 mEq/L suggests an acidosis characterized by excessive organic or inorganic acids, such as lactic acidosis or DKA

▶ A normal anion gap occurs in hyperchloremic acidosis and renal tubular acidosis

◆ Osmolality

▶ Serum osmolality (normal value: 280 to 295 mOsm/kg) is a measure of the number of particles in serum

- Elevated serum osmolality (greater than 295 mOsm/kg) is found in conditions produced by excessive diuresis (such as DI and DKA); HHNS results in an extremely high serum osmolality (usually greater than 350 mOsm/kg)
  - Decreased serum osmolality (less than 280 mOsm/kg) is found in certain hypervolemic conditions such as SIADH
- ▶ Urine osmolality (normal range: 50 to 1,400 mOsm/kg; average range: 500 to 800 mOsm/kg) is a measure of the number of particles in urine
  - Elevated urine osmolality is seen in SIADH
  - Decreased urine osmolality is seen in DI
- ◆ Glucose (normal value for fasting specimen: 70 to 110 mg/dl)
  - ▶ The glucose level can provide a quick assessment of metabolic status
  - ▶ A glucose level greater than 300 mg/dl indicates severe hyperglycemia in patients with HHNS; glucose levels may be 600 mg/dl or higher
  - ▶ A glucose level less than 70 mg/dl usually indicates hypoglycemia
  - ▶ Glycosylated hemoglobin (hemoglobin A_{1C}) is a measurement of the percentage of erythrocytes irreversibly glycosylated; it's a much stabler measurement than plasma glucose, which is affected by metabolic processes; hemoglobin A_{1C} levels indicate diabetes control history 5 to 8 weeks before the measurement. Goal is hemoglobin A_{1C} level of less than 7%
  - ▶ Specific hormone assays may also help differentiate the disorder's cause
- ■ Diagnostic tests
  - ◆ Radiologic studies (such as X-ray, scans, computed tomography, magnetic resonance imaging, arteriography, and bone mineral densitometry) can help identify precipitating factors in endocrine disorders
    - ▶ X-rays of the skull, chest, and abdomen may identify tumors responsible for increased, inhibited, or ectopic secretion of hormones, such as ADH, prolactin, or cortisol
    - ▶ The radioactive iodine uptake test may identify abnormal uptake of iodine by the thyroid
  - ◆ Electrocardiograms (ECGs) can identify arrhythmias associated with a metabolic disturbance such as an elevated potassium level and the tachyarrhythmias associated with dehydration; continuous ECG monitoring is recommended for patients with metabolic disturbances related to endocrine dysfunction
  - ◆ Arterial blood gas (ABG) analysis can be used to determine the extent and physiologic basis of acidosis or alkalosis; metabolic acidosis with a pH less than 7.25 is associated with DKA
  - ◆ Visual field testing is used to determine deficits

❖ Diabetes insipidus
- ■ Description
  - ◆ Patients with DI are unable to concentrate urine because of insufficient or impaired ADH production or activity

◆ Three types of DI exist

❱ Neurogenic (hypothalmic), or central, DI results from organic brain lesions that cause insufficient amounts of ADH to be synthesized, transported, or released from the posterior pituitary gland

● Organic lesions of the hypothalamus, infundibular stem, or posterior pituitary gland can result from primary brain tumors, hypophysectomy, cerebral aneurysms, thrombosis, other vascular disorders, or closed head trauma

● Organic brain lesions may also result from infections or immunologic disorders

❱ Nephrogenic DI is usually an acquired disorder that causes an inadequate kidney response to ADH; nephrogenic DI is typically caused by disorders and drugs affecting the kidneys and is relatively rare

● Disorders that may lead to nephrogenic DI include pyelonephritis, amyloidosis, sarcoidosis, destructive neuropathies, polycystic disease, intrinsic renal disease, multiple myeloma, and sickle cell disease

● Nephrotoxic agents that can lead to nephrogenic DI include phenytoin, lithium carbonate, ethanol, demeclocycline, general anesthetics, and methoxyflurane

❱ Dipsogenic DI (primary polydipsia) results from the ingestion of large volumes of water, which depresses ADH, leading to polyuria

● Dipsogenic DI may be idiopathic or associated with psychoses

● Autoimmune disorders, such as multiple sclerosis and sarcoidosis, and drugs, such as lithium and tricyclic antidepressants, may cause dipsogenic DI

◆ The impairment of ADH activity seen in DI causes immediate excretion of large amounts of dilute urine, resulting in increased plasma osmolality and decreased urine osmolality

◆ In conscious patients, the hypothalamic thirst mechanism is stimulated and induces polydipsia

■ Clinical signs and symptoms

◆ Polyuria of 5 to 20 L/24 hours

◆ Polydipsia

◆ Tachycardia and hypotension

◆ Decreased skin turgor and dry mucous membranes

◆ Rapid, shallow respirations

■ Laboratory values

◆ Elevated serum osmolality (greater than 295 mOsm/kg) and serum sodium level (hypernatremia)

◆ Decreased urine osmolality (less than 500 mOsm/kg; may be as low as 30 mOsm/kg)

◆ Low urine specific gravity (1.001 to 1.005)

◆ Decreased urine sodium concentration (less than 20 mEq/L)

■ Diagnostic tests

◆ In a patient with DI, a decreased urine output resulting from the vasopressin test confirms the diagnosis of neurogenic DI

◆ The water deprivation test differentiates psychogenic polydipsia from DI and may be used in conjunction with direct measurements of plasma vasopressin

◆ The hypertonic saline (5%) infusion test can differentiate neurogenic, nephrogenic, and dipsogenic DI

  ◆ Plasma osmolality as it responds to hypertonic saline is assessed

    ▶ In neurogenic DI, ADH level is very low after hypertonic saline solution; in nephrogenic DI, ADH level is elevated; in dipsogenic DI, ADH level is normal to low

■ Medical management

  ◆ Establish I.V. access for a dehydrated patient

  ◆ Administer oral or I.V. hypotonic fluids

  ◆ Restrict oral and I.V. fluid intake when administering the water deprivation test

    ▶ Explain the fluid restrictions to the patient, visitors, and other health care providers

    ▶ Obtain hourly body weight and urine osmolality measurements and vital sign readings during the test

    ▶ Consider discontinuing the test if the patient experiences a more than 3% to 5% weight loss; the test is discontinued when there's an hourly increase of less than 30 mmol/kg for three successive tests

  ◆ Administer ADH in central DI replacement therapy

    ▶ Administer aqueous vasopressin (Pitressin) I.V. or subcutaneously (S.C.)

    ▶ Administer lypressin intranasally

    ▶ Administer desmopressin acetate S.C. or intranasally or I.V.

  ◆ Administer pharmacological agents in nephrogenic DI

    ▶ Chlorpropamide stimulates ADH release and augments tubular response to ADH

    ▶ Thiazide diuretics and sodium restriction enhances water reabsorption

■ Nursing management

  ◆ Document the patient's medical history, noting risk factors that predispose the patient to DI, including medications and recent neurosurgery

  ◆ Assess the patient's level of knowledge of the disease process; knowledge deficits must be addressed to increase awareness of early disease onset and to prevent a recurrence of DI

  ◆ Assess skin turgor and hydration of skin, mucous membranes, and eyeballs; these assessments are good indicators of hydration status, especially in patients who are unable to communicate

  ◆ Obtain an accurate baseline weight to help evaluate patient response to therapy

  ◆ Meticulously monitor input and output; note the amount, color, and specific gravity of urine

  ◆ In neurosurgical patients, monitor input and output for 7 to 14 days postoperatively; neurogenic DI resulting from head trauma may appear to resolve, then reappear permanently if undetected and untreated

◆ Monitor serum electrolyte, glucose, and hemoglobin levels and hematocrit

  ❱ A normal glucose level eliminates DKA and HHNS as the causes of polyuria, polydipsia, and dehydration

  ❱ An elevated hemoglobin level and hematocrit may indicate hemoconcentration, a sign of dehydration

◆ Monitor pulse rate, ECG activity, and blood pressure; sinus tachycardia and hypotension may indicate hypovolemia; and the vasopressant effect of ADH replacement therapy may predispose patients (especially those with underlying coronary artery disease) to angina

◆ Monitor for the adverse effects of exogenous vasopressin administration: edema, low urine output, hyponatremia, headache, nasal congestion, nausea, slight increase in blood pressure, personality changes, and changes in level of consciousness (LOC)

◆ Water intoxication is also a possible adverse effect of high-dose exogenous vasopressin therapy and may occur with ADH therapy if excess fluids are ingested

◆ Administer thiazide diuretics as prescribed; these medications induce mild sodium depletion and reduce the solute load, enhancing water reabsorption, and may be effective in nephrogenic DI

◆ Restrict dietary sodium in nephrogenic DI to induce sodium depletion; a 250-mg (11-mEq) daily sodium diet can effectively reduce urine output by 40% to 50%

◆ After the initial hypovolemia is resolved, educate the patient about risk factors, medication administration, adverse effects, and the potential for recurrence of symptoms; this helps prevent the severe complications associated with DI

❖ **Syndrome of inappropriate secretion of antidiuretic hormone**

  ■ Description

   ◆ SIADH is characterized by plasma hypotonicity and hyponatremia resulting from the aberrant or sustained secretion of ADH

    ❱ SIADH is caused by failure of the negative feedback system; ADH secretion continues despite low plasma osmolality and expanded volume

    ❱ The continuous release of ADH from the posterior pituitary gland causes the renal tubules and collecting ducts to increase their permeability to water and to promote water reabsorption

    ❱ Uninhibited ADH secretion ultimately leads to water retention and intoxication; symptoms usually resolve with the correction of hyponatremia

   ◆ Several predisposing factors for SIADH exist

    ❱ Ectopic ADH production associated with leukemia and bronchogenic (small cell), prostatic, or pancreatic cancer or Hodgkin's disease

    ❱ CNS disorders, such as brain trauma from injury, neoplasms, infections, or vascular lesions

    ❱ ADH stimulation secondary to hypoxemia or decreased left atrial filling pressure; this may be caused by respiratory tract infections, heart failure, and the use of positive end-expiratory pressure (PEEP) during mechanical ventilation

▶ Use of medications that increase or potentiate ADH secretion, including nicotine, tricyclic antidepressants, chemotherapeutic drugs, exogenous ADH therapy, lismapril, metoclopramide, morphine, and selective serotonin reuptake inhibitors

▶ Other causes include acquired immunodeficiency syndrome (AIDS) and AIDS-related complex, senile atrophy, myxedema, and idiopathic causes

◆ SIADH is confirmed by comparison of serum and urine osmolalities, with serum osmolality being considerably lower than urine osmolality

■ Clinical signs and symptoms

◆ Symptoms of hyponatremia (serum sodium level less than 135 mEq/L): low urine output; dark, concentrated urine; thirst; impaired taste; dulled sensorium and fatigue; dyspnea on exertion; weight gain without edema; headache; and nausea

◆ Symptoms of severe hyponatremia (serum sodium level less than 115 mEq/L): confusion, lethargy, muscle twitching, and seizure activity

◆ Severity of symptoms is also related to the duration of SIADH; acute development of SIADH (less than 48 hours) causes more severe symptoms

■ Laboratory values

◆ Serum sodium level: less than 135 mEq/L

◆ Serum osmolality: decreased, less than 275 mOsm/kg

◆ Urine specific gravity and urine osmolality: increased; 1.035 and 800 mOsm/kg, respectively, after 12 hours with nothing by mouth

◆ Serum ADH level: inappropriately elevated

■ Diagnostic tests

◆ Normal kidney, adrenal, and thyroid function test results

◆ Water-loading test with elimination of less than one-half of the fluid challenge

■ Medical management

◆ Restrict combined I.V. and oral fluid intake to 1,000 ml or less every 24 hours; I.V. and oral intake are usually calculated based on urine output plus insensible losses

◆ Administer hypertonic sodium chloride solution (such as 3% sodium chloride) to patients with severe hyponatremia; this is controversial because it may precipitate heart failure, fluid overload, and cerebral demyelination syndrome

◆ Monitor serial electrolyte levels at least every 4 hours for response to fluid and electrolyte interventions; replace as indicated

◆ Administer furosemide to increase urine output

◆ Administer potassium supplements

■ Nursing management

◆ Assess for precipitating factors: recent head trauma, medication use, known history of cancer or cancer treatment, and the use of PEEP; the onset of SIADH may be related to known precipitating events or previously undetected patient problems, such as ADH-secreting tumors, particularly bronchogenic cancer

◆ Observe the patient for CNS changes, including headache, personality changes, confusion, irritability, dysarthria, lethargy, and impaired memory; assessment of neurologic status provides important information about the level of impairment from water intoxication and hyponatremia

◆ Observe the patient for alterations in activity, including restlessness, weakness, tremor, muscle twitches, seizure activity, excess fatigue, gait disturbances, and sleep pattern disturbances; changes in activity level must be noted to address the patient's safety needs

◆ Assess for nutritional alterations, including nausea, anorexia, vomiting, and sudden weight gain without edema; changes in nutritional status are further evidence of electrolyte imbalance and water intoxication onset

◆ Percuss for deep tendon reflexes; commonly delayed in a severely hyponatremic patient

◆ Meticulously record hourly intake and output, urine specific gravity, body weight, hydration status, and cardiovascular and neurologic status; hourly assessments provide the most accurate determination of treatment efficacy and the onset of adverse effects

◆ Monitor the patient carefully for symptoms of hypernatremia, such as serum sodium levels greater than 145 mEq/L, edema, and hypertension after treatment is initiated

⬤ A sudden increase in the serum sodium level can cause brain damage and heart failure

⬤ Osmotic demyelination syndrome can develop in patients with chronic hyponatremia who have had time to become adapted to the state

◆ Maintain the patient on bed rest, and institute seizure precautions and safety measures to prevent self-injury; severe hyponatremia increases the risk of seizure activity, physical injury, and hypoxemia

◆ Frequently reorient the patient to his surroundings, explain all procedures and treatments, and reassure him that he's progressing well

⬤ Diminished cognitive functioning is a frightening experience

⬤ Frequent reorientation can help prevent injury and assist the patient in conserving energy for recovery

❖ **Diabetic ketoacidosis**
  ■ Description
    ◆ DKA develops when there's an absolute or relative deficiency of insulin and an increase in stress
      ⬤ The lack of circulating insulin produces an accumulation of glucose in the blood that exceeds the renal threshold, spilling glucose into the urine
      ⬤ Excess serum glucose produces osmotic diuresis, extracting water from the vascular space and causing rapid dehydration
      ⬤ Because of insulin deficiency and elevated counterregulatory hormones (such as glucagon, epinephrine, cortisol, and GH), the liver be-

gins to break down fats and protein to provide energy to glucose-deprived cells; this process is called gluconeogenesis and involves production of glucose from nonglucose sources

▶ Ketone bodies—the end products of fat metabolism (lipolysis)—form in the liver, accumulate in the bloodstream, and can spill into the urine and contribute to metabolic acidosis

▶ The by-products of fatty acid oxidation (keto acids, acetoacetic acid, and beta-hydroxybutyric acid) form acetone, which is responsible for the fruity odor noted on the patient's breath

▶ To compensate for metabolic acidosis, the lungs attempt to eliminate the excess carbonic acid by hyperventilating carbon dioxide (Kussmaul's respirations)

▶ The body attempts to buffer excess cellular hydrogen ions with proteins, phosphate, and bicarbonate (HCO_3^-); leading to HCO_3^- depletion in ABG values

▶ As hydrogen ions enter the cell, potassium ions are driven into the extracellular space (in ion exchange); elevated serum potassium levels in the range of 4.5 to 6.5 mEq/L are commonly seen in patients with DKA

◆ Patients with type 1 diabetes mellitus and those newly diagnosed with diabetes are at greatest risk for DKA

▶ Complications can result in mortality from untreated hyperglycemia and include profound hypovolemic shock; inadequate organ and tissue perfusion with subsequent thrombus formation, infarction, or both; electrolyte imbalance with associated arrhythmias; and prolonged, uncorrected acidosis that may result from underlying, undetected sepsis

◆ The most common stressors that precipitate DKA are infections, trauma, surgery, myocardial infarction, emotional stress, and failure to take insulin when needed

◆ A growing cause of DKA in adolescent females is the decrease or elimination of insulin for weight loss

■ Clinical signs and symptoms

◆ History may include poor compliance with the diabetic regimen, disrupted use of the continuous insulin infusion device, and medications, such as thiazide diuretics, diazoxide, phenytoin, or glucocorticoids

◆ Diminished LOC

◆ Polyuria, polydipsia, vomiting, anorexia

◆ Decreased skin turgor, dry mucous membranes, acetone breath odor

◆ Tachycardia, hypotension, fever

◆ Tachypnea, Kussmaul's respirations

◆ Abdominal tenderness on palpation

■ Laboratory values

◆ Serum glucose: greater than 250 mg/dl

▶ Metabolic acidosis

▶ Positive serum and urine ketones

▶ Azotemia

▶ Hypocalcemia

▶ Hyperosmolality

▶ Elevated urine glucose levels

◆ Electrolytes: initially, hypokalemia, eukalemia, or hyperkalemia and hyponatremia; then hypokalemia

◆ Blood urea nitrogen (BUN): elevated in severely dehydrated patients

◆ Serum osmolality: 295 to 330 mOsm/kg

◆ Hematocrit and white blood cell count: elevated

◆ Serum ketones: significantly elevated

◆ Anion gap: greater than 12 mEq/L

◆ ABG values: pH less than or equal to 7.20; HCO_3^- less than 10 mEq/L; decreased partial pressure of carbon dioxide level

◆ Glycosuria, ketonuria, elevated acetone, proteinuria, decreased urine sodium level, and urine specific gravity greater than 1.025

■ Medical management

◆ Establish I.V. access

▶ Administer rapid-acting I.V. regular insulin (bolus followed by continuous infusion)

▶ Switch to S.C. insulin 1 to 2 hours before stopping continuous infusion

▶ Monitor serum glucose hourly; adjust insulin dosage as indicated

◆ Administer I.V. fluids and electrolytes (such as potassium chloride) according to serum electrolyte levels and hydration status

◆ Obtain serum electrolyte levels and ABG measurements hourly

◆ Administer sodium bicarbonate therapy for patients with an arterial pH less than 7.10

■ Nursing management

◆ Assess for risk factors, including previously diagnosed diabetes, history of other endocrine disorders, recent reports of physical or emotional stress, and inadequate diabetic self-care practices; at least one-third of hospitalizations for DKA are associated with poor glucose control related to knowledge deficit and psychosocial distress

◆ Note blurred vision, abdominal pain, decreased LOC, lethargy, fatigue, weakness, polyuria, nocturia, nausea, vomiting, abdominal bloating and cramping, polyphagia, polydipsia, and recent weight loss; cognitive and perceptual dysfunction as well as elimination and nutritional status are important indicators of the duration of illness and degree of dehydration

◆ Inspect for flushed and dry skin, dry mucous membranes, decreased skin turgor, sunken eyeballs, and medical identification information noting that the patient has diabetes; early detection of the physical signs and symptoms of diabetes can help in the rapid diagnosis of DKA, prompt treatment of dehydration and hyperglycemia, and prevention of multiple organ damage from dehydration

◆ Check for tachycardia, hypotension, tachypnea, Kussmaul's respirations, and an acetone breath odor

◆ Assess intake and output, urine specific gravity, central venous pressure or pulmonary artery wedge pressure, skin turgor, and mucous membranes every hour; hourly assessments provide the most comprehensive information on hydration status and patient response to treatment

◆ Administer regular insulin I.V. to correct hyperglycemia at 0.15 U/kg of body weight

▶ I.V. insulin produces the stablest and most predictable reductions in serum glucose levels

◆ After the I.V. insulin bolus administration, begin an insulin infusion by an infusion pump at 0.1 U/kg/hour in adults

◆ Use a diabetic flow sheet to monitor hourly glucose levels, serum laboratory values (sodium, potassium, blood, urea, BUN, creatinine), and ABG values; this form helps to identify changes and trends in the patient's condition; it also prevents potential complications of hyperchloremic acidosis and hypoglycemia and the adverse effects of sodium bicarbonate therapy

◆ Dextrose 5% to 10% may be added to I.V. fluids, and insulin may be reduced, according to plasma glucose level

◆ Maintain insulin infusion until ketones are absent from blood or urine

▶ Because the plasma glucose level generally falls before ketogenesis is reversed, the insulin infusion should be maintained at a low rate to prevent rebound hyperglycemia (the Somogyi effect) and acidosis

▶ The rationale is that if ketones are still present, then acidosis isn't completely resolved

◆ Administer fast and intermediate-acting insulin S.C. at least 2 hours (sometimes 4 to 6 hours) before discontinuing the I.V. insulin infusion; because the half-life of I.V. insulin is short, insulin S.C. administration before discontinuing I.V. infusion helps prevent rebound hyperglycemia and acidosis

◆ As the patient's condition improves, teach him about DKA's precipitating factors and the need for more careful monitoring and control of his diabetes, including correct insulin management, dosage measurement and administration, rotation of injection sites, glucose monitoring, and sick day management

❖ **Hyperglycemic hyperosmolar nonketotic syndrome**
   ■ Description
      ◆ HHNS, like DKA, is a condition of hyperglycemia and profound dehydration resulting from insulin deficiency

▶ HHNS results when there's enough circulating insulin to prevent lipolysis, but the amount of insulin is insufficient to offset the gluconeogenic and insulin resistance effects of the elevated counterregulatory hormones

▶ The resulting elevated blood glucose level produces osmotic diuresis, leading to intracellular and extracellular dehydration

▶ As in DKA, sodium, potassium, and phosphorus are excreted through diuresis

▶ Severe dehydration results in hypoperfusion of the kidneys and altered glomerular filtration, leading to azotemia and acute tubular necrosis

❯ Impaired renal function exacerbates hyperglycemia

❯ If uncorrected, the high serum osmolality seen in HHNS leads to severe confusion, coma, and death

◆ HHNS is distinguished from DKA by the lack of ketosis and acidosis

◆ Risk factors for HHNS include type 2 diabetes, impaired glucose tolerance, advanced age, tube feedings and TPN, history of hypertension and coronary artery disease, pancreatitis, use of certain medications (thiazide diuretics, steroids, epinephrine, and phenytoin), and certain medical treatments (dialysis and burn therapy)

■ Clinical signs and symptoms

◆ Lethargy, fatigue

◆ Severe confusion, generalized seizure disorder, positive Babinski's reflex, and nystagmus

◆ Rapid, shallow respirations

◆ Poor skin turgor and dry mucous membranes

◆ Tachycardia, hypotension, and arrhythmias

■ Laboratory values

◆ Serum glucose: greater than 600 mg/dl

◆ Electrolyte levels vary with hydration state; severe electrolyte losses (sodium, chloride, phosphate, magnesium, potassium) occur with osmotic diuresis

◆ Serum osmolality: greater than or equal to 320 mOsm/kg

◆ BUN: greater than or equal to 20 mg/dl

◆ HCO_3^- level: normal

◆ Serum ketones: absent or minimal

◆ pH: 7.30 to 7.50

◆ Anion gap: less than 12 mEq/L

■ Medical management

◆ Establish I.V. access and rapidly replace fluids, using crystalloid and colloid solutions; administer approximately 2 L of half-normal saline solution or normal saline solution during the first hour

◆ Administer potassium and phosphorus replacement solutions, as indicated by laboratory findings

◆ Administer insulin therapy by bolus and I.V. infusion; insulin doses administered to a patient with HHNS are lower than those for a patient with DKA

◆ Adjust I.V. fluids (such as dextrose) according to glucose levels

■ Nursing management

◆ Identify risk factors—such as impaired cognition, advanced age, type 2 diabetes, and pancreatitis—that predispose the patient to HHNS; although DKA and HHNS are similar, HHNS is usually a more serious medical emergency

◆ Assess for diminished skin turgor, dry mucous membranes, excessive thirst, frequent voidings of dark and concentrated urine, altered LOC, and seizure activity; because dehydration is typically more severe in HHNS than in DKA, the extent of dehydration is a priority assessment

◆ Check for hypotension and tachycardia, signs of hypovolemia

◆ Assess for shallow, rapid respirations; Kussmaul's respirations shouldn't be present

◆ Monitor ECG for arrhythmias; hyperkalemia and hypovolemia can produce ECG changes that should resolve with medical treatment

◆ Auscultate breath sounds every 1 to 2 hours; rapid administration of a saline solution to a debilitated, elderly patient significantly increases the risk of pulmonary edema

◆ Monitor electrolyte levels; keep in mind that an elderly patient may take longer to reach normal fluid and electrolyte levels due to metabolic alterations associated with aging

◆ Accurately record hourly intake and output; these measurements are the most efficient method of assessing patient response to fluid replacement and of detecting adverse effects of fluid overload

◆ Use a diabetic flow sheet to monitor hourly blood glucose levels, serum laboratory values, ABG values, and intake and output; hourly glucose checks help prevent development of hypoglycemia; other laboratory values are useful in assessing the patient's response to therapy

◆ Maintain the patient on strict bed rest, and instruct him and family members not to massage the lower extremities; these actions reduce the possibility of dislodging a thrombus formed by hemoconcentration and hyperviscosity of the blood

◆ Educate the patient and family members about risk factors for HHNS as well as signs and symptoms of hyperglycemia; early detection of blood glucose alterations and dehydration helps ensure prompt treatment to prevent severe dehydration and hospital readmission

◆ Teach the patient appropriate diabetic self-care management techniques, including the correct administration of oral and S.C. antidiabetic medications, signs and symptoms of hypoglycemia and hyperglycemia, proper glucose monitoring techniques, and sick day management

◆ Discuss dietary management of diabetes, which is essential for optimal glucose control

❖ **Acute hypoglycemia**
  ■ Description
      ◆ Acute hypoglycemia is characterized as a glucose level less than 70 mg/dl, resulting from endogenous, exogenous, or functional causes
      ◆ Also called "insulin reaction" or "insulin shock," acute hypoglycemia most often occurs in patients with type 1 diabetes, although it can also occur in type 2 diabetes treated with insulin or insulin secretagogues
      ◆ Predisposing factors for the development of acute hypoglycemia fall into three categories
          ▶ Exogenous hypoglycemia is caused by insulin excess, insulin secretagogue, oral antidiabetic agents (for example, sulfonylureas and meglitinides), and the use of alcohol or other drugs (for example, salicylates in large doses and pentamidine)
          ▶ Endogenous hypoglycemia is caused by pancreatic and other tumors and inborn metabolic errors

◗ Functional hypoglycemia is caused by dumping syndrome, spontaneous reactive hypoglycemia, other endocrine deficiency states, and prolonged muscular exercise

◆ In acute hypoglycemia, glucose production—by means of food intake or liver gluconeogenesis—lags behind glucose utilization

◆ Because glucose is the preferred fuel of the CNS, hypoglycemia produces changes in LOC and elevated levels of counter-regulatory hormones (glucagon, epinephrine, cortisol, and GH)

◆ Patients taking beta-adrenergic blocking agents (such as propranolol) may not be symptomatic; these agents also inhibit glycogenolysis, which may impair recovery from hypoglycemia

◆ In exogenous hypoglycemia and functional hypoglycemia, symptoms generally follow a pattern related to eating, exercise, and administration of insulin or oral hypoglycemic agents; in endogenous hypoglycemia such as insulinoma, the onset of hypoglycemic events isn't precipitated by any factors

■ Clinical signs and symptoms
  ◆ Tachycardia and tachyarrhythmias
  ◆ Diaphoresis
  ◆ Fatigue, irritability, headache, altered responsiveness, coma
  ◆ Tremor, nervousness, weakness, seizures
  ◆ Nausea, hunger
  ◆ Slurred speech

■ Laboratory values
  ◆ Blood glucose less than 70 mg/dl
  ◆ Abnormal electrolyte levels, osmolality, urine specific gravity, and ABG values (if the patient has been unresponsive for a prolonged period)

■ Medical management
  ◆ Administer glucose
    ◗ Infuse dextrose 10% in water until blood glucose level reaches 100 to 200 mg/dl
    ◗ In an unresponsive patient with severe hypoglycemia, administer dextrose 50% in water I.V.
    ◗ In a conscious patient, administer 15 to 20 g of oral glucose
  ◆ Obtain capillary or plasma glucose sample 15 to 20 minutes after administration of glucose, and treat again as necessary

■ Nursing management
  ◆ Inspect for cool, clammy, pale skin; assess the patient's LOC and sensory and motor function; check for tremors and seizure activity (adrenergic stimulation is a compensatory reaction that produces the neurologic and cardiovascular changes associated with hypoglycemia)
  ◆ Check for medical identification information, which may indicate that the patient uses insulin or oral insulin secretagogues; acute hypoglycemia is seen most often in patients with diabetes, and medical identification information can help identify hypoglycemia in an unconscious patient

◆ Palpate and auscultate for tachycardia, tachyarrhythmias, and low blood pressure; these cardiac indicators provide clues about the patient's levels of shock and adrenergic stimulation

◆ Monitor the patient's neurologic and cardiovascular status closely; hypoglycemia can cause arrhythmias, extend infarcts, and produce seizures

◆ Use a diabetic flow sheet to record all glucose administration, responses to treatment, and capillary blood glucose values; accurate assessment of the trends during recovery or relapse is essential in preventing further hypoglycemic or hyperglycemic complications

◆ Institute seizure precautions to prevent injury: have suction equipment available at the bedside, place an oral airway at the head of the bed, keep padded side rails up on the bed, and ensure that oxygen is readily available

◆ Compare the patient's neurologic status against capillary blood glucose level measurements; a rapid, dramatic return to alertness should occur when the glucose level is corrected; if the patient remains unresponsive, suspect cerebral edema

◆ When the patient is stabilized, educate him about medication administration, hypoglycemic symptoms, and diet therapy; knowledge of the overall treatment regimen can facilitate self-care and help prevent future complications

◆ Tell the patient to carry a rapid-acting sugar source (such as hard candy or glucose tablets or gel) at all times and to wear medical identification; these actions will help ensure prompt treatment if a hypoglycemic episode recurs

◆ Dietary management to help delay glucose absorption and gastric emptying

    ▶ Small, frequent meals
    ▶ Ingestion of complex carbohydrates, fiber, and fat
    ▶ Avoidance of simple sugars, alcohol, and fruit drinks

Review questions

1. A 63-year-old male fell from a scaffold about 6:30 this morning, breaking his arm and leg. When he was admitted 2 hours later, his vital signs were as follows: temperature, 98° F (36.6° C); blood pressure, 150/94 mm Hg; pulse rate, 102 beats/minute; and respiratory rate, 24 breaths/minute. On questioning, his speech is slurred, and he can't recall the events leading up to his accident but does say he was running late this morning. He has a history of type 2 diabetes. An appropriate immediate nursing action is to:

○ **A.** discuss the importance of eating breakfast when taking insulin and insulin secretagogues.

○ **B.** make sure he's well covered because he's shaking and seems to be cold.

○ **C.** obtain a capillary blood glucose level to rule out hypoglycemia.

○ **D.** ask his spouse if he had been drinking alcohol this morning.

Correct answer: C The patient's symptoms are consistent with hypoglycemia as well as a head injury.

2. A 43-year-old female patient is recovering from a hypophysectomy performed 6 days ago for an aggressive pituitary tumor. She's being treated with thyroid and cortisol replacement. Her intake and output levels have been reasonable to date. This morning, she complains of thirst, and she was incontinent three times during the night. The nurse should:

○ **A.** make sure there are extra bed linens available.

○ **B.** insert an indwelling catheter.

○ **C.** test the patient's urine for ketones.

○ **D.** determine the patient's urine specific gravity.

Correct answer: D A complication of hypophysectomy is diabetes insipidus, which may be detected noninvasively by determining the patient's urine specific gravity.

3. A 16-year-old female has had type 1 diabetes mellitus for 12 years. She is admitted for the third time in 6 months with DKA. Her mother is distraught and states that she doesn't know why her daughter stops taking her insulin and feels very guilty about the incidents. The nurse should:

○ **A.** reassure the patient's mother that adolescents are often rebellious.

○ **B.** explore the patient's feelings about her weight and self-image.

○ **C.** educate the patient on the importance of being consistent with her insulin dose.

○ **D.** suggest a nutritional consultation to teach the patient and her mother carbohydrate counting.

Correct answer: B Adolescence is a difficult time for the patient as well as the family; viewing the situation from the patient's perspective can help guide the nurse in determining the cause of repeated DKA and reduce further episodes.

4. An 83-year-old male admitted this afternoon with a serum glucose level of 1,646 mg/dl was diagnosed with HHNS. He also has chronic obstructive pulmonary disease and recently began steroid therapy. He has received 4 L of half-normal saline solution I.V. this evening and seems to have developed difficulty breathing and shallow respirations. The most appropriate nursing action is to:

○ **A.** increase his steroids.

○ **B.** auscultate his lungs for crackling.

○ **C.** discontinue his I.V. fluids.

○ **D.** put an extra pillow under his head.

Correct answer: B The patient may be experiencing fluid overload as a complication of therapy. Auscultating the patient's lungs is the first step in determining the cause of his respiratory problem so that appropriate treatment may be given.

5. A 59-year-old male with small cell carcinoma of the lung recently developed pneumonia. His laboratory results (serum sodium, 118 mEq/L; serum osmolality, 270 mOsm/kg) indicate hyponatremia. His urine specific gravity is 1.037 and urine osmolality is 880 mOsm/kg. The patient is diagnosed with SIADH. His wife, who's visiting, comes to the nurse in tears because he gets very upset with everything she tries to do for him. The appropriate nursing action is to:

○ **A.** send his blood for a serum sodium level.

○ **B.** tell her he's irritable because of his cancer, and make a psychiatric referral.

○ **C.** tell her his irritability is related to his low sodium level and will resolve with treatment.

○ **D.** test his urine specific gravity.

Correct answer: C The patient's symptoms are consistent with his diagnosis and altered laboratory values. Appropriate reassurance should be given to the family.

Hematologic and immunologic disorders

❖ **Anatomy**
- **Spleen**
  - ◆ The spleen is surrounded by a fibromuscular capsule that extends inward as trabeculae and forms partitions within the organ
    - ◆ Smooth muscle in the surrounding capsule and trabeculae cause contractions that force additional blood cells into the circulation
  - ◆ The internal structure of the spleen is composed of two types of tissue
    - ▶ White pulp, randomly distributed throughout the spleen, contains lymph nodes and lymph strands
    - ▶ Red pulp, the majority of spleen tissue, consists of reticular tissue and cells that make and store red blood cells (RBCs)
- **Liver**
  - ◆ Divided into a larger right lobe and a smaller left lobe by the falciform ligament, the liver is attached to the diaphragm and moves with respiration
  - ◆ The liver is protected by the lower right rib cage and supplied with blood by the hepatic artery
  - ◆ The lobules that form the functional units of the liver are interconnected by cords of hepatic cells; each lobule is surrounded by several portal triads consisting of a hepatic artery, hepatic vein, and biliary duct branch
- **Bone marrow**
  - ◆ Productive bone marrow is located in the vertebrae, skull, rib cage, ilium, and proximal long bones
  - ◆ The amount of productive bone marrow gradually decreases as a person ages
- **Thymus gland**
  - ◆ The thymus gland is located behind the sternum in the upper part of the chest
  - ◆ A large, two-lobed organ in infants and children, the thymus gland shrinks during adolescence; by adulthood, it's nonfunctional and replaced by fibrous connective tissue and fat
  - ◆ The thymus gland has a cortex and a medulla
    - ▶ The cortex is composed of clusters of lymphocytes (thymocytes) but has no nodes
    - ▶ The medulla contains loose thymocytes and Hassall's corpuscles

- Lymph system
  - Lymph fluid is similar in composition to plasma and contains large quantities of leukocytes in the form of lymphocytes
  - Lymph capillaries are small, dead-end vessels that merge to form lymph vessels, including the right lymphatic duct and the thoracic duct; lymph capillaries are larger and have thinner walls and more valves than venous capillaries
  - Lymph nodes consist of oval bodies of lymph tissue encapsulated by fibrous tissue; internally, the nodes are a matrix of connective tissue forming small compartments that contain lymphocytes
    - Lymph nodes are located along the lymph vessels and concentrated in the cervical, axillary, and inguinal areas
    - Clusters of lymph nodes are found in the lungs, near the aorta, and in the intestinal mesentery

- ❖ Physiology
  - Spleen
    - The white pulp in the spleen produces antibodies, lymphocytes, and monocytes and stimulates B cell activity
    - The red pulp acts as a blood reservoir (holding 150 to 250 ml of blood), breaks down damaged RBCs, and produces, stores, and destroys platelets
  - Liver
    - The liver plays a significant role in the host defense against infection; Kupffer's cells, located throughout the liver, destroy bacteria in the blood
    - The liver also breaks down RBCs for bile production and destroys toxic substances that enter the circulatory system
    - The liver manufactures plasma clotting factors (factor VIII, vitamin K) and antithrombin
    - All blood from the GI tract passes through the liver before returning to general circulation
  - Bone marrow
    - Bone marrow produces the precursors of RBCs and white blood cells (WBCs)
    - Erythrocytes, granulocytes, and thrombocytes are produced only in the bone marrow; bone marrow is also a site for lymphocyte and monocyte production
    - Bone marrow can remove very small protein toxins from circulation
  - Thymus gland
    - The thymus gland produces thymic hormone, which stimulates the body's immune capabilities
    - It also regulates cellular immunity and T cell activity
  - Lymph system
    - Lymph fluid contains glucose, amino acids, urea, and creatinine; it doesn't circulate but flows toward the heart as increased interstitial pressure forces fluid into the lymphatic system
    - Lymph capillaries carry lymph fluid to larger vessels
    - Lymph vessels filter the intercellular fluids, returning proteins to the blood

◗ The right lymphatic duct drains lymph from the right upper quadrant of the body and head to the right subclavian vein
◗ The thoracic duct drains lymph from the rest of the body to the left subclavian vein
◆ Lymph nodes produce lymphocytes, monocytes, and plasma cells
◗ They also filter and remove foreign substances, dying cells, and microorganisms from the lymph fluid
◗ They produce globulins from the breakdown of cells and antibodies

■ Erythropoiesis
◆ Erythropoietin stimulates the stem cells in the red bone marrow to produce mature RBCs; it's secreted by the kidneys when the partial pressure of arterial oxygen drops below normal
◆ RBCs (erythrocytes) are nonnucleated, round, biconcave cells with a life span of approximately 120 days
◗ The stroma, or inner part of an RBC, is the point of attachment for hemoglobin; hemoglobin production requires iron, vitamin B_{12}, and folic acid
◗ The stroma contains the antigens that determine blood type
◆ RBCs are highly permeable to hydrogen ions, chloride ions, water, and bicarbonate ions
◆ Aged or damaged RBCs are removed from the circulation by the liver and spleen

■ Clotting factors and coagulation
◆ Clotting factors are proteins and other substances, numbered I to XIII, which form a fibrin matrix at sites of blood vessel or tissue injury (See *Understanding clotting,* page 142)
◆ The more common factors are:
◗ Factor I, fibrinogen
◗ Factor II, prothrombin
◗ Factor III, tissue thromboplastin or tissue factor
◗ Factor IV, calcium
◗ Factor VIII, antihemophilic factor
◆ Hemostasis occurs through vascular constriction, platelet plug formation at the injury site, initiation of the coagulation cascade, and subsequent limitation of hemostasis to damaged blood vessels

■ Leukopoiesis
◆ Leukopoiesis refers to the formation and development of various types of WBCs
◆ WBCs (leukocytes) are the body's principal defense against foreign substances and infectious organisms
◗ WBCs can move between multiple infection sites
◗ They're capable of reproducing rapidly and altering their structure to fit the situation
◆ Five types of leukocytes exist
◗ Neutrophils play a role in phagocytosis
◗ Eosinophils help in the detoxification of allergens, phagocytosis, antiparasitic action, and anaphylaxis

Understanding clotting

When a blood vessel is severed or injured, clotting begins within minutes to stop loss of blood. Coagulation factors are essential to normal blood clotting. Absent, decreased, or excess coagulation factors may lead to a clotting abnormality. Coagulation factors are commonly designated by Roman numerals.

Arriving at clotting through two pathways

Clotting may be initiated through two different pathways, the intrinsic pathway or the extrinsic pathway. The intrinsic pathway is activated when plasma comes in contact with damaged vessel surfaces. The extrinsic pathway is activated when tissue thromboplastin, a substance released by damaged endothelial cells, comes in contact with one of the clotting factors. All the factors in the cascade must be activated in the order shown.

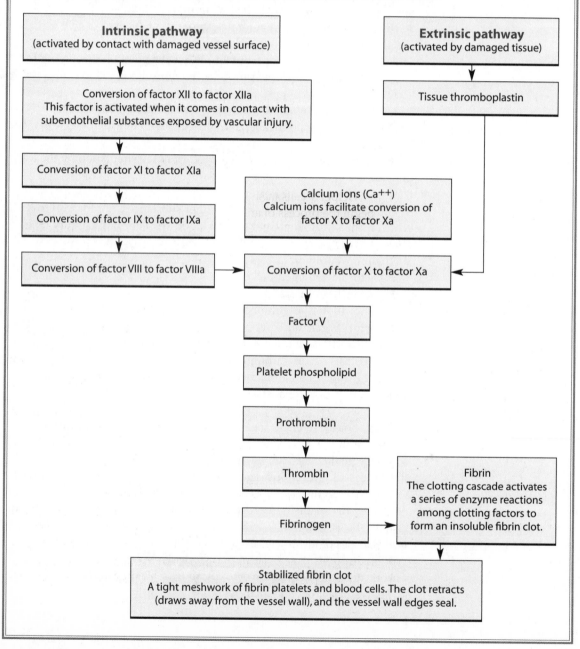

Lymphocytes and their functions

Although three types of lymphocytes exist, they aren't produced in the same amounts in all bodies. The chart below provides approximate percentages of the three groups of lymphocytes, along with their functions.

Type of lymphocyte	Normal count	Function
T cells	60% to 80%	Active in immune responses and immunoregulation
B cells	10% to 15%	Produce antibodies; destroy antigens
Null cells	5% to 15%	Attack and eliminate infected cells

▶ Basophils play a role in allergies, hypersensitivity reactions, and chronic infections; basophils secrete heparin and histamine
▶ Monocytes—produced in the bone marrow, lymph nodes, and spleen—function in phagocytosis
▶ Lymphocytes are produced in the bone marrow and divided into three groups (see *Lymphocytes and their functions*)
  ● T cells are produced in response to antigens and play a role in cellular immunity; there are four T cell subtypes:
    − Helper T cells (also known as T_H or T_4 cells) help B cells and begin the process of antigen destruction
    − Suppressor T cells (also known as T_S or T_8 cells) stop the immune response and destroy abnormal cells
    − Cytotoxic T cells (also known as T_C or killer T cells) identify and directly or indirectly attack (lyse) infected cells
    − Memory T cells recall and respond to previously encountered antigens; they initiate a more rapid response
  ● B cells produce antibodies and play a role in humoral immunity
  ● Null cells are undifferentiated killer cells that help prevent cancer
■ Immunity
  ◆ Immunity is the body's ability to resist or combat invading organisms
  ◆ There are three types of immunity
    ▶ Innate immunity is derived from the body's inherent immune mechanisms; examples of innate immunity are the resistance of the skin, acidic secretions of the stomach, enzymes of the digestive tract, phagocytosis by blood cells, and the production of natural antibodies
    ▶ Passive immunity is a temporary form of acquired immunity produced by the injection of antibodies or sensitized lymphocytes; passive immunity can be acquired, for example, through injection of gamma globulin, tetanus toxoid, or antivenin (for snake bites)
    ▶ Active immunity is a type of acquired immunity in which the body creates its own antibodies in response to invasion by foreign organisms; humoral immunity and cellular immunity are the two types of active immunity

- A humoral immune response produces immunoglobulins for specific antigens; macrophages present these antigens to the B lymphocytes; in turn, the B cells differentiate into plasma cells, which then produce antibodies for those specific antigens
  - A cellular immune response results in the sensitization of T cells to specific antigens, such as viruses, fungi, cancer cells, and transplanted organs and tissues

■ Immunoglobulins
  ◆ Immunoglobulins are protein substances synthesized by lymphocytes and plasma cells
  ◆ Each of the five types of immunoglobulins function as antibodies
    ▶ Immunoglobulin G (IgG) comprises 80% of circulating antibodies and has primarily antibacterial and antiviral properties
    ▶ Immunoglobulin A comprises 10% to 15% of circulating antibodies and is found primarily in the mucous membranes; it protects against antigen adherence and invasion
    ▶ Immunoglobulin M comprises 5% to 10% of circulating antibodies and is the first antibody to respond to bacterial and viral invasions
    ▶ Immunoglobulin D comprises less than 0.1% of circulating antibodies and activates B cells
    ▶ Immunoglobulin E (IgE) comprises less than 0.01% of circulating antibodies and produces the symptoms of allergic reactions
  ◆ Hypersensitivity reactions are classified by the time between exposure and reaction, the immune mechanism involved, and the site of the reaction
    ▶ Type I reactions are mediated by IgE that reacts to common allergens, resulting in local or systemic effects
    ▶ Type II immediate hypersensitivity reactions are mediated by antibody and complement (for example, mismatched blood transfusion or drug reactions)
    ▶ Type III immediate hypersensitivity results from antigen-antibody immune complexes that react with normal tissue, causing damage (for example, serum sickness or drug reactions)
    ▶ Type IV delayed hypersensitivity reactions occur days after antigen exposure and result from migration of immune cells; for example, contact dermatitis, measles rash, tuberculosis skin test, and transplant graft reactions

❖ Hematologic and immunologic assessment
  ■ Noninvasive assessment techniques
    ◆ Assess the patient's history for signs and symptoms of fatigue, weakness, lethargy, malaise, fever, chills, sweats, dyspnea, and pain; the patient's family history, social history, habits, and medications can affect hematologic and immunologic systems
    ◆ Inspect for enlarged lymph nodes, edema, erythema, red streaks on the skin, lesions, petechiae, hematomas, urticaria, shortness of breath, evidence of bleeding from any site, swelling of joints, and fever

◆ Palpate superficial lymph nodes for enlargement, consistency, mobility, tenderness, and size; use the fingertips of your second, third, and fourth fingers
 ▶ A hard, discrete node may indicate a malignant tumor
 ▶ A tender node usually indicates inflammation
 ▶ A palpable supraclavicular node on the left side often indicates a malignant tumor in the chest or abdomen
◆ Assess abdomen for hepatomegaly, splenomegaly, and enlarged lymph nodes of the axilla or groin; assess the musculoskeletal system for pain on palpation
◆ Auscultation may reveal tachycardia, hypotension, orthostatic changes, tachypnea, crackles, rhonchi, or decreased breath sounds
■ Key laboratory values
 ◆ WBC count (normal: 6,000 to 10,000 cells/µl)
 ◆ Differential WBC count: neutrophils (normal: 54 to 70 cells/µl), eosinophils (normal: 1 to 5 cells/µl), basophils (normal: 0 to 1 cell/µl), monocytes (normal: 1 to 8 cells/µl), and lymphocytes (normal: 25 to 40 cells/µl)
 ▶ Shift to the left indicates an infection, reflected by an increase in immature neutrophils (bands)
 ▶ Shift to the right usually indicates pernicious anemia or hepatic disease, reflected by an increase in mature, hypersegmented neutrophils
 ▶ Degenerative shift indicates bone marrow depression, reflected by an increased number of bands and a low WBC count
 ▶ Regenerative shift indicates stimulation of the bone marrow, as seen in pneumonia and appendicitis, and is reflected by an increased number of WBCs, bands, and myelocytes
 ◆ Bleeding time measures how long it takes platelets to adhere to the broken blood vessel and form the platelet plug in the primary phase of hemostasis (normal is 3 to 10 minutes but depends on the measurement method)
 ◆ Thrombin time (TT) measures how long it takes thrombin (factor IIa) to convert to fibrinogen (factor I) and then into fibrin (factor Ia). Normal value is 7 to 12 seconds but may be markedly prolonged in the presence of heparin
 ◆ Prothrombin time (PT) measures the clotting ability of the extrinsic coagulation cascade (factor VII) and the common pathway (factor X or Stuart factor), factor V (proaccelerin), factor II (prothrombin), and factor I (fibrinogen); normal PT is 11 to 13 seconds; the PT is used to monitor warfarin (Coumadin) therapy
 ◆ Partial thromboplastin time (PTT) is a more sensitive measure of clotting ability and the common pathway factors X, V, II, and I; normal PTT is 30 to 45 seconds; the PTT is used to monitor heparin therapy
 ◆ International Normalized Ratio (INR) is a comparative rating of PT ratios in which the measured PT is adjusted by the International Reference Thromboplastin; normal INR is 0.9 to 1.1; the INR is a more uniform way of monitoring warfarin therapy

◆ Fibrin split products (FSP) measures levels of fibrin degradation products, with a normal result of negative at a 1:4 dilution. D-dimers also reflect fibrin degradation but are a more specific test for disseminated intravascular coagulation (DIC) due to specificity for fibrinolysis (normal is less than 250 mg/ml)

◆ Coombs' test determines the presence of hemolyzing antibodies and is used to diagnose various hemolytic anemias

> ▶ A direct Coombs' test detects the presence of IgG in RBCs
> ▶ An indirect Coombs' test detects the presence of IgG in plasma

◆ Human immunodeficiency virus (HIV) tests, for antibodies, include the enzyme-linked immunosorbent assay (ELISA) and the Western blot (more specific and sensitive)

◆ Blood typing detects ABO and Rh antigens present on RBCs and is necessary for compatibility testing with blood transfusions; a more specific blood typing test detects human leukocyte antigens and is necessary for compatibility testing before some types of tissue transplantation (such as bone marrow)

■ Diagnostic testing

◆ Radiologic testing

> ▶ Ultrasound may be used to estimate the spleen's size and shape
> ▶ A liver-spleen scan can detect their size and function
> ▶ A gallium scan can detect malignant tissue, especially of lymphoid origin
> ▶ A lymphangiogram uses radioactive dye to visualize the lymph system, especially the nodes

◆ Biopsy of bone marrow or lymph nodes to evaluate for pathology

◆ Skin testing to determine hypersensitivities (or hyposensitivities) to specific antigens

■ **Organ transplantation**

■ Description

◆ Organ transplantation has become a fairly common procedure

◆ The kidneys, heart, lungs, pancreas, and liver as well as various tissues can be transplanted

◆ Patients who undergo organ transplantation receive high dosages of immunosuppressant medications to prevent rejection of the transplanted organ; most patients spend a significant amount of time in the intensive care unit (ICU) during the postoperative period

◆ In cases where a beating heart donor is required (as in heart, lung, and liver transplants), the donor's brain death may need to be determined (see *Determination of brain death*)

■ Medical management

◆ Maintain the patient on mechanical ventilation, as needed

◆ Prescribe analgesic and sedative medications

◆ Administer I.V. fluids

◆ Prescribe antibiotics and immunosuppressant medications

■ Nursing management

Determination of brain death

These factors must be present to declare brain death:

- Generalized flaccidity
- No spontaneous muscle movement
- No posturing or shivering
- No spontaneous breathing or breathing movements for 3 minutes after disconnection from a ventilator
- Flat electroencephalogram (This isn't absolutely required when the patient is connected to life-support devices)
- No blood flow on brain scan or angiogram

- No cranial nerve reflexes
  - No pupil responses (fixed; may be dilated or constricted)
  - Absent corneal reflex
  - Absent response to upper and lower airway stimulation
  - Absent cold caloric response
  - Absent doll's eyes
- Negative responses not caused by induced hypothermia or central nervous system depressant medications

---

◆ Monitor cardiac output and vital signs (blood pressure, heart rate and rhythm, respiratory rate, and temperature) every 5 minutes while the patient is rewarmed, every 15 minutes until stable, and then every hour for 12 hours; frequent and thorough monitoring of vital signs allows early detection of complications and prompt treatment

◆ Monitor hemodynamic parameters, including mean arterial pressure, pulmonary artery pressure, pulmonary artery wedge pressure (PAWP), and central venous pressure (CVP); these parameters are critical indicators of cardiac function and help assess left ventricular function, fluid status, and arterial perfusion of vital organs

◆ Monitor respiratory function and check endotracheal tube placement and patency; most patients are intubated after a heart transplant

◆ Check the settings on the ventilator, and ensure that it's working properly; as a result of anesthesia and opioid analgesics administration, postoperative patients are dependent on the ventilator for adequate oxygenation and reduced cardiac workload

◆ Monitor urine output every hour; output less than 30 ml/hour is a sign of possible heart failure, kidney failure, or hypovolemia

◆ Monitor the amount and color of chest tube drainage; more than 100 ml of drainage per hour during the first 24 hours may indicate abnormal bleeding

◆ Assess the patient's neurologic status every 1 to 2 hours for the first 24 hours; abnormal neurologic findings may indicate temporary or permanent disruption of central nervous system function related to anesthesia, use of the bypass machine, intraoperative stroke, or decreased cardiac output

◆ Monitor laboratory blood values, including complete blood count (CBC), serum electrolytes, blood urea nitrogen (BUN), creatinine, WBC count with differential, and arterial blood gas analysis; significant changes in key blood values may indicate hemorrhage, bleeding disorders, kidney failure, decreased respiratory function, or infection

◆ Check for signs and symptoms of infection, including fever, chills, tachycardia, weakness, fatigue, and localized pain; the use of immuno-suppressant medications increases the patient's risk of infection and may mask its signs

◆ Assess for signs and symptoms of organ rejection, including decreased cardiac output, abnormal heart rhythms, chest pain, and enlargement of the heart; many patients experience some type of rejection episode approximately 1 week after transplantation; early detection allows for prompt treatment with increased doses of immunosuppressant medications

◆ After extubation, encourage the patient to cough and deep breathe every hour to loosen and mobilize secretions and to prevent atelectasis and pneumonia

◆ Reduce the patient's exposure to infectious organisms by placing him in a private room, restricting visitors to the immediate family, using proper hand-washing technique, and wearing a mask and gloves for invasive procedures

◆ Change dressings according to facility protocol, and check the surgical site for signs of infection, such as redness, warmth, and purulent drainage

◆ Obtain culture specimens from draining wounds or incisions; successful antibiotic treatment depends on accurate identification of the invasive microorganisms

◆ Provide adequate rest periods; sleep deprivation reduces the body's ability to cope with stress and may lead to disorientation and uncooperative behavior

◆ Reorient the patient to his surroundings frequently to reduce anxiety and stress

◆ Allow family members to visit as much as possible, based on the patient's condition; the family is usually the patient's primary support system and vital to his recovery

❖ **Disseminated intravascular coagulation**
   ■ Description
      ◆ A common complication of many severe illnesses, DIC is a pathophysiologic process resulting from the presence of thrombin in the systemic circulation, which causes microthrombi to form throughout the circulatory system (see *Deciphering DIC*)
         ▶ The body responds to this diffuse coagulation with a massive release of fibrinolytic factors
         ▶ The result is the depletion of thrombin available for normal clotting and the circulation of an excessive amount of fibrinolytic enzymes, thus producing massive bleeding
      ◆ Although any severe illness that induces a decrease in blood pressure can cause DIC, the condition is commonly secondary to severe trauma, extensive burns, cancer, obstetric problems, sepsis, and autoimmune reactions
   ■ Clinical signs and symptoms

Deciphering DIC

This simplified flowchart shows the pathophysiology of disseminated intravascular coagulation (DIC). Circulating thrombin activates both coagulation and fibrinolysis, leading to paradoxical bleeding and clotting.

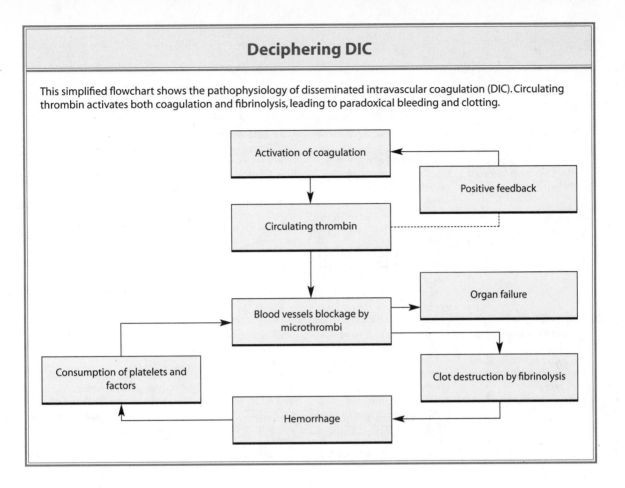

- ◆ Excessive and unusual bleeding from the gums, mucous membranes, and from sites, such as venipuncture, tubes, drains, and wounds, and excess blood in stools and urine
- ◆ Petechiae, purpura, ecchymosis, hematoma
- ◆ Laboratory findings indicate prolonged PT, decreased fibrinogen, increased fibrin split products, increased D-dimers, and prolonged TT
- ■ Medical management
  - ◆ Transfuse whole blood and blood products, including platelets, plasma, and packed cells as necessary (see *Blood products,* pages 150 to 152)
  - ◆ Administer heparin in the early stages of the disease to prevent microclotting
  - ◆ Amniocaproic acid may be given to inhibit fibrinolysis
  - ◆ Antithrombin III is also approved for use in DIC
- ■ Nursing management
  - ◆ Assess mental status, orientation, and level of consciousness (LOC); check for complaints of headache, dizziness, and behavioral changes; patients with DIC are at increased risk of intracranial bleeding, which can lead to cerebral hypoxemia and changes in neurologic status
  - ◆ Assess cardiovascular status, including blood pressure, heart rate, CVP, PAWP, and cardiac output; ongoing assessments can help identify

(Text continues on page 152.)

Blood products

Blood component	Indications	ABO and Rh compatibility	Nursing considerations
Whole blood ● Complete blood with no additional processing after collection (except testing)	● Symptomatic chronic anemia ● Prevention of morbidity from anemia in patients at greatest risk for tissue hypoxia ● Active bleeding with signs and symptoms of hypovolemia ● Preoperative hemoglobin < 9 g/dl with possibility of major blood loss ● Sickle cell disease (red cell exchange)	● ABO identical: Type A receives Type A Type B receives Type B Type AB receives Type AB Type O receives Type O ● Rh match necessary	● Keep in mind that whole blood is seldom administered. ● Use a blood administration set to infuse blood within 4 hours. ● Administer only with 0.9% normal saline solution. ● Closely monitor patient volume status during administration for risk of volume overload.
Packed red blood cells (RBCs) ● Same as whole blood except most of the plasma removed	● Symptomatic chronic anemia ● Prevention of morbidity from anemia in patients at greatest risk for tissue hypoxia ● Active bleeding with signs and symptoms of hypovolemia ● Preoperative hemoglobin < 9 g/dl with possibility of major blood loss ● Sickle cell disease (red cell exchange)	● ABO compatibility: Type A receives Type A or O Type B receives Type B or O Type AB receives Type A, B, AB, or O Type O receives Type O ● Rh match necessary	● Use a blood administration set to infuse blood within 4 hours. ● Administer only with 0.9% normal saline solution. ● Keep in mind that an RBC transfusion isn't appropriate for anemias treatable by nutritional or drug therapies.
Platelets ● Platelet sediment from whole blood	● Bleeding due to critically decreased circulating platelet counts or functionally abnormal platelets ● Prevention of bleeding due to thrombocytopenia ● Platelet count < 50,000/µl before surgery or a major invasive procedure	● ABO identical when possible ● Rh-negative recipients should receive Rh-negative platelets when possible	● Use a filtered component drip administration set to infuse. ● If ordered, administer prophylactic pretransfusion medications, such as antihistamines or acetaminophen, to reduce chills, fever, and allergic reactions. ● Use single donor platelets if the patient needs repeated transfusions due to risk for allergic reaction to foreign leukocyte antigens that may be present on leukocytes and platelets. ● Keep in mind that platelets shouldn't be used to treat autoimmune thrombocytopenia or thrombocytopenic purpura unless patient has a life-threatening hemorrhage.

Blood products *(continued)*

Blood component	Indications	ABO and Rh compatibility	Nursing considerations
Fresh frozen plasma (FFP) ● Uncoagulated plasma separated from RBCs and rich in clotting factors	● Bleeding ● Coagulation factor deficiencies ● Warfarin reversal ● Thrombotic thrombocytopenic purpura	● ABO compatibility required ● Rh match not required	● Use a blood administration set to infuse rapidly. ● Monitor the patient for signs of hypocalcemia because the citric acid in FFP may bind to calcium. ● Remember that FFP must be infused within 24 hours of being thawed.
Cryoprecipitate ● Insoluble plasma portion of FFP containing fibrinogen, Factor VIII:c, Factor VIII:vWF, Factor XIII, and fibronectin	● Bleeding associated with hypofibrinogenemia or dysfibrinogenemia ● Significant factor XIII deficiency (prophylactic or treatment)	● ABO compatibility preferred but not necessary ● Rh match not required	● Use a blood administration set to infuse. ● Add 0.9% normal saline solution to each bag of cryoprecipitate as necessary to facilitate transfusion. ● Keep in mind that cryoprecipitate must be administered within 6 hours of thawing. ● Before administering, check laboratory study results to confirm deficiency of a specific clotting factor present in cryoprecipitate. ● Be aware that patients with hemophilia A or von Willebrand's disease should be treated with cryoprecipitate only when appropriate factor VIII concentrates aren't available.
Factor VIII concentrate ● Recombinant genetically engineered product, derivative obtained from plasma	● Hemophilia A ● von Willebrand disease	● Not required	● Administer by I.V. injection, using a filter needle or the administration set supplied by the manufacturer.
Albumin 5% (buffered saline); albumin 25% (saltpoor) ● A small plasma protein prepared by fractionating pooled plasma	● Volume lost due to burns, trauma, surgery, or infection ● Hypoproteinemia (with or without edema)	● Not required	● Use the administration set supplied by the manufacturer, and set rate based on patient condition and response. ● Keep in mind that albumin isn't to be used to treat severe anemia. ● Administer cautiously in cardiac and pulmonary disease because heart failure may result from volume overload.

(continued)

Blood products *(continued)*

Blood component	Indications	ABO and Rh compatibility	Nursing considerations
Immune globulin • Processed human plasma from multiple donors that contains 95% IgG, < 2.5% IgA, and a fraction of IgM	• Primary immune deficiencies • Secondary immune deficiencies • Kawasaki syndrome • Idiopathic thrombocytopenia purpura • Neurologic disorders (Guillain-Barre syndrome, dermatomyositis, myasthenia gravis)	• Not required	• Reconstitute the lyophilized powder with 0.9% sodium chloride injection, 5% dextrose, or sterile water. • Administer at the minimal concentration available and at the slowest practical rate.

potential underlying bleeding and facilitate the evaluation of the patient's response to fluid and blood replacement

◆ Monitor peripheral circulation by checking skin color and temperature and quality of pulses; the presence of acrocyanosis indicates microthrombi within the peripheral circulation and blood vessels

◆ Check for transfusion reactions, which can result from the rapid administration of large quantities of blood and blood products (see *Transfusion reactions*)

◆ Monitor blood loss and relevant laboratory test results, including CBC, PTT, PT, and FSP; changes in these key laboratory values provide an indication of the patient's status and his response to treatment

◆ Assess pulmonary status; the highly vascular pulmonary system—a prime area for increased bleeding—may cause decreased lung compliance and respiratory distress if bleeding occurs there

◆ Assess renal status; urine output less than 30 ml/hour may indicate hypovolemia, kidney damage, or microemboli in the kidneys

◆ Assess the mobility of all extremities; thrombosis and bleeding into the joints and muscles may require that the patient limit movement to reduce the risk of injury

◆ Measure blood loss in urine, nasogastric and chest tube drainage, stools, and wound drainage; the multiple-organ effect of DIC requires a careful balance of fluids; both overhydration and underhydration are dangerous, and appropriate fluid replacement depends on accurate blood loss measurements

◆ Administer blood and fluid replacement therapy using appropriate techniques; monitor vital signs before, during, and after blood administration to detect transfusion reactions

◆ Prevent further bleeding by protecting the patient's skin from breakdown; use soft toothbrushes for oral care, suction only when necessary, avoid use of a blood pressure cuff and intramuscular and subcutaneous injections; any tissue damage can result in massive bleeding

Transfusion reactions

Type of reaction	Cause	Clinical signs and symptoms	Time of onset	Treatment
Febrile (nonhemolytic) • most common transfusion reaction	• Antigen-antibody reaction to a component of the blood product (white blood cells, platelet, protein)	• Anxiety • Chills • Flushing • Fever (rise in temperature greater than 1° C) • Muscle pain • Nausea and vomiting	• Immediately or within 6 hours of the transfusion	• Immediately stop transfusion. • Notify practitioner and blood bank—draw blood samples if indicated. • Administer medications, as ordered.
Mild allergic	• Allergic reaction to a plasma-soluble antigen that is in the blood	• Flushing • Hives • Itching	• Up to 1 hour after the transfusion	• Stop transfusion if fever occurs. • If no fever, slow transfusion and contact practitioner. • Notify practitioner and blood bank—draw blood samples if indicated. • Administer medications, as ordered. • Continue to monitor patient.
Anaphylaxis	• Allergic reaction seen in patients who are sensitized to IgA	• Abdominal cramps • Anxiety • Cyanosis • Diarrhea • Dysphagia • Dyspnea • Facial edema • Stridor or wheezing • Urticaria • In extreme cases, shock or cardiopulmonary arrest may occur	• Immediately	• Stop transfusion. • Administer saline through the I.V. • Notify practitioner and blood bank—draw blood samples if indicated. • Administer medications, as ordered. • Administer oxygen, as indicated. • Follow emergency protocols, as needed.
Acute hemolytic	• ABO group incompatibility	• Back pain • Chest pain • Chills • Dyspnea • Fever • Flushing • Hypotension • Nausea and vomiting • Tachycardia • Tachypnea • In extreme cases, shock or cardiopulmonary arrest	• Usually within 15 minutes from start of transfusion • May occur at any time during transfusion	• Stop transfusion. • Administer saline through the I.V. • Notify practitioner and blood bank—draw blood samples if indicated. • Administer medications and fluids, as ordered. • Continue to monitor and assess patient.

♦ Administer heparin, as prescribed; sometimes heparin is used in the early stages of the disease, but it has no value in the later stages; although heparin reduces the depletion of thrombin by preventing clot formation, its use in the treatment of DIC is controversial

♦ Instruct the patient to avoid sneezing, vigorous coughing, and the Valsalva maneuver; any stress to blood vessels throughout the body can cause increased bleeding

♦ Because the lungs are generally affected in DIC, maintain pulmonary status through proper oral hygiene, encouragement of deep breathing, and use of incentive spirometry; use nasal and endotracheal suctioning only as needed

♦ Promote good skin care through frequent turning, use of air mattresses, and relief of pressure over bony prominences; in patients with DIC, even minor skin breakdown can cause significant blood loss

♦ Assess the patient's and family's understanding of the disease; DIC is usually fatal, and they should be prepared for this possibility

♦ Allow the patient to express his fears and anxiety; this helps him reduce stress and conserve strength

❖ **Sickle cell crisis**
  ■ Description
    ♦ Congenital, inherited, hemolytic anemia that results from a defective Hb molecule
      ▶ The defective molecule causes RBCs to become roughened and sickle shaped with increased fragility
    ♦ The sickle-shaped RBCs become tangled in blood vessels, causing tissue oxygen starvation and possible necrosis
    ♦ Factors that may lead to a sickle cell crisis include deoxygenation, cold exposure, acidosis, and infection
  ■ Clinical signs and symptoms
    ♦ The patient may complain of severe abdominal, thoracic, muscular, or bone pain
    ♦ He may have fever, pale lips or nail beds, and lethargy
    ♦ There may also be increased jaundice and darkened urine
  ■ Laboratory findings
    ♦ Stained blood smear shows sickle-shaped RBCs
    ♦ Hemoglobin electrophoresis shows HbS
    ♦ RBC count is low; WBC and platelet counts are elevated
    ♦ Hemoglobin drops suddenly
    ♦ Erythrocyte sedimentation rate and RBC survival time are decreased
  ■ Medical management
    ♦ Transfuse packed RBCs to enhance tissue oxygenation
    ♦ Administer fluid to help increase RBC mobility
    ♦ Give analgesics and antipyretics as needed
    ♦ Hydroxyurea to help prevent future sickle cell crisis
  ■ Nursing management
    ♦ Assess pain frequently and provide adequate pain relief; a sickle cell crisis can be very painful, and many patients need high doses of opioids

◆ Apply a warm compress to painful areas; don't use a cold compress because it may aggravate the condition

◆ Keep the patient warm and comfortable

◆ Administer antipyretics to control fever

◆ Administer fluids as ordered to help decrease the viscosity of the blood cells; encourage the patient to increase oral intake as tolerated

◆ Keep the patient on bedrest during the acute phases of the sickle cell crisis

◆ Administer oxygen; this increases the amount of available oxygen in the blood and helps prevent hypoxia

◆ Administer vaccines to the patient to help prevent infection, which may precipitate further crisis

◆ Assess patient for liver failure; as clumps of RBCs become lodged in the vessels of the liver, circulation decreases and may cause liver failure

❖ **Immunosuppression**
■ Description

◆ Immunosuppression occurs when the patient is at increased risk for infection due to a defect in the immunological system

◆ Immunosuppression can be a complication of an underlying disease, the result of various drugs affecting the hematologic and immunologic systems (nonsteroidal anti-inflammatory drugs, steroids, and immunosuppressive drugs), or genetic

■ Clinical signs and symptoms

◆ The patient may complain of malaise, chills, night sweats, sore throat, dyspnea, and pain with urination or defecation

◆ On inspection, temperature exceeds 101° F (38.3° C), and the patient appears short of breath

◆ The patient may have loss of skin integrity, typically at I.V. and central venous catheter sites

◆ Tachycardia, hypotension, crackles, rhonchi, and lymphadenopathy may be present

■ Laboratory findings

◆ Cultures are positive for unusual or opportunistic organisms

■ Medical management

◆ Antibiotics to treat documented infection and possibly to prevent infection

◆ Reduction in use of the drug that is causing the immunosuppression, even though flare-up of the underlying disease process may occur

◆ Supportive treatment

■ Nursing management

◆ Monitor vital signs

◆ Administer I.V. fluids and monitor intake and output

◆ Institute compromised host precautions if the patient is neutropenic

◆ Institute nursing management for the specific underlying disorder causing the immunosuppression

HIV infection classification system

The Centers for Disease Control and Prevention's revised classification system for human immunodeficiency virus (HIV) infected adolescents and adults categorizes patients on the basis of three ranges of CD4$^+$ T-lymphocyte counts along with three clinical conditions associated with HIV infection.

The classification system identifies where the patient lies in the progression of the disease and helps to guide treatment.

Ranges of CD4$^+$ T-lymphocytes
• *Category 1:* CD4$^+$ cell count greater than or equal to 500
• *Category 2:* CD4$^+$ cell count 200 to 499
• *Category 3:* CD4$^+$ cell count less than 200

Clinical categories
• *Category A* (conditions present in patients with documented HIV infection): Asymptomatic HIV infection persistent, generalized lymph node enlargement, or acute (primary) HIV infection with accompanying illness or history of acute HIV infection
• *Category B* (conditions present in patients with symptomatic HIV infection): Bacillary angiomatosis, oropharyngeal or persistent vulvovaginal candidiasis, fever or diarrhea lasting more than 1 month, idiopathic thrombocytopenic purpura, pelvic inflammatory disease (especially with a tubo-ovarian abscess), and peripheral neuropathy
• *Category C* (conditions present in patients with acquired immunodeficiency syndrome): Candidiasis of the bronchi, trachea, lungs, or esophagus; invasive cervical cancer; disseminated or extrapulmonary coccidioidomycosis; extrapulmonary cryptococcosis; chronic intestinal cryptosporidiosis; cytomegalovirus (CMV) disease affecting organs other than the liver, spleen, or lymph nodes; CMV retinitis with vision loss; encephalopathy related to HIV; herpes simplex involving chronic ulcers or herpetic bronchitis, pneumonitis, or esophagitis; disseminated or extrapulmonary histoplasmosis; chronic, intestinal isosporiasis; Kaposi's sarcoma; Burkitt's lymphoma or its equivalent; immunoblastic lymphoma or its equivalent; primary brain lymphoma; disseminated or extrapulmonary *Mycobacterium avium* complex or *M. kansasii;* pulmonary or extrapulmonary *M. tuberculosis;* any other species of *Mycobacterium* (disseminated or extrapulmonary); *Pneumocystis carinii* pneumonia; recurrent pneumonia; progressive multifocal leukoencephalopathy; recurrent *Salmonella* septicemia; toxoplasmosis of the brain; wasting syndrome caused by HIV

❖ Acquired immunodeficiency syndrome
  ■ Description
    ◆ Immunodeficiency disorders, such as acquired immunodeficiency syndrome (AIDS), result from defects in one or more immune system components
    ◆ HIV causes AIDS by attacking T cells, reducing their ability to destroy foreign organisms that enter the body. It's believed that everyone infected with HIV will eventually develop AIDS (see *HIV infection classification system*)
    ◆ More than two-thirds of HIV-infected patients develop respiratory failure, often caused by *Pneumocystis carinii,* and require extensive and specialized care, typically in the ICU
  ■ Clinical signs and symptoms
    ◆ Recurrent high fevers, night sweats
    ◆ Tachycardia, hypotension, crackles, rhonchi
    ◆ Rapid, unplanned weight loss
    ◆ Swollen lymph nodes
    ◆ Constant fatigue
    ◆ Diarrhea and diminished appetite
    ◆ White spots and sores in the mouth

◆ Opportunistic infections due to the decreased immunity of the body; can affect any body system
- ▶ Bacterial
  - • Tuberculosis
  - • Salmonellosis
- ▶ Fungal
  - • Coccidioidomycosis
  - • Candidiasis
  - • Cryptococcosis
- ▶ Protozoan
  - • *Pneumocystis carinii* pneumonia
  - • Toxoplasmosis
  - • Coccidiosis
- ▶ Viral
  - • Herpes simplex virus
  - • Cytomegalovirus
  - • Herpes zoster
- ▶ Neoplasms
  - • Kaposi's sarcoma
  - • Malignant lymphomas

■ Diagnostic tests
  ◆ HIV infection is confirmed by laboratory tests indicating seroconversion
  ◆ AIDS is defined by the Centers for Disease Control and Prevention (CD) as laboratory confirmation of HIV infection, a CD4+ T cell count of 200 cells/ml, and coexistence of one or more "indicator" diseases

■ Medical management
  ◆ Administer antibiotics and anticancer medications
  ◆ Administer zidovudine (Retrovir), interferon, and other medications approved for the treatment of AIDS
  ◆ Treat cancers that develop as a result of AIDS surgically or with radiation therapy

■ Nursing management
  ◆ Assess for signs and symptoms of infections, including chills, fever, tachycardia, generalized weakness, and open or draining wounds; in an immunosuppressed patient, fever may be the only clinical sign
  ◆ Reduce the patient's exposure to infectious organisms by placing the patient in a private room, restricting the number of visitors, using proper hand-washing technique, and wearing a mask and gown for invasive procedures
  ◆ Monitor fluid and electrolyte status to prevent drying of the skin and mucous membranes, which can increase the risk of infection
  ◆ Assess skin condition and observe for irritation or breakdown; use measures to redistribute pressure on the skin, including turning, special mattresses, and heel and elbow protectors; immunosuppression and malnutrition increase the risk of skin breakdown and formation of pressure ulcers

◆ Check for the development of urinary tract infection (UTI), which is indicated by burning on urination and cloudy, strong-smelling urine; UTIs are a common complication of AIDS and can lead to sepsis

◆ Monitor for intravascular infection at the site of I.V. catheters and lines; these infections can lead to septicemia and are frequently fatal in immunosuppressed patients

◆ Monitor laboratory values, including BUN, creatinine, electrolytes, CBC, and WBC count with differential; significant changes in the patient's condition can be determined by making comparisons to baseline values

◆ Monitor nutritional intake, weight, and daily intake and output; GI functioning is generally impaired by the disease process and the medications used to treat it, making adequate nutritional intake difficult; malnutrition can worsen the immunosuppression

◆ Implement measures to control diarrhea, including pharmacologic measures, special diets, and frequent, small, low-residue meals

◆ Check for unusual or excessive bleeding; bone marrow depression and suppression of liver function can occur, leading to bleeding tendencies

◆ Obtain culture specimens using appropriate techniques; successful antibiotic treatment depends on identification of the invasive microorganisms; keep in mind, however, that many nosocomial pathogens are resistant to standard antibiotics

◆ Help the patient maintain good oral hygiene; immunosuppressed patients are at increased risk of developing stomatitis from the disease and drugs used to treat it

◆ Assess for signs of anxiety, which can lead to increased stress and further immune system suppression; to reduce anxiety, explain all procedures, reassure the patient, and encourage him to participate in his care as much as possible

◆ Assess the patient's knowledge of the disease process, and actively involve friends and family in his care

◆ Discuss the treatment regimen and discharge planning with the patient and family members; accurate information about the disease can decrease anxiety and increase cooperation with treatment

◆ Establish an atmosphere of mutual trust and caring; encourage expression of feelings, identify stressors, and develop strategies for dealing with stress

❖ Leukemias
■ Description

◆ Leukemias are cancers that develop when immature WBCs grow without restraint, accumulating in the bone marrow and blood

◆ This accumulation of abnormal leukemic WBCs interferes with the production of normal RBCs, WBCs, and platelets

◆ Leukemias are classified according to the type of WBC that's most prevalent and whether the condition is acute or chronic

  ◗ Acute lymphocytic or lymphoblastic
  ◗ Acute nonlymphocytic or myelogenous

> ▶ Chronic lymphocytic
> ▶ Chronic myelogenous

◆ Patients with leukemia are usually treated in the oncology unit, but complications of leukemia (such as overwhelming sepsis and acute tumor lysis syndrome) may require treatment in the ICU

■ Clinical signs and symptoms
   ◆ Anemia, fatigue, malaise
   ◆ Thrombocytopenia
   ◆ Bone pain
   ◆ Lymphadenopathy, splenomegaly, hepatomegaly
   ◆ Headache, fever
   ◆ Stroke
   ◆ Nausea, vomiting
   ◆ Bleeding (joint swelling, ecchymosis, hemorrhage), petechial rash, easy bruising
   ◆ Weight loss
   ◆ Tachycardia, hypotension

■ Diagnostic findings
   ◆ Laboratory findings may show very high or very low total WBC count with immature blast cells seen on differential and low RBC and platelet counts; if acute tumor lysis syndrome is present, uric acid levels exceed 7.2 mg/dl, potassium levels exceed 5.3 mg/dl, phosphate exceeds 4.5 mg/dl, and calcium is less than 8.6 mg/dl; bone marrow biopsy helps guide diagnosis and treatment

■ Medical management
   ◆ Chemotherapy with a combination of drugs
   ◆ Admission to ICU with low WBC (less than 1,200 cells/μl), low platelet count (less than 20,000 cells/μl), indications of increased intracranial pressure, or active infection
   ◆ Transfusion of whole blood, packed cells, plasma, and other blood products
   ◆ Bone marrow transplantation (graft-versus-host rejection)
   ◆ Radiation therapy

■ Nursing management
   ◆ Monitor mental status (LOC, orientation), hematologic status (joint pain and swelling, ecchymosis, and active bleeding in stools, urine, or gums), and infection
   ◆ Monitor fluid and electrolyte balance, as the patient is being given large amounts of fluid and blood products
   ◆ Monitor and control adverse effects of chemotherapy and radiation therapy
   ◆ Maintain a strict aseptic environment (protective isolation) when the patient is in the acute disease stages
   ◆ Administer medications as ordered, particularly antibiotics and blood products
   ◆ Monitor and control pain with pain medications, biofeedback, imaging, and other pain-control measures

◆ Increase fluid intake to 2 to 3 L/day; this helps flush chemotherapeutic drugs from the system to prevent renal damage

◆ Perform active and passive range-of-motion exercises on all joints to maintain mobility and prevent contractures

◆ Provide proper oral care; advise the patient to use a soft toothbrush and mouth rinses; suction only when necessary

◆ Promote the patient's appetite; allow a choice of meals, as desired, to ensure adequate intake of essential nutrients

◆ Assess the patient's and family's understanding of the disease; provide education about treatments, complications, and prognosis

◆ Reduce the patient's and family's anxiety by encouraging them to express feelings, fears, and concerns

Review questions

1. The nurse is caring for a 32-year-old patient experiencing organ rejection after a kidney transplant. Which of the following signs will the patient likely exhibit?

○ **A.** Decreased serum creatinine and BUN levels

○ **B.** Elevated transaminase level

○ **C.** Increased urine output

○ **D.** Elevated serum creatinine and BUN levels

Correct answer: D In kidney dysfunction, serum creatinine and BUN levels rise, and urine output declines. An elevated transaminase level is a sign of liver dysfunction.

2. A 24-year-old patient is being aggressively treated for acute leukemia. The nurse should also anticipate:

○ **A.** hemodialysis.

○ **B.** leukapheresis after chemotherapy.

○ **C.** fluid overload.

○ **D.** grief counseling.

Correct answer: A Hemodialysis is commonly used to prevent acute tumor lysis that may occur with aggressive treatment of leukemia.

3. A coworker who has been battling infection with HIV is admitted to the ICU for acute respiratory failure attributed to *Pneumocystis carinii*. The family is devastated, and the staff is also having difficulty dealing with the situation. The best course of action would be to:

○ **A.** transfer the patient to another unit.

○ **B.** rotate staff to care for the patient.

○ **C.** assign primary care nursing to the patient.

○ **D.** schedule a staff meeting to discuss the situation.

Correct answer: D Discussing feelings openly and collaborating on a plan of care would be in the best interest of the patient and staff.

4. A patient's laboratory work reveals prolonged PT, decreased fibrinogen, increased FSP, increased D-dimers, and prolonged TT. These findings are consistent with:

○ **A.** acute leukemia.

○ **B.** acute tumor lysis syndrome.

○ **C.** thrombocytopenia.

○ **D.** DIC.

Correct answer: D Prolonged PT, decreased fibrinogen, increased FSP, increased D-dimers, and prolonged TT are laboratory findings consistent with DIC.

5. Successful management of a patient with DIC may include all of the following except:

○ **A.** treating the underlying disorder.

○ **B.** administering heparin.

○ **C.** limiting transfusions of blood and blood products.

○ **D.** administering fluids.

Correct answer: C Successful management of DIC requires prompt recognition and treatment of the underlying disorder and careful administration of fluids. Active bleeding may require administration of blood, fresh frozen plasma, platelets, or packed RBCs. Heparin is used in the early stages of the disease.

Neurologic disorders

❖ Anatomy and physiology
  ■ Skull
    ◆ The brain is protected from superficial injury by the skull's bony structure
    ◆ A substantial blow to the skull can cause shifting of the brain itself, resulting in laceration or contusion of the brain tissues, or fracture of the bony segments, with the resultant fragments being propelled into brain tissue
    ◆ The skull is composed of eight flat, irregular bones fused at sutures
      ❙ The frontal bone overlies the anterior aspect, or frontal lobe, of the brain
      ❙ The occipital bone overlies the posterior aspect, or occipital lobe, of the brain
      ❙ Two temporal bones overlie the inferolateral aspect, or temporal lobe, of the brain
      ❙ Two parietal bones overlie the superolateral aspect, or parietal lobe, of the brain
      ❙ The sphenoid bone is located at the base of the skull in front of the occipital and temporal bones and has at its center the sella turcica, in which the pituitary gland is located
      ❙ The ethmoid bone (cribriform plate) fits into a notch in the frontal bone and forms the roof of the nasal fossa and the floor of the cranial cavity
    ◆ At the base of the skull is a large opening, the foramen magnum, through which the brain stem extends and becomes continuous with the spinal cord
  ■ The meninges
    ◆ The meninges, composed of the dura mater, arachnoid mater, and pia mater, lie immediately below the skull and provide an additional layer of protection for the brain and spinal cord
    ◆ The dura mater consists of two layers, which form the venous sinus between them
      ❙ The outer layer forms a tough, fibrous periosteum that adheres to the cranial bones
      ❙ The inner layer, or meningeal dura, extends into the cranium and forms rigid membrane plates that support and separate various brain structures

▶ The outer dura separates from the meningeal dura to form sinuses that assist with venous drainage from the brain

▶ The meningeal dura has several extensions

   ● The falx cerebri is located between the right and left hemispheres of the brain

   ● The tentorium cerebelli supports the occipital lobe and covers the upper surface of the cerebellum

      – Structures above the tentorium cerebelli are called supratentorial

      – Structures below the tentorium cerebelli are called infratentorial or described as the posterior fossa

   ● The falx cerebelli extends along the division of the lateral lobes of the cerebellum

   ● The diaphragm sella canopies the sella turcica and thus encloses the pituitary gland

▶ The dura mater is separated from the next meningeal layer, the arachnoid, by a thin subdural space; this area is vulnerable to trauma because of the presence of a network of unsupported veins; if lacerated, these tiny veins form a subdural hematoma

◆ The arachnoid mater is a fragile membrane that surrounds the brain

▶ The arachnoid mater is separated from the pia mater by the relatively wide subarachnoid space, which contains cerebrospinal fluid (CSF), connective tissues, and cerebral arteries (circle of Willis) and veins

▶ The arachnoid villi connect the subarachnoid space to the sagittal and transverse sinuses

   ● These structures facilitate the reabsorption of CSF from the subarachnoid space into the sinuses

   ● Impedance of CSF reabsorption by the arachnoid villi is called communicating hydrocephalus; conditions that impede CSF reabsorption include hemorrhage in the subarachnoid space and bacterial or viral meningitis

◆ The pia mater is the innermost layer of the meninges

▶ It adheres to the entire surface of the brain and spinal cord following its sulci and gyri

▶ The pia mater contains the arterial blood supply for the tissues of the brain and is part of the choroid plexus (the structure that manufactures CSF)

■ Brain

◆ The cerebrum is the largest segment of the brain and consists of two cerebral hemispheres separated by a longitudinal fissure and joined by the corpus callosum; each hemisphere is divided by anatomic demarcations into four paired lobes: the frontal, parietal, temporal, and occipital lobes

▶ The left cerebral hemisphere is dominant for verbal, linguistic, mathematical, and analytic functions in most people; the nondominant hemisphere is more concerned with geometric, spatial, visual, and musical function

▶ The frontal lobes underlie the frontal bone and are separated from the parietal lobes by the central sulcus, or fissure of Rolando, and from the temporal lobes by the lateral cerebral sulcus, or fissure of Sylvius; the frontal lobes have several functions
  • They control voluntary motor functions
  • They control some autonomic nervous system (ANS) functions
  • They play a role in cognition, memory, language, personality, and higher intellectual functions
▶ The parietal lobe is posterior to the frontal lobe and separated by the central sulcus; it's responsible for sensory function, sensory association areas, and higher-level processing of general sensory modalities (such as stereognosis)
▶ The temporal lobe underlies the temporal bone; it's responsible for hearing, sensory speech in the dominant hemisphere, vestibular sense, behavior, and emotion
▶ The limbic area is anatomically integrated with the temporal lobe to form the borders of the lateral ventricles; the limbic lobe contains the uncus, hippocampus, primary olfactory cortex, and amygdaloid nucleus; the limbic lobe has several functions
  • It initiates actions of self-preservation
  • It stimulates emotions
  • It stores short-term memory
  • It interprets smell
▶ The occipital lobe is the most posterior of the cerebral lobes; it plays a role in vision by translating visual stimuli into integrated meaning
◆ The cerebral cortex forms the outer layer of the cerebrum
  ▶ It's composed of unmyelinated cells (gray matter)
  ▶ The myelinated tracts (white matter) below the cerebral cortex function in the transmission of impulses from the cerebral cortex to the rest of the brain
    • The commissural fibers create a tract of communication between the cerebral cortex of one hemisphere and the corresponding parts in the other hemisphere; the largest of these tracts is the corpus callosum. The commisural fibers transfer learned discrimination, sensory experience, and memory from one cerebral hemisphere to the other
    • Projection fibers create a tract of communication between the cerebral cortex and the lower brain and spinal cord; these tracts consist of ascending or afferent tracts, which are located primarily in the thalamus, and descending or efferent tracts, which are found in the motor area of the cortex
◆ The diencephalon is positioned at the top of the brain stem, where the olfactory nerve (cranial nerve I) and the optic nerve (cranial nerve II) begin; it consists of the thalamus, hypothalamus, subthalamus, and epithalamus
  ▶ The thalamus, which forms the lateral walls of the third ventricle, has several functions
    • It relays motor and sensory information

- It conveys all sensory information (except olfactory) to the appropriate area of the cerebral cortex
  - It coordinates the functions of the parietal lobe of the cerebrum and cerebral cortex for both sensory and motor stimuli
    - It processes basic brain functions and more complex behavior
  ▶ The hypothalamus, located below the thalamus, forms the floor and anterior wall of the third ventricle; it's responsible for regulating temperature, autonomic responses, water and food intake, behavioral responses, and hormonal secretions
◆ The ANS consists of parasympathetic and sympathetic responses
  ▶ Parasympathetic responses stimulate the body to slow down activities and conserve energy
  ▶ Sympathetic responses, also known as fight-or-flight responses, stimulate the body to increase activities and consume energy
◆ The pituitary gland is located below the hypothalamus in the sella turcica (see chapter 4, Endocrine disorders)
◆ The basal ganglia make up the central gray matter of the cerebrum and lie between the white matter of the cerebrum and the thalamus
  ▶ These fibers are primarily motor tracts and influence the ability to produce smooth, coordinated, voluntary movements and to maintain balance
◆ The brain stem is continuous with the spinal cord and extends through the foramen magnum of the skull; it consists of the medulla oblongata, pons, midbrain, and reticular formation
  ▶ The medulla oblongata is the site where decussation (crossing) of motor tracts occurs; at this level, stimulation from one side of the brain affects movement on the contralateral side of the body
    - Involuntary swallowing, hiccuping, coughing, vomiting, heart rate, arterial vasoconstriction, and respirations are wholly or partly controlled by the medulla
    - The respiratory center, which is located in the medulla, acts in concert with the apneustic and pneumotaxic centers of the pons to control respiratory rhythm
    - Also arising in the medulla are the beginnings of the reticular formation and cranial nerves VIII (acoustic), IX (glossopharyngeal), X (vagus), XI (spinal accessory), and XII (hypoglossal)
  ▶ The pons is located immediately superior to the medulla
    - It's a major relay station for the transmission of impulses from the cerebellum to the cerebral cortex; this contributes to smooth body movements
    - The apneustic respiratory center, which is located in the pons, controls the length of inspiration and expiration
    - Cranial nerves V (trigeminal), VI (abducens), and VII (facial and acoustic) originate in the pons
  ▶ The midbrain forms the connection between the pons and the diencephalon
    - It relays voluntary motor activity
    - It's the site of origin of cranial nerves III (oculomotor) and IV (trochlear)

- It also is the location of the extrapyramidal tracts that control the involuntary tone of flexor muscles (rubrospinal) and the involuntary reflex motor movements resulting from auditory or visual stimuli (tectospinal)
  - The aqueduct of Sylvius is also located in the midbrain
- ◗ The reticular formation is located in the central core of the brain stem and projects into the cerebral cortex, thalamus, spinal cord, and cerebellum
  - All sensory input to the brain stem is relayed through the reticular formation on its way to the cerebral cortex
  - Composed of motor and sensory tracts, the reticular formation has both excitatory and inhibitory capacities
  - The ascending reticular activating system is essential for arousal from sleep, alert wakefulness, focused attention, and perceptual association; the descending reticular system may inhibit or facilitate motor neurons of the skeletal musculature
- ◆ The cerebellum is located at the posteroinferior aspect of the cerebrum
  - ◗ Equilibrium, spatial orientation, coordination of movement, and proprioception are integrated functions of the cerebellum
  - ◗ Dysfunction of or injury to the cerebellum can result in ataxia and dysarthria
- ■ Ventricular system of the brain
  - ◆ The ventricles of the brain consist of four connected compartments filled with CSF
  - ◆ The largest ventricles, called the lateral ventricles, are paired, with one ventricle located within each of the cerebral hemispheres; the lateral ventricles connect with the third ventricle through the foramen of Monro
    - ◗ Each lateral ventricle consists of a body, frontal horn, temporal horn, and occipital horn
    - ◗ The frontal horn of the lateral ventricle is most frequently selected as the site for intracranial pressure (ICP) monitoring
  - ◆ The third ventricle is centrally located, immediately above the midbrain and between the thalamic structures of the diencephalon; it's linked to the fourth ventricle by the aqueduct of Sylvius
  - ◆ The fourth ventricle is situated behind the pons and medulla and in front of the cerebellum; within the fourth ventricle are two openings (known as the foramen of Luschka and the foramen of Magendie) that allow CSF to flow into the subarachnoid space for reabsorption by the arachnoid villi
  - ◆ CSF is formed almost wholly by the choroid plexus located in the four ventricles; a scant amount is secreted by the ependymal cells that line the ventricles and the spinal cord and by the capillaries of the pia mater
    - ◗ CSF is an odorless, colorless, clear substance that contains a small amount of protein (5 to 25 mg/dl) and glucose (50 to 75 mg/dl, or approximately 60% of serum glucose)
    - ◗ CSF provides support for the central nervous system (CNS), cushions the CNS against trauma, and assists in the removal of waste products and delivery of nutrients

◗ Approximately 500 ml (20 ml/hour) of CSF are produced daily; no feedback mechanism regulates CSF production

  ● An obstruction of the cerebral aqueducts within the ventricular system, such as from a tumor or blood clot, blocks the flow of CSF and causes noncommunicating hydrocephalus

◗ CSF is thought to be a filtrate of blood resulting from active transport and osmotic pressure; key elements in CSF production include blood pressure, serum osmolality, and cerebral metabolism

◗ Normal CSF pressure at the level of the lumbar cistern in a recumbent position is 80 to 180 mm H_2O; in the cerebral ventricle, normal CSF pressure is 3 to 15 mm Hg

◗ CSF flows through a closed system from secretion in the lateral cerebral ventricles through the foramen of Monro to the third ventricle, which secretes more CSF; it then travels through the aqueduct of Sylvius to the fourth ventricle, where more CSF is added; it continues through the foramina of Magendie and Luschka to the subarachnoid space

  ● From the subarachnoid space, CSF travels down the spinal cord and up over the surface of the brain to be reabsorbed by the arachnoid villi

  ● The arachnoid villi empty into the intracerebral and meningeal veins, which drain into the venous sinuses

  ● The venous sinuses drain into the internal jugular vein and back into central venous circulation

◆ ICPs (static and dynamic) are exerted by the volume of intracranial contents

  ◗ The Monro-Kellie doctrine describes the volume-pressure relationship within the brain and the pathologic condition associated with increased ICP

    ● This doctrine asserts that the skull is a rigid compartment of limited space

    ● This space is filled to capacity by three components—brain tissue, blood, and CSF—all of which have a fairly constant volume

    ● An increase in any one component necessitates a concomitant decrease in one of the other components, or cerebral edema and increased ICP will result

  ◗ Herniation of cerebral tissues is caused by compression and displacement of areas of the brain against the bony cranial compartment or its structures; increased ICP caused by tumors, hemorrhage, or cerebral edema produces this displacement

    ● Supratentorial herniation involves the structures located above the tentorial notch: the cerebral hemispheres, basal ganglia, and diencephalon

      — Cingulate (transflex herniation) develops when one cerebral hemisphere is shifted laterally, forcing the cingulate gyrus under the falx cerebri; the lateral shifting compresses and displaces the large cerebral veins of that hemisphere

      — Central (transtentorial) herniation occurs when increased, diffuse pressure is exerted downward, forcing the cerebral structures down through the tentorial opening and resulting in rostral-caudal herniation. It is often preceded by uncal and cingulate herniation

— Early rostral-caudal herniation is characterized by a decreased level of consciousness (LOC); normal respiratory control, but an atypical respiratory pattern with frequent sighs or yawns; and small, but equally reactive pupils; as the herniation continues and more structures become compressed, deep coma, pathologic respiratory patterns, and pupillary and reflex changes associated with brain stem involvement occur

— Uncal herniation is the lateral compression of cerebral tissues downward through the tentorial opening; lateralizing signs present with uncal herniation differentiate it from central herniation; in uncal herniation, the typically decreased LOC is accompanied by a unilaterally dilated pupil, signifying the beginning of brain stem involvement and rapid deterioration to fixed and dilated pupils, flaccidity, and coma and brain death

- Infratentorial herniation involves structures located below the tentorial notch: the cerebellum and lower brain stem

— Infratentorial herniation develops when a tumor, abscess, or hemorrhage forces the cerebellum and brain stem to shift laterally, upward through the tentorial opening, or downward through the foramen magnum

— Lumbar puncture in a patient with high ICP may cause a rapid downward shift of cerebral tissues that leads to infratentorial herniation; signs of compression usually are unilateral, and deterioration is rapid

- Transcranial herniation involves the cerebral tissues throughout the cranial vault; it's caused by cerebral extrusion through a skull fracture, craniotomy site, or opening in the skull from a bullet wound

▶ Cerebral edema causes an increase in extracellular or intracellular tissue volume after brain insult

- Vasogenic cerebral edema results from disruption of the blood-brain barrier, causing extracellular edema; this, in turn, causes osmotic pressure gradients in the cerebral vessels that move water from the intravascular space to the cerebral interstitium that increase the edema; vasogenic edema may be caused by trauma, infection, abscess, hypoxia, or tumor

- Cytotoxic cerebral edema results from failure of the sodium-potassium pump, which allows potassium to leave the cell while sodium, chloride, and water enter the cell and cause it to swell; this intracellular edema can be caused by hypoxic states, administration of hypotonic fluids (such as dextrose 5% in water), other hyposmotic conditions, and certain diseases (such as Reye's syndrome)

- Interstitial (hydrocephalic) cerebral edema is extracellular edema that results from a buildup of CSF pressure within the ventricular system, producing transudation of CSF into the periventricular areas; hydrocephalus can be acute or chronic and may be communicating (nonobstructive) or noncommunicating (obstructive)

— Communicating hydrocephalus is caused by increased production or decreased absorption of CSF; causes include meningeal tumors, congenital malformations, and infection

— Noncommunicating hydrocephalus is caused by adhesions or mechanical obstructions in or adjacent to the ventricular system; causes include subarachnoid hemorrhage and infection

▶ Venous outflow has a role in determining ICP

• The two major outflow vessels for venous cerebral blood are the internal jugular veins and the basal cerebral veins

• ICP can be increased if these outflow tracts are impeded, which can result from

— Placing the head of the bed in a flat position

— Rotating the head to one side or neck flexion

— Engaging in any activity that increases intra-abdominal or intrathoracic pressure, such as the Valsalva maneuver, coughing, suctioning, use of positive end-expiratory pressure during mechanical ventilation, and positioning the patient in the prone position or with hips flexed more than 90 degrees

▶ Compliance is a measure of adaptive capacity of the brain and is the term used to describe the mechanisms that maintain fairly constant ICP in the face of increased volume (normal range is 0 to 15 mm Hg, ideally 10 mm Hg)

• Compliance mechanisms include

— Relocation of CSF from the intracranial cavity to the spinal space

— Constriction of cerebral blood vessels to decrease circulating blood volume

— Decreased production or increased reabsorption of CSF

— Expansion of the skull to accommodate increased volume (in children whose cranial sutures have not yet fused)

• Compliance is effective only to a certain degree; compliance is most effective when volume increases slowly, allowing compensatory mechanisms time to adjust

• Once compliance mechanisms reach their limit of effectiveness, small increases in volume result in significant increases in ICP

▶ Cerebral perfusion pressure (CPP) is a measure of the pressure gradient between the systemic mean arterial pressure (MAP) and the opposing ICP

• CPP is a measure of the ability to sufficiently perfuse cerebral tissues; it's calculated as follows: CPP = MAP − ICP

• Normal CPP is 80 to 100 mm Hg; a CPP of at least 60 mm Hg is necessary to sustain cerebral tissues

• Autoregulation fails with a CPP of 40 mm Hg or less, and irreversible hypoxic states occur when the CPP is 30 mm Hg or less

▶ Decompensation occurs when a patient can no longer compensate for changes in MAP or ICP; there are four stages of compensation-decompensation

- Stage I: intracranial volume increases without a concomitant increase in ICP as a result of active compliance mechanisms; no changes are evident in vital signs or LOC; compensation is present
- Stage II: intracranial volume increases with a concomitant increase in ICP; compliance mechanisms are reaching end-stage effectiveness, and slight changes in vital signs, LOC, and motor functions may be evident; compensation is beginning to fail
- Stage III: ICP approaches arterial blood pressure, and compliance methods are no longer effective; Cushing's triad and decreased LOC are present; decompensation begins
- Stage IV: autoregulation fails; cerebral blood flow (CBF) is greatly decreased or absent; decompensation is present, and death results if the condition isn't immediately reversed

■ Blood-brain barrier
  ◆ The existence of the blood-brain barrier is based on the theory of "tight junctions" among the capillary endothelium cells of the brain
  ◆ The blood-brain barrier protects delicate neurons by keeping out certain substances by means of selective permeability
    ▶ The blood-brain barrier is easily permeable to oxygen, water, glucose, and carbon dioxide; ions and other substances are taken up more slowly
    ▶ The homeostatic environment of the neurons is maintained by metabolic levels and ionic composition of tissue and fluids
  ◆ The blood-brain barrier can be altered by trauma, induction of some toxic elements, intracranial tumor, and brain irradiation

■ Circulatory system of the CNS
  ◆ Approximately 80% of the blood flow to the CNS is supplied by the carotid arteries and 20% by the vertebral arteries; blood returns by way of the venous system
  ◆ The external carotid artery supplies blood to the scalp, face, skull, and middle meningeal artery; laceration of the middle meningeal artery, which lies between the dura and the skull, causes an epidural hematoma
  ◆ The internal carotid artery proceeds up through the base of the skull, where it connects to the anterior aspect of the circle of Willis, a ring of anastomotic vessels
    ▶ Immediately before connecting to the circle of Willis, the internal carotid artery branches into the ophthalmic artery
    ▶ The ophthalmic artery supplies blood to the optic nerves and eyes
  ◆ The two vertebral arteries travel posteriorly after branching from the subclavian arteries, proceeding upward through the cervical spine, where they enter the skull through the foramen magnum
    ▶ The vertebral arteries come together at the level of the posterior rim of the pons to form the basilar artery
    ▶ The basilar artery supplies blood to the brain stem and the cerebellum before branching into paired posterior cerebral arteries (that form the posterior portion of the circle of Willis)
    ▶ The circle of Willis consists of an anterior communicating artery, paired posterior communicating arteries, and paired anterior, posterior, and middle cerebral arteries

- The anterior cerebral arteries supply blood to the medial surfaces of the frontal and parietal lobes
  - The middle cerebral arteries supply blood to the surface of the frontal, parietal, and temporal lobes; basal ganglia; internal capsule; and thalamic nuclei
  - The posterior communicating arteries supply blood to the medial and inferior aspects of the occipital lobes and the medial and lateral aspects of the temporal lobe
- ◆ The venules move venous blood from the capillaries to the paired cerebral veins
  - ▶ The venous sinuses, established through the cranium, drain venous blood from the cerebral veins
  - ▶ The venous blood then returns to the heart through the internal jugular veins
- ◆ The resistance of the cerebral arterioles is regulated by the vascular system to produce a constant flow, regardless of the systemic arterial pressure
  - ▶ The mechanism that produces this constant flow during changes in CPP is called autoregulation
  - ▶ When the systemic MAP falls below 50 mm Hg or rises above 150 mm Hg, autoregulation fails and the CBF mirrors systemic pressures; hypotension may cause cerebral ischemia
  - ▶ CBF varies with changes in CPP and diameter of the cerebrovascular bed; CPP = MAP – ICP (Normal values: MAP, 80 to 100 mm Hg; ICP, 5 to 10 mm Hg; and CPP, 70 to 95 mm Hg)
- ◆ Arterial blood gases (ABGs) have strong vasoactive properties
  - ▶ Hypercapnia (high carbon dioxide content) causes vasodilation, which increases circulating cerebral blood volume and, in turn, raises ICP
  - ▶ Hypocapnia (low carbon dioxide content) causes vasoconstriction, which decreases circulating blood volume
    - Induced hypocapnia, such as in hyperventilation, causes cerebral vasoconstriction and is an effective method of decreasing ICP
    - Prolonged hypocapnia (characterized by partial pressure of arterial carbon dioxide [$Paco_2$] less than 20 mm Hg) produces cerebral ischemia
  - ▶ Hypoxemia (characterized by low partial pressure of arterial oxygen [Pao_2]) causes vasodilation, which increases CBF and, in turn, raises ICP; Pao_2 less than 50 mm Hg exposes the brain to ischemia due to low circulating Pao_2 and increased ICP
- ■ Spinal cord
  - ◆ The spinal cord extends from the brain stem at the level of the foramen magnum to the level of the first or second lumbar vertebra, where it tapers and forms the conus medullaris
  - ◆ At the level of the conus medullaris, 31 pairs of nerve roots—known as the cauda equina (horse's tail)—exit from the spinal cord and travel down the intervertebral foramen

◆ Bony support for the vertebral column is provided by 33 vertebrae: 7 cervical (C1 through C7), 12 thoracic (T1 through T12), 5 lumbar (L1 through L5), 5 sacral (S1 through S5), and 4 coccygeal

◆ Twenty-four intervertebral disks provide flexible support for the spinal cord

◆ The spinal cord contains 31 pairs of spinal nerves: 8 cervical, 12 thoracic, 5 lumbar, 5 sacral, and 1 coccygeal

▶ The first 7 pairs of cervical nerves exit above the similarly numbered cervical vertebrae

▶ The eighth cervical nerve pair exits below the seventh cervical vertebra and above the first thoracic vertebra (there is no eighth cervical vertebra)

▶ Each vertebral nerve pair after the eighth one exits below the similarly numbered vertebra

◆ A horizontal cross section of the spinal cord shows a central core of gray matter in the shape of an H, surrounded by myelinated white matter

▶ The white matter of the spinal cord contains ascending and descending tracts that conduct impulses to and from the brain; these tracts are labeled with names that identify their origin and destination

● The prefix identifies the tract's origin in the spinal tract, and the suffix identifies its destination

● The prefix *spino* denotes an ascending sensory tract; for example, the spinothalamic tracts are ascending sensory tracts that conduct impulses upward to the thalamus

● The suffix *spinal* denotes a descending motor tract; for example, the corticospinal tracts are descending motor tracts that originate in the cortex

▶ Each projection of the gray matter (the "H") forms an anterior (ventral) or posterior (dorsal) horn for the left and right sides of the spinal cord

● The anterior horns contain motor cells

● The posterior horns contain axons from the peripheral sensory neurons

● Lateral horns arising at the level of T1 to L2 contain sympathetic fibers, and those of S2 to S4 contain parasympathetic fibers of the ANS

■ Nervous system cellular functions

◆ The neuron is the basic structural unit of the nervous system

◆ Neurons consist of a cell body, dendrites, and an axon

▶ The cell bodies form the gray matter of the brain, brain stem, and spinal cord; ganglia are cell bodies in the peripheral nervous system that lie close to the CNS

● The cell body contains the nucleus which stores deoxyribonucleic acid (DNA) and ribonucleic acid (RNA) and synthesizes RNA

● The cell body also contains the Golgi apparatus, which stores protein, lysosome-intracellular scavengers, and structures that synthesize cell membrane

- Nissl bodies within the cell body store RNA and synthesize protein
▶ Dendrites are short fibers that branch outward from the cell body
- Dendrites receive stimuli moving toward the cell body
- Each cell body may contain several dendrites
▶ Axons are fibers that branch outward from the cell body in varying lengths; some are several feet long
- Axons transmit stimuli away from the cell body
- Each cell body contains only one axon
- Some axons are covered by a protein-lipid complex known as a myelin sheath
  - The myelin sheath is produced by Schwann cells in the peripheral nervous system and by oligodendroglia in the CNS
  - The sheath isn't a continuous covering but is broken at intervals by nodes of Ranvier
  - The sheath acts as an insulator for the conduction of nerve impulses, allowing for efficient conduction of nerve impulses from one node of Ranvier to the next
  - Demyelinization of the sheath disrupts conduction of nerve impulses away from the neuron, as seen in degenerative diseases such as multiple sclerosis
◆ Neuroglial cells protect, structurally support, and nourish neurons
▶ Unlike neurons, neuroglial cells retain mitotic function; this may cause CNS neoplasms
▶ Four types of neuroglial cells exist
- Astrocyte cells help form the blood-brain barrier
- Ependymal cells are found in the choroid plexus of the ventricular system
- Microglial cells are phagocytic cells found in white matter
- Oligodendroglial cells make up the myelin sheath for axons in the CNS
◆ A nerve impulse can be defined as a physiochemical change in the nerve fibers, which is self-propagating when initiated
▶ Transmission of nerve impulses in neurons begins with depolarization of the cell membrane
▶ Depolarization begins with an impulse from another cell in the form of a chemical stimulus
▶ The chemical stimulus triggers the release of neurotransmitters from the bouton terminal (or presynaptic terminal) at the end of the axon; the impulse then crosses the synaptic cleft to reach the postsynaptic membrane of another nerve cell's dendrite (or cell body)
▶ The speed of nerve impulse transmission depends on the nerve's degree of myelinization (or lack thereof)
- In unmyelinated nerve cells, the impulse must travel the length of the nerve fiber
- In myelinated nerve cells, the impulse travels faster by jumping from one node of Ranvier to the next
  - The velocity of transmission of the nerve impulse in myelinated nerves increases because less energy is expended

– The conduction of nerve impulse from node to node is known as saltatory conduction

◆ Neurotransmitters are classified as excitatory or inhibitory

▶ Excitatory neurotransmitters foster the transmission of a nerve impulse across the synaptic cleft

▶ Inhibitory neurotransmitters chemically block or slow the transmission of a nerve impulse by increasing the negativity of the cell, thus increasing the cell's resistance to depolarization

◆ Impairment of the synaptic pathway causes increased transmission of some impulses and faulty, or no transmission, of others

▶ Myasthenia gravis, a disease characterized by weakness and rapid exhaustion of skeletal muscles after exertion, is caused by diminished receptors for the neurotransmitter acetylcholine on the postsynaptic membrane

▶ Parkinsonism, a disease characterized by tremors, rigidity, and fragmentary or incomplete voluntary movements, is caused by a deficiency of dopamine in the basal ganglia, resulting in unsuppressed activity of excitatory neurotransmitters

❖ Neurologic assessment

■ Description

◆ A neurologic assessment consists of key components that are meaningful only if evaluated together

▶ LOC

▶ Motor function

▶ Pupil and eye signs

▶ Vital signs

▶ Comprehensive history of events prior to hospitilization

◆ Another component, often of clinical significance, is the medical history of the patient and family; these may indicate further testing

■ LOC

◆ The two principal elements in assessing LOC are alertness and awareness

▶ Assessment of alertness is an evaluation of the reticular activating system and its link to the thalamus and cerebral cortex

▶ Assessment of awareness is an evaluation of the patient's orientation to person, place, and time; awareness requires a higher level of brain function than alertness

◆ Changes in LOC are generally subtle but frequently the first signs of neurologic deterioration

◆ The Glasgow Coma Scale (GCS) is the tool most commonly used to assess LOC

▶ On this scale, a score of 15 is best, 3 is the lowest, and 7 or below denotes coma; however, more important than a particular score is recognition of subtle changes from an individual's baseline LOC in a series of scores over time

▶ The GCS assesses LOC only; it can't be used to rate motor deficits of one side of the body in comparison with the other, pupillary changes and comparisons, or aphasia

Glasgow Coma Scale

The Glasgow Coma Scale provides an easy way to describe the patient's baseline mental status and to help detect and interpret changes from baseline findings. The ability to respond to verbal, motor, and sensory stimulation is assessed, with findings graded by the scale. If the patient is alert, can follow simple commands, and is oriented to person, place, and time, his score will total 15 points. A decreased score in one or more categories may signal an impending neurologic crisis. A total score of 7 or less indicates severe neurologic damage.

Characteristic	Response	Score
Eye opening response	● Spontaneous	4
	● To verbal command	3
	● To pain	2
	● No response	1
Best motor response	● Obeys commands	6
	● To painful stimuli	
	– Localizes pain; pushes stimulus away	5
	– Flexes and withdraws	4
	– Abnormal flexion	3
	– Extension	2
	– No response	1
Best verbal response (Arouse patient with painful stimuli, if necessary)	● Oriented and converses	5
	● Disoriented and converses	4
	● Uses inappropriate words	3
	● Makes incomprehensible sounds	2
	● No response	1
		Total: 3 to 15

▶ The scale doesn't clearly differentiate between extremities, so lateralizing signs that may be of primary and emergent importance aren't accounted for

▶ The scale also doesn't reflect the quality of the auditory commands given by the rater

   ● Commands should be simple, clear, and given in the absence of other verbal or tactile stimuli; this avoids misinterpretation of reflexes as responses to the commands

   ● A command frequently used but open to misinterpretation is the request that a patient clasp and release his hands; to avoid random reflex responses, a more appropriate command is to ask the patient to show a particular finger or thumb or to turn his palms up or down

   ● In patients who are unable to follow commands, the rater often must use noxious stimuli to assess motor function

     – Examples of acceptable noxious stimuli are pressure applied to the patient's nail bed with a hard, dull object (such as a pen), pinching the trapezius muscle, firmly patting the sternal area, and pinching the sensitive inner aspect of the thigh or arm (see *Glasgow Coma Scale*)

Cranial nerves and their functions

Each cranial nerve has one or more specific functions. These functions can be described as motor or sensory; some cranial nerves have both. The chart below details the location of each cranial nerve as well as its function.

Cranial nerve	Location	Function	Assessment
I. Olfactory	Diencephalon (olfactory tract), with interpretation in temporal lobe	Smell	Test smell sense with different strong odors; test each nostril separately
II. Optic	Diencephalon (optic chiasm), with interpretation in occipital lobe	Sight	Tested indirectly by pupillary light reflexes, Snellen chart
III. Oculomotor	Midbrain	Movement of eye, movement of eyelids, and pupillary constriction	Direct light reflex (brisk, sluggish, nonreactive); moves eyes up and down; consensual light reflex (present, absent); moves eyes to noxious stimuli; observe shape of pupil
IV. Trochlear	Midbrain	Movement of eyes	Observe movement of eyes in all directions
V. Trigeminal	Pons	Facial sensations and mastication	Corneal reflex; apply pressure to supraorbital ridge, and observe for grimacing
VI. Abducens	Pons	Movement of eyes	Move eyes up and down; move eyes to noxious stimuli
VII. Facial	Medulla and caudal pons	Taste, facial expression, and secretion of saliva and tears	Observe patient raise eyebrows, smile, frown; assess strength against resistance; taste test
VIII. Acoustic	Medulla, with interpretation in temporal lobe	Hearing and balance	Ocucephalic reflex (doll's eyes); oculovestibular reflex (caloric irrigation); test hearing acuity; Weber and Rinne tests
IX. Glossopharyngeal	Medulla, with interpretation of taste in temporal lobe	Taste, swallowing, gag reflex, secretion of saliva, and phonation	Gag reflex; speech; swallowing; hoarseness; carotid sinus reflex; observe palatine arch while patient says "ah"
X. Vagus	Medulla	Pain and temperature sensations near the ears; gag reflex, coughing, swallowing; and visceral sensations from the abdomen and thorax	Same as glossopharyngeal
XI. Spinal accessory	Medulla and C1 to C5	Movement of head and shoulders	Observe movements of head and shoulders; inspection of size and symmetry; test strength
XII. Hypoglossal	Medulla	Movement of tongue	Observe tongue protrusion; check alignment and strength

Remembering cranial nerve functions

Use the two mnemonic phrases below to recall the cranial nerves and their motor, sensory, or mixed functions. Read each phrase vertically: the first letter of each word in the phrase corresponds to the name of the cranial nerve or its function.

Cranial nerve	Mnemonic for name	Mnemonic for function
I. Olfactory	On	Some (sensory)
II. Optic	Old	Say (sensory)
III. Oculomotor	Olympus'	Marry (motor)
IV. Trochlear	Towering	Money (motor)
V. Trigeminal	Tops	But (both)
VI. Abducens	A	My (motor)
VII. Facial	Finn	Brother (both)
VIII. Acoustic	And	Says (sensory)
IX. Glossopharyngeal	German	Bad (both)
X. Vagus	Viewed	Business (both)
XI. Spinal accessory	Some	Marry (motor)
XII. Hypoglossal	Hops	Money (motor)

    — Examples of unacceptable noxious stimuli are applying pressure to the supraorbital area, rubbing the sternal area with the knuckles, and pinching the nipples, breasts, groin, or testicles

■ Motor function

    ◆ The assessment of motor function includes evaluation of motor tone, strength, posturing, and the ability to follow commands appropriately

    ◆ Observe size and contours of muscles; palpate muscles; then test strength, tone, and reflexes (stretch and superficial)

    ◆ Coordinated motor function requires an intact motor cortex, basal ganglia, and descending motor pathways (including the corticospinal tract, extrapyramidal tract, cerebellum, lower motor neurons, neuromuscular junctions, and skeletal muscle)

    ◆ Because the bulk of corticospinal neurons decussate in the medulla, motor impairment on one side of the body reflects deficits in the ipsilateral side of the brain

    ◆ Assessment of the 12 pairs of cranial nerves can help in identifying the area of injury in a neurologically impaired patient (see *Cranial nerves and their functions*); the cranial nerves have motor (III, IV, VI, XI, and XII), sensory (I, II, and VIII), or mixed (V, VII, IX, X) functions (see *Remembering cranial nerve functions*)

◆ The Romberg test can be used to evaluate cerebellar intactness, balance, and proprioception; in this test, the patient stands with his feet together, closes his eyes, and would normally be able to remain erect; abnormal responses to the test are significant swaying from side to side or falls. To test for proprioception, the examiner pulls the patient's big toe up or down with the patient's eyes closed; the patient should be able to tell which direction his toe is pointing without looking

◆ Assessment of Babinski's reflex determines intactness of corticospinal tract

   ▶ This test involves stroking the lateral part of the sole and ball of the foot

   ▶ A normal adult response is plantar flexion, an abnormal response is dorsiflexion of the big toe (normal in infants)

◆ Meningeal irritation can cause muscle spasm or abnormal posturing

   ▶ Nuchal rigidity describes the involuntary muscle spasm that prevents a patient from putting chin to chest

   ▶ Opisthotonos is an extreme spasm of the spinal muscles, causing drastic extension of the spine; it's also seen in tetanus and decerebrate posturing

   ▶ A positive Kernig's sign is resistance to extension, and pain, as the leg is flexed at a 90-degree angle (if the thigh is already flexed at a 90-degree angle to the hip); this sign may be seen with tumors of the cauda equina, herniated disks, and meningeal irritation

   ▶ Brudzinski's sign is an involuntary flexion of the hip and knees produced by flexion of the neck; it indicates meningeal irritation

   ▶ Abnormal posturing includes flexor spasm and extensor spasm

   • Decorticate posturing manifests as abnormal flexion and internal rotation in the upper extremities, with accompanying extension of the lower extremities; it indicates an interruption in a corticospinal pathway by a lesion in the cerebral hemisphere, basal ganglia, or diencephalon

   • Decerebrate posturing manifests as abnormal extension (adduction and hyperpronation) of the upper extremities and the lower extremities; it indicates injury to the brain stem

   • Sensory function is tested using bilateral dermatomes; spinothalamic tracts may be tested with light touch, pain, and temperature; deep sensory modalities of the posterior columns (fasciculus gracilis and fasciculus cuneatus) may be tested with vibration and proprioception; cortical discrimination tests determine the patient's discrimination of objects

■ Pupil and eye signs

◆ Assessment of pupil size, shape, equality, and degree of response to light stimuli is valuable, primarily because it may delineate the path of innervation from the ANS

   ▶ Sympathetic innervation of the pupil starts in the hypothalamus and runs the length of the brain stem

   • Intact sympathetic stimulation causes pupillary dilation; pupils are normally equally round and reactive to light and accommodation

- Disrupted sympathetic control manifests as pinpoint, nonreactive pupils; causes include conditions with pathologic brain stem involvement or lesions of the pons that interrupt sympathetic pathways before they enter the brain stem
▶ The parasympathetic response is controlled by the oculomotor nerve (cranial nerve III), which exits the brain stem at the level of the midbrain and tentorial notch
  - Intact parasympathetic stimulation causes pupillary constriction
  - Disrupted parasympathetic control, which occurs when increased ICP compresses the oculomotor nerve against the tentorial notch, results in dilated, nonreactive pupils absent of consensual response
    − A unilaterally dilated pupil, absent of light response, in a patient at risk for increasing ICP signifies possible brain herniation
    − Patients who have undergone cardiopulmonary resuscitation (CPR) may show anoxic pupillary dilation, which carries a grave prognosis if it lasts more than a few minutes; however, patients who receive mydriatic agents (for example, atropine) during CPR may have dilated pupils from the medication and don't necessarily have a poor prognosis
◆ Pupil reactivity may be the most important clinical sign in the differentiation of metabolic coma from structural injury coma; in the presence of metabolic disturbances, pupil reactivity remains relatively intact
  ▶ Pupils should always be assessed relative to baseline or previous assessments and relative to each other
  ▶ Pupil reactivity and size can be affected by medications and previous injuries or surgery to the eye; the patient's medication and medical history should be considered before inferences are made from pupillary signs
◆ The function of three cranial nerves—the oculomotor (III), trochlear (IV), and abducens (VI)—can be assessed by evaluating the ability of an eye to move through the six points of the cardinal fields of gaze
  ▶ This assessment can be performed only if the patient is alert and cooperative
  ▶ Unconscious patients can be assessed for intactness of cranial nerve function by evaluating the oculocephalic (doll's eyes) reflex and the oculovestibular reflex; these reflexes are used to assess the intactness of cranial nerves III through VIII and reflect brain stem integrity; tests of these reflexes shouldn't be performed on a conscious patient
    - In the oculocephalic reflex, the nurse holds the patient's eyelids open while briskly turning the head to one side; this test shouldn't be performed if a cervical injury is suspected
      − If the reflex is intact, the eyes move in the direction away from which the head is turned (doll's eyes are present); this normal reflex indicates intact brain stem function
      − If the eyes drift in an irregular manner or move in opposite directions when the head is turned (doll's eyes are abnormal), the patient has some degree of brain stem impairment

– If the eyes move with the head as it's turned and maintain the same position as though fixed in place (doll's eyes are absent), significant brain stem impairment has occurred
- In the oculovestibular reflex, 20 to 50 ml of cold water is instilled into the external auditory canal with a large-bore syringe
  – The normal response is nystagmus with movement toward the ear into which the water was instilled, indicating intact brain stem function
  – Movement away from the stimulated ear is an abnormal response, indicating some brain stem impairment
  – No movement in any direction is an absent reflex, indicating significant brain stem injury

■ Vital signs
  ◆ Changes in vital signs, like changes in pupillary response, are late signs of neurologic deterioration compared with changes in the LOC
  ◆ In a neurologically injured patient, vital signs may reflect changes in autoregulation; for example, intracranial injury often results in loss of cerebral autoregulation
  ◆ Autoregulation is a compensatory mechanism whereby the cerebral vessels constrict or enlarge in response to increasing or decreasing arterial pressure
    ▶ When autoregulation fails, the cerebral vessels relax and allow the volume in the cerebral tissues to mirror the systemic arterial pressure
      • In the face of failed autoregulation, increased systemic arterial pressure increases blood flow to the brain
      • Increased blood flow to the brain increases volume in the cranial vault, resulting in increased ICP
    ▶ In the brain stem, the center for regulation of blood pressure loses its ability for autoregulation when injury to the brain increases ICP and causes medullary hypoxia
      • As a result, arterial pressure increases in an attempt to raise oxygenation by means of increased perfusion
      • Increased perfusion results in increased ICP, which produces parasympathetic stimulation of the lower brain stem with ensuing bradycardia
      • If left unchecked, this results in destruction of the medullary centers and causes signs of decompensation, hypotension, tachycardia, and respiratory arrest
  ◆ Cushing's triad consists of three clinically significant signs of decreased CPP and cerebral ischemia
    ▶ These signs are increased systolic blood pressure with widening pulse pressure, bradycardia, and irregular respiratory function
    ▶ In an attempt to increase cerebral perfusion, the heart rate slows; this in turn increases the stroke volume and raises systolic blood pressure
  ◆ Temperature dysfunctions can arise from disruption of the sympathetic pathways between the hypothalamus and the peripheral vessels; these

can result from spinal cord injury or infection and cause a deleterious chain of effects

> ▶ Elevated temperature increases the metabolic rate
> ▶ An elevated metabolic rate causes increased levels of carbon dioxide
> ▶ Increased levels of carbon dioxide cause dilation of the cerebral vasculature
> ▶ Increased dilation leads to cerebral edema and elevated ICP

◆ Respiratory patterns are closely associated with, and should be assessed in conjunction with, clinical assessment of vital signs and LOC

> ▶ Cheyne-Stokes respirations are characterized by periodic waxing and waning of respiratory excursion, with alternating periods of apnea and hyperpnea; they usually result from upper brain stem lesions
> ▶ Central neurogenic hyperventilation may be caused by middle brain stem lesions; this respiratory pattern is characterized by sustained, deep, rapid hyperpnea with resultant hypocapnia; ABG values show elevated PaO_2, elevated pH, and decreased $PaCO_2$
> ▶ A protracted peak inspiration pattern is characteristic of apneustic breathing; in the absence of unopposing stimuli from the pneumotaxic center (which normally limits the rate of inspiration), the apneustic center continues unchecked, resulting in this respiratory pattern
> ▶ Cluster breathing, characterized by irregular clusters of breaths followed by irregular pauses, indicates lower brain stem herniation
> ▶ Ataxic breathing, or Biot's respirations, may result from medullary lesions or rapid cerebellar or pontine hemorrhage; this respiratory pattern is characterized by an irregular rate and depth of respirations, accompanied by irregular periods of apnea
> ▶ Kussmaul's respirations, characterized by slow, deep, and labored breathing, are a sign of metabolic acidosis—not neurologic dysfunction

❖ **Diagnostic tests**
■ Noninvasive diagnostic tests

◆ Computed tomography (CT) scans can be used to assess hydrocephalus, infarction, tumors, atrophy, abscess, and cerebral swelling; when used with contrast media (making the scan an invasive test), CT provides greater visualization of cerebral vasculature and thus can help identify congenital malformations and aneurysms; CT scans are also used to evaluate the spine (myelography)

> ▶ Skull radiograph may be used in diagnosing fractures and skull abnormalities, but these have been replaced with skull series CTs
> ▶ Spine series X-ray may be used to diagnose fractures, dislocations, or degenerative abnormalities; a CT may be used as an adjunct to further delineate abnormalities

◆ Magnetic resonance imaging (MRI) is used to evaluate cerebral edema, infection, bone lesions, infarction, and blood vessels by providing views not seen on a CT scan

◆ An EEG monitors brain wave activity through electrodes placed on the scalp

▶ The EEG is useful for determining the focus of seizure activity or cause of coma and can indicate an area of lesions

▶ The EEG may be used in determining brain death or to monitor patients in barbiturate comas

◆ Evoked potentials are another diagnostic tool using surface electrodes; patient response to visual, auditory, and tactile stimulation is measured along a specific neuronal pathway and graphically depicted using computer analysis

▶ Visual responses aid in the evaluation of posttraumatic injury

▶ Auditory responses help in the evaluation of brain stem function, multiple sclerosis, auditory lesions, and coma

▶ Tactile responses are useful in the evaluation of peripheral nerve disease and lesions of the brain and spinal cord involving demyelinated neurons

◆ Electromyography (EMG) is a useful diagnostic tool for muscular dystrophies, myasthenia gravis, amyotrophic lateral sclerosis, and peripheral nerve dysfunctions; through electrical stimulation of specific muscle groups, EMG can help differentiate neuromuscular junction disease from lower motor neuron disease

◆ Nerve conduction velocity may be used in the diagnosis of peripheral neuropathies and nerve conduction (with the use of needle electrodes)

■ Invasive diagnostic tests

◆ Digital subtraction angiography uses computerized fluoroscopy to visualize cerebral vessels and carotid blood flow

▶ After a baseline scan is made, contrast dye is injected, and a second scan is done; the computer then "subtracts" the first scan from the second, providing greater definition of the targeted vasculature

▶ As with CT scans that require contrast media, angiographic contrast dye is hypertonic and may temporarily reduce cerebral edema; however, in the absence of actions to correct the condition's cause, cerebral edema will return

▶ Magnetic resonance angiography (MRA) helps depict flow relationship in vessels and identify abnormalities

◆ Cerebral angiography is used to diagnose malformations of the cerebral vasculature; it requires injection of radiopaque dye into the cerebral circulation

▶ Cerebral angiography may indicate tumors, if vessel displacement is observed, or may identify arteriovenous malformations (AVMs) and aneurysms

▶ It's also used to diagnose vessel thrombosis, arterial spasm, cerebral edema, and herniation

◆ Positron emission tomography (PET) measures tissue uptake of a radionuclide that's inhaled or administered I.V.

▶ PET assesses tissue metabolism and CBF

▶ Uptake of the isotope by different regions of the brain may reveal hemorrhage, infarction, abscess, or tumor

◆ Brain scans involve use of an I.V. radionuclide and measurement of its uptake by the brain; areas of greater uptake indicate disturbances in the blood-brain barrier, such as in contusions, tumors, hemorrhage, infarction, and abscess

◆ Lumbar puncture requires the insertion of a hollow needle into the subarachnoid space of the spine, generally at the L4 or L5 level; this test is usually performed to obtain CSF samples, measure CSF pressure, administer medications, or to prepare the patient for other diagnostic studies (such as myelography)

  ❯ During the lumbar puncture, CSF pressure is measured (normal pressure is 50 to 200 cm H_2O), and samples of CSF are taken and evaluated for the presence of blood cells, protein, glucose, electrolytes, and microorganisms

  ❯ Lumbar puncture is contraindicated in patients with increased ICP resulting from space-occupying lesions of the brain or acute head trauma

    • In these patients, the release of pressure in the subarachnoid space below the brain may force the brain to herniate through the foramen magnum

    • Cisternal puncture is an alternate method of obtaining access; complications include injury of the brain stem, shock, hemorrhage, and infection

◆ CBF and metabolism abnormalities may be assessed by transcranial Doppler study, xenon isotope inhalation, stable xenon CT, single photon emission tomography, PET, and jugular venous oxygen saturation

◆ ICP can be monitored using one of several methods

  ❯ In the intraventricular method, a catheter is inserted into the anterior or occipital horns of the lateral ventricle; a three-way stopcock, attached to the catheter, permits ICP monitoring by a pressure transducer and drainage of CSF

    • Advantages of this method are that it allows direct measurement of ICP and instillation of medication or contrast media to visualize the size and patency of the ventricular system

    • Disadvantages include risk of infection, hemorrhage, CSF loss, difficulty inserting the catheter into collapsed ventricles, midline shifting, and marked cerebral edema

  ❯ In the intraparenchymal method, a fiber-optic–tipped probe is inserted through a twist drill hole into the skull and placed into the parenchyma of the brain; the probe is connected to a monitor providing a readout; it can also be attached to a standard pressure monitor to see waveforms

    • An advantage of this method is easy placement, independent of ventricular size or position

    • Disadvantages include inability to re-zero once placed and fragility of the fiber-optic probe, which can break, bend, or become dislodged

  ❯ A subarachnoid screw—a screw with a hollow core—is inserted into the subarachnoid space by means of a burr hole, usually over the frontal lobe area; a three-way stopcock attached to the screw allows ICP monitoring by pressure transducer and CSF drainage

- Advantages of this method are that it permits direct measurement of ICP, the screw is easy to insert, and the infection rate is lower than in ventricular monitoring
- Disadvantages include risk of infection, possibility of inaccurate measurements if the screw lumen becomes occluded, and requirement of a firm skull (this method usually can't be used on patients under age 6); the screw is also more easily dislodged than a catheter

▶ In the epidural sensor method, a fiber-optic sensing device is inserted through a burr hole into the space between the skull and the dura and the sensor membrane placed against the dura

- Advantages of this method are that it's less invasive than other methods, and the device is easy to insert
- Disadvantages include lack of a route for CSF drainage and questionable accuracy, as readings are higher than those obtained by other methods (inaccurate readings may result if the dura is compressed or thickened, or with increased surface tension)

▶ Somewhat similar to an arterial hemodynamic waveform, a normal ICP waveform has a sharp upward slope, followed by a more gradual downward slope with a dicrotic notch; an abnormal ICP waveform may be one of three types (See *Interpreting ICP waveforms*)

- A waves
- B waves
- C waves

■ Key laboratory values
   ◆ The laboratory tests with the most clinical significance in a patient with neurologic problems are ABG analysis, CSF analysis, and toxicology (alcohol and drug screens)
   ◆ Other laboratory tests, such as complete blood count (CBC), chemistries (including osmolality), electrolytes, clotting profile (prothrombin time, partial thromboplastin time, D-dimer, fibrinogen), and urinalysis are used to rule out other diseases that may produce neurologic symptoms

❖ Nursing care common to all neurologic disorders
   ■ Assessment of changes in neurologic status
      ◆ Check for alterations in LOC
      ◆ Check pupillary and eye signs
      ◆ Monitor vital signs, including quality of respirations and heart rhythm
      ◆ Assess motor and sensory abilities
      ◆ Assess cranial nerve status
   ■ Maintenance of adequate ventilatory status
      ◆ Maintain airway; suction as necessary to keep airway patent
      ◆ Prevent aspiration
      ◆ Treat hypoxemia
   ■ Maintenance of adequate cerebral perfusion
      ◆ Maintain adequate blood pressure
      ◆ Maintain adequate heart rate
      ◆ Treat hypovolemia, hypervolemia, hypoxemia

Interpreting ICP waveforms

Three waveforms—A, B, and C—are used to monitor intracranial pressure (ICP). A waves are an ominous sign of intracranial decompensation and poor compliance, B waves correlate with changes in respiration, and C waves correlate with changes in arterial pressure.

Normal waveform
- Steep upward systolic slope followed by a downward diastolic slope with a dicrotic notch.
- This waveform is continuous and indicates an ICP between 0 and 15 mm Hg (normal pressure).

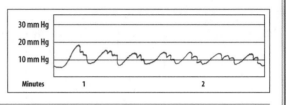

A waves
- Reach elevations of 50 to 100 mm Hg, persist for 5 to 20 minutes, then drop sharply, signaling exhaustion of the brain's compliance mechanisms.
- A waves signify a reduction in cerebral perfusion pressure with ensuring hypoxia and decompensation.
- Ominous sign and require emergency treatment.

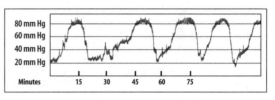

B waves
- Sharp and rhythmic with a sawtooth pattern, occur every 1½ to 2 minutes and may reach elevation of 50 mm Hg.
- The clinical significance of B waves isn't clear; however, the waves correlate with respiratory changes and may occur more frequently with decreasing compensation.

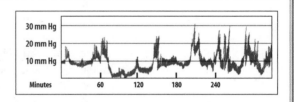

C waves
- Rapid and rhythmic but not sharp and last 1 to 2 minutes with an ICP of 20 to 50 mm Hg.
- Clinically insignificant and may fluctuate with respirations or systemic blood pressure changes.

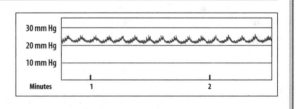

♦ Institute measures to keep CPP within the normal range (ICP for monitoring and draining, barbiturate coma, chemical paralysis and hyperventilation with ventilator, medications such as mannitol to reduce ICP)
♦ Avoid factors that can increase ICP (see *Factors that increase ICP*, page 186)
■ Prevention of complications associated with decreased mobility
♦ Maintain patent airway with suctioning, percussion, and positioning
♦ Position the patient to prevent aspiration
♦ Turn the patient frequently, and use special mattresses to prevent pressure ulcers from developing over bony prominences
♦ Maintain adequate nutrition and hydration without fluid overload

---

Factors that increase ICP

Decreasing venous return from the brain
- Increased intrathoracic pressure
    - Positive pressure mechanical ventilation
    - Positive end-expiratory pressure
    - Valsalva maneuver
- Neck flexion, hyperextension, or rotation
- Tracheostomy ties or cervical collar that are too tight

Increased metabolic rate
- Increased body temperature
- Seizures

Positioning
- Prone
- Trendelenburg
- Hip flexion > 90 degrees

Stress
- Bright lights
- Noise
- Noxious stimuli
- Pain
- Upsetting conversations

Ventilation or oxygenation problems
- Deep breathing
- Hypercapnia
- Hypoxia
- Obstructed airway
- Suctioning

- ◆ Minimize risk of infection
- ◆ Maintain joint range of motion
- ◆ Assess for phlebitis
- ■ Maintenance of normal temperature
    - ◆ Use thermic blankets and continuous monitoring
    - ◆ Investigate the cause of temperature elevations
- ■ Education of patient and family members
    - ◆ Orient the patient and family members to the environment and routine of care
    - ◆ Communicate calmly and clearly
    - ◆ Explain procedures before they're implemented
    - ◆ Explain the reasons for interventions

❖ **Encephalopathy**
- ■ Description
    - ◆ Neurologic degeneration that results from buildup of toxic metabolic products, structural changes in the brain, changes in blood flow to the brain, changes in the electrical activity of the brain, changes in the supply or utilization of neurotransmitter substances, or other cellular changes that alter neurologic function
    - ◆ Not a disease in itself but the result of other systemic diseases or disorders of the brain; hypoxia, ischemia, metabolic changes, infectious diseases, and structural changes can all lead to encephalopathy
- ■ Clinical signs and symptoms
    - ◆ Signs and symptoms will vary widely (memory problems to behavioral disorders and depressed LOC), but the hallmark sign is altered mental state
    - ◆ Neurologic changes are consistent with cause of encephalopathy

◆ Family history, social history, and medical history can help determine findings
■ Diagnostic tests
◆ Laboratory tests, radiological findings, and MRI results will vary depending on the cause of the encephalopathy
■ Medical management
◆ Treatment varies according to type and severity of encephalopathy
◆ Treating the underlying cause
◆ Supportive treatment
■ Nursing management
◆ Nursing care will vary depending on the cause of the encephalopathy and medical treatment indicated
◆ Supportive treatment for oxygenation, circulation, nutrition, and metabolism as necessary
◆ Care determined by exact neurologic deficits

❖ Head trauma
■ Description
◆ Head trauma is caused by acceleration-deceleration, rotation, or missile injuries
▶ Acceleration-deceleration injuries occur when the skull strikes (or is struck by) an object
• The brain is carried by force of movement until it strikes the inside of the skull (coup injury)
• If the impact is strong enough, the force that hasn't yet dissipated pitches the brain in the reverse direction, where it strikes the opposite side of the skull (contrecoup injury)
▶ Rotation injuries, which occur in conjunction with acceleration-deceleration injuries, result in tearing or shearing of tissues
▶ Missile injuries are direct penetrating injuries such as those that occur from a bullet wound; the mortality rate is greater than 90% in the United States, and two-thirds of patients never reach the hospital
◆ Whatever the cause of injury, traumatic head injuries are classified according to the ensuing loss of function
▶ Concussions are the mildest form of brain injury and are characterized by brief loss of consciousness
• The patient experiences headache, dizziness, and possibly nausea and vomiting
• Postconcussion syndrome is common and may include memory problems, headache, dizziness, information processing problems, visual disturbances, coordination problems, and lethargy
▶ Contusions are closed head injuries that cause small, diffuse, venous hemorrhage (bruising); they usually occur in the frontal lobe; unconsciousness usually is prolonged with evident neurologic deficits
▶ Diffuse axonal injury is the result of white matter shearing, associated with disruption of axons and neuronal pathways in the hemispheres, diencephalon, and brain stem. It's believed that all head trauma involves changes consistent with diffuse axonal disruption; signs

may include presence of coma and profound neurologic, psychological, or personality defects; treatment is supportive

▶ Cerebral lacerations are tears in the brain tissue caused by shearing forces
  • Lacerations generally cause a greater amount of hemorrhage than contusions and may affect arterial and venous vessels
  • Lacerations tend to cause a deteriorating state unless the bleeding and increased ICP are treated promptly

▶ Intracranial hemorrhage occurs in one-third of severely head-injured patients, with the clinical course and outcome varying with the size and type of mass (see "Intracranial hemorrhage," pages 201 to 204)

◆ Trauma to the head can fracture the skull

▶ In a linear skull fracture, the skull is broken, but the bone isn't displaced; this type of fracture generally requires no treatment unless a concomitant injury to the cerebral vasculature has occurred

▶ In a depressed skull fracture, the skull is broken, and the bone is displaced downward toward the brain; this type of fracture usually requires surgical intervention to raise the bony fragments and repair any cerebral injury

▶ Focal neurologic deficits depend on the location and extent of cerebral involvement

▶ Scalp lacerations should be shaved, cleaned, and dressed, with surgery repair in 24 to 48 hours

▶ In a compound skull fracture, the break in the skull exposes the brain; if the dura has been lacerated, CSF may leak out
  • This type of fracture is associated with a high risk of infection and meningitis
  • Treatment involves the use of antibiotics, debridement of the wound, and subsequent closure of the skull

▶ In a basilar skull fracture, the skull is fractured at the base of the brain, and injury to the cervical spine is likely; the fracture is repaired surgically, and the neck is immobilized to prevent further damage to the area; Battle's sign (bruising behind the ears at the mastoid process), raccoon eyes (bruising around the eyes), otorrhea (CSF leaking from the ears), and rhinorrhea (CSF leaking from the nose) may be present as well as pneumocephalus resulting in meningitis or cranial nerve injuries

▶ In a comminuted skull fracture, the skull is splintered, and the bony fragments must be removed surgically

◆ Clinical signs and symptoms

▶ Severity of head injury is based on the LOC after resuscitation, based on the GCS

▶ Suspect head injury in patients who were in a motor vehicle crash or experienced other trauma to the head

▶ Mild head injury patients (GCS of 13 to 15) may have persistent complaints of headache, visual disturbances, memory problems (short term), short attention span, altered information processing, and dizziness

Care of the craniotomy patient

Indications
- Various treatments
  - Ventricular shunting
  - Excision of tumor or abscess
  - Hematoma evacuation
  - Aneurysm clipping

Key assessments
- Neurological status
- Maintain CPP 70 to 100 mm Hg
- Maintain airway, oxygenation, ventilation
- Maintain fluid balance
- Control pain

Complications
- Cerebral hemorrhage
- Cerebral ischemia or infarct
- Diabetes insipidus or syndrome of inappropriate antidiuretic hormone
- Intracranial hypertension
- Infection
- Leaking CSF
- Seizures

Nursing management
- Continuously monitor neurological status for any changes
- Monitor incision site for signs of infection, and give antibiotics as ordered
- Monitor intake and output and urine specific gravity
- Monitor ICP if monitoring system in place
- Control pain with analgesics as needed
- Institute seizure precautions and have emergency equipment available
- Keep environment quiet with minimal stimuli
- Elevate head of bed 30 degrees
- Monitor patient's oxygenation level and maintain arterial oxygen saturation ≥ 95%

❿ Moderate head injury (GCS of 9 to 12) patients may present confused, open eyes only to commands or painful stimuli, and may follow commands or only localize to painful stimuli; most have an abnormal CT

❿ Severe head injury patients (GCS of 3 to 8) are usually in a coma, defined as no eye opening, no verbal response, and inability to follow commands

❿ In addition to LOC as described by the GCS and depending on the type, location, and extent of injury, the patient may experience altered light reflexes, cranial nerve deficits, focal neurologic deficits (hemiparesis and dysphagia), signs of increased ICP, CSF drainage, Battle's sign (ecchymosis behind the ears), hemotympanum, and raccoon's eyes (ecchymotic periorbital areas); other obvious signs of head trauma (bleeding, lacerations) may be present as well

■ Diagnostic tests
   ◆ A brain scan or CT scan may be performed to pinpoint the area of injury
   ◆ An MRI scan may also be used to determine the location and extent of a head injury
   ◆ Skull X-rays and cervical or complete spine X-rays may show evidence of injury
   ◆ Cerebral angiogram may be done in gunshot or stab wounds, severe head injury, or suspected vasospasm or infarction
   ◆ Transcranial Doppler study may reveal vasospasm

■ Medical management
   ◆ Expect surgical intervention for injury repair, ventriculostomy placement, or ICP monitor insertion (See *Care of the craniotomy patient*)

◆ Control ICP with osmotic diuretics, hyperventilation, CSF drainage, steroids, and/or barbiturate therapy

◆ Reduce cerebral metabolic rate with sedatives, antipyretics, and paralytic agents

◆ Maintain blood pressure to ensure adequate cerebral perfusion

■ Nursing management

◆ Assess for additional defining characteristics, test drainage for halo (the presence of a yellow ring, indicating CSF fluid infiltrate) and glucose (CSF contains glucose, mucus doesn't), and note other clinical signs and symptoms

◆ Monitor for signs of intracranial infections

◆ In confirmed CSF leakage, don't put anything into the nose or ears, but allow fluid to run freely onto a dry sterile dressing

◆ Maintain lumbar drain, if present, as ordered

◆ Place the patient away from cranial defect, and assess nerve function

◆ Employ nursing interventions appropriate to affected cranial nerve; for example, prevent corneal abrasion of cranial nerve V or VII if deficits are detected

◆ Maintain airway, ICP, and cardiovascular system as assessments and medical status warrant; maintain adequate fluid balance and CPP

◆ Prevent patient complications of physical mobility; collaborate with physical therapists, occupational therapists, and speech therapists as the patient's condition warrants

❖ **Aneurysms**
 ■ Description

◆ An aneurysm is a dilated area or an outpouching in an artery wall that weakens the vessel wall

◆ Aneurysms are classified as saccular or berry (bulging or ballooning of the vessel wall with a stemlike attachment to the vessel), fusiform (a usually large atherosclerotic outpouching), dissecting (blood leaking from a tear in the intima of the vessel wall into the layers of the arterial wall), or mycotic (an infected lesion or embolism of the arterial wall)

◆ 95% of cerebral aneurysms are of the saccular type, formed close to the circle of Willis at the bifurcation of the arteries

◆ Traumatic injury to a vessel can also cause an aneurysm to form

◆ Some aneurysms are congenital defects; of these, a small percentage are caused by AVMs

❯ AVMs occur when a miscommunication develops between arteries, veins, and capillaries, resulting in shunting of arterial blood directly into the venous system, bypassing the capillaries

❯ This "stealing" of blood causes ischemia and atrophy in the tissues from which the arterial blood is shunted

❯ The higher-than-normal pressures exerted on the venous side by the arterial flow create engorgement of the veins into which the arterial blood is shunted

 ■ Clinical signs and symptoms

Grades of subarachnoid hemorrhage

The five grades of subarachnoid hemorrhage are based on the severity of the neurologic symptoms.

Grade I: Slight headache, slight nuchal rigidity, or asymptomatic

Grade II: Moderate headache, nuchal rigidity, and slight neurologic deficits

Grade III: Confusion, drowsiness, and mild neurologic deficits

Grade IV: Stupor, moderate hemiparesis, and beginning of decerebrate posturing

Grade V: Comatose, decerebrate or decorticate posturing, and clinical deterioration

- ◆ Sometimes asymptomatic, or the patient may have symptoms before or after the rupture or bleeding
- ◆ Severe headaches, vomiting, photophobia, and nuchal rigidity; loss of consciousness (due to aneurysm rupture)
- ◆ Signs and symptoms associated with meningeal irritation
- ◆ Headaches or seizures resulting from enlargement of the vessels and ischemic changes associated with AVM
  - ▶ AVM has a 20% mortality
  - ▶ Rupture of the aneurysm causes hemorrhage into the subarachnoid space (see *Grades of subarachnoid hemorrhage*)
- ◆ Varying focal neurologic signs and deficits, depending on the site of the aneurysm or intracranial hemorrhage
- ■ Diagnostic tests
  - ◆ Cerebral aneurysm is most often diagnosed with a CT scan
  - ◆ Lumbar puncture isn't performed if there are signs of increased ICP; if performed, the lumbar puncture shows bloody or xanthochromic (yellow) CSF, with elevated protein and cell counts and, usually, elevated CSF pressure
  - ◆ MRI reveals evidence of hemorrhage but isn't the study of choice; CT provides greater visualization of vasculature and can help identify aneurysms
  - ◆ MRA may noninvasively diagnose the aneurysm
  - ◆ Transcranial Doppler studies may reveal increased blood flow velocity
  - ◆ CBF studies can reveal decreased flow if vasospasm is present or if brain damage has occurred
- ■ Medical management
  - ◆ Resect the affected vessel, or surgically repair the vessel
  - ◆ In patients with AVM, consider surgical intervention to clamp the diverting arteries if the area of AVM isn't so deep into the brain as to make it inaccessible
  - ◆ Treat complications; rebleeding, hydrocephalus, and vasospasm are common complaints

▶ Rebleeding is related to the body's natural fibrinolytic process; as the clot that sealed the initial bleeding undergoes fibrinolysis, the risk of rebleeding increases; it's most common in the first day or two after the rupture and in those who haven't had surgical clipping

▶ The chief consequence of cerebral vasospasm is ischemia in large areas of the cerebral hemispheres, leading to cerebral infarction and death

● Another treatment option is the use of calcium channel blockers (nimodipine), serotonin antagonists (reserpine), and beta-adrenergic agents (isoproterenol [Isuprel]) in tandem with a smooth-muscle relaxant (aminophylline)

● Hypervolemic hemodilution hypertension (triple-H therapy) can also be used to treat vasospasm after surgical clipping

− During this treatment, the patient is given fluid and volume expanders to achieve decreased hematocrit level to about 30%, an increased cardiac output to 6.5 to 8.4 L/min, central venous pressure to 8 to 10 mm Hg, or pulmonary artery wedge pressure 12 to 16 mm Hg. If unsuccessful, add a vasopressor (dopamine), or alternatives of phenylephrine (Neo-Synephrine) or norepinephrine (Levophed); dobutamine may also be added to increase cardiac output; the goal of therapy is CPP greater than 70 mm Hg and systolic blood pressure of 160 to 180 mm Hg

− Two potential complications of this therapy are rebleeding of an unstable aneurysm and the development of pulmonary edema and complications associated with fluid overload

− Acute onset of hydrocephalus may occur, causing a sudden rise in ICP, which is treated with ventriculostomy

■ Nursing management

◆ Prevent and control conditions that contribute to increased ICP

◆ Assess neurologic status (compare with baseline values), and determine the grade of subdural hemorrhage

◆ Maintain a patent airway; hypoxia may cause brain cell death, and hypercapnia may cause increased ICP and decreased cerebral perfusion

◆ Maintain the patient on bed rest with the head of the bed elevated 15 to 30 degrees to facilitate venous drainage; position the patient with his neck midline, avoid crossing his legs, and use pillows under his knees to allow for free blood flow to decrease the possibility of thrombus formation

◆ Ensure that the patient has adequate rest periods; activity increases metabolic demands as well as ICP

❖ **Acute spinal cord injuries**

■ Description

◆ Injuries to the spinal cord are classified by the area and mechanism of injury

◆ The area of injury refers to the level of the spine (cervical, thoracic, or lumbar) where the injury occurred; the higher the level, the greater the degree of injury

◆ Mechanisms of injury include hyperflexion, hyperextension, rotation, axial loading or compression, and penetration by a knife or bullet; these mechanisms result in fractures, dislocations, or subluxations of the bony areas as well as stretching, crushing, or vascular compromise to the spinal cord itself; disease processes may also result in acute loss of function

   ▶ Hyperflexion is most commonly seen in cervical injuries (C5 to C6); most often the cause is sudden deceleration, with the resulting dislocated or subluxated intervertebral disk (or bone fragments) compressing the spinal cord nerve roots

   ▶ Hyperextension is commonly seen in whiplash injuries; it results from backward and downward movements that stretch the spinal cord, disrupt disks, and tear ligaments

   ▶ Rotation occurs in combination with flexion or extension injuries; rotational forces tear spinal ligaments, resulting in displacement of disks and compression of nerve roots

   ▶ Axial loading or compression results from an impact great enough to cause the intervertebral disks to burst; this injury is seen in falls from heights and generally results in complete neurologic damage below the level of injury

   ▶ A penetrating injury, such as a knife or bullet wound, usually causes complete transection of the spinal cord

■ Clinical signs and symptoms

◆ The signs and symptoms associated with acute spinal cord injuries depend on the level of vertebral damage (see *Consequences of spinal cord injuries,* page 194); changes may result from decreased spinal cord perfusion as a consequence of lost autoregulation, edema, decreased tissue oxygenation, and release of vasoactive substances (dopamine, serotonin, or norepinephrine)

◆ Although the level of vertebral and spinal nerve damage can be used as a guide, anatomic and functional levels of injury also bear consideration

◆ The anatomic level of injury refers to damage of the upper or lower motor neurons; the upper motor neurons descend from the brain to the spinal cord and begin and end with the CNS; the lower motor neurons originate in the anterior horns of the spinal cord and end in the muscle tissues

   ▶ Damage to a specific motor neuron results in pathologic signs, such as a positive Babinski's reflex, muscle spasticity, or muscle flaccidity

   ▶ If damage to an upper motor neuron occurs above the level of decussation at the medulla, contralateral dysfunction is seen; if damage occurs below the level of decussation for upper or lower motor neurons, ipsilateral dysfunction occurs

◆ The functional level of injury refers to the extent of disruption of normal spinal cord functions; functional injuries are classified as complete or incomplete

   ▶ A complete injury generally involves permanent loss of motor and sensory function in the nerve fibers distal to the injury; complete in-

Consequences of spinal cord injuries

The signs and symptoms accompanying spinal cord injury can help diagnose the extent of the injury. Likewise, knowing the level of injury and the body areas affected can help the critical care nurse plan appropriate interventions. The chart below details the motor function, sensation, and outcome for certain levels of spinal cord injury. Keep in mind that the motor function and sensation of a particular level of spinal cord injury also includes any features noted in the levels above.

Level of injury	Motor function	Sensation	Outcome
C4 or above	Movement of head and upper neck; respiratory paralysis	Full sensation to head and upper neck	Quadriplegia; patient may require mechanical ventilation
C4 to C5	Control of head, neck, shoulders, trapezius, and elbow flexion	Shoulders, back, anterior chest, and lateral upper arms	Quadriplegia and possible phrenic nerve involvement resulting in loss of respiratory function; patient requires assistive devices for limited participation in activities of daily living (ADLs)
C5 to C6	Index finger and thumb, some extension of wrist, phrenic nerve intact	Index finger and thumb	Quadriplegia with diaphragmatic breathing; patient has increased ability to help with some ADLs
C6 to C7	Elbow extension	Middle and ring fingers	Quadriplegia with biceps intact; diaphragmatic breathing; patient is capable of some finger commands and some ADLs, feeding, and dressing
C7 to T1	Hand movement	Complete hand and medial arm	Paraplegia with varying loss of intercostal and abdominal muscle function; patient has greater independence
T1 to T2	Upper extremity control	Some upper trunk sensation above the nipple line	Paraplegia; patient has full use of hands and arms with no trunk control
T3 to T8	Back and chest to nipple line	Some trunk sensation below the nipple line, increasing as the injury occurs lower in the spinal cord (autonomic dysreflexia may occur with injuries at the level of T4 to T6 and above)	Patient has some trunk control
T9 to T10	Muscles of the trunk and upper thigh	Intact to below the waist	Bowel and bladder reflex
T11 to L1	Most leg and some foot movement	Lower leg and dorsal foot	Leg brace, ambulation
L1 to L2	Reflex centers for lower legs, feet, and perineum	Bowel, bladder, and sexual function	Below L2 is cauda equina injury; mixed picture of motor and sensory loss; continued dysfunction of bowel, bladder, and sexual reflexes if S2 to S4 spinal nerves are involved

juries at the level of the cervical spine result in quadriplegia, and those at the level of the thoracic or lumbar spine result in paraplegia

- Complete transection of the spinal cord can result in spinal or neurogenic shock, with immediate loss of all motor and sensory function below the level of injury; this is irreversible
  - Complete transection causes loss of motor neuron function, as evidenced by the absence of reflex activity and flaccid paralysis below the level of injury
  - All sensation of temperature, vibration, touch, proprioception, and pain are lost below the level of injury
  - Loss of autonomic function results in lowered and unsteady arterial blood pressure and an inability to perspire
  - Loss of vascular tone causes venous pooling and warm, dry skin prone to heat loss, thus lowering body temperature
  - Bradycardia is present because of the lack of parasympathetic opposition; if hypotension accompanies bradycardia in a patient with a spinal cord injury, spinal shock is likely; if hypotension accompanies tachycardia, hemorrhagic shock should be suspected
- Spinal shock lasts between 1 and 6 weeks, at which point 50% of patients regain some degree of spinal cord function; as reflexes return, a hyperactive state is seen with spastic paralysis of the upper motor neurons and continued flaccidity of the lower motor neurons

▶ In an incomplete injury, function of a portion of the spinal cord remains intact; a patient may suffer from one of several types of incomplete injuries

- Damage to the anterior horns of the spinal cord involves the motor tracts, spinothalamic (pain perception) tracts, and corticospinal (temperature perception) tracts
  - Anterior cord damage generally is seen in flexion and dislocation injuries of the cervical cord
  - Pain and temperature sensations and motor function are lost at the level below the injury
  - Touch, proprioception, pressure, and vibration senses remain intact
  - Babinski's reflex is pathologically positive, and spastic paralysis is seen
- Damage to the posterior horns of the spinal cord results in loss of proprioception and sensation of light touch
  - Pain and temperature sensations and motor function remain intact
  - Posterior cord injuries, which are rare, generally are associated with hyperextension of the cervical spine
- Damage to the central gray matter of the spinal cord results in significant loss of upper-extremity motor function with an accompanying but less significant loss of lower-extremity motor function
  - Some patients don't experience loss of lower-extremity motor function; this results from the central placement of the upper

motor neurons in the cord and the peripheral placement of the lower motor neurons

— Central cord injuries typically are seen in hyperextension of the cervical spine and in older patients in whom degenerative changes of the vertebrae and disks allow central cord compression to occur

● Damage to one side of the cord, called Brown-Séquard syndrome or transverse hemisection, results in ipsilateral loss of motor function

— It also causes ipsilateral loss of touch, proprioception, pressure, and vibration sensations; and contralateral loss of pain and temperature sensations

— Brown-Séquard's syndrome is caused by penetrating wounds, such as bullet or knife wounds that transect one side of the cord; this syndrome is also seen in surfers who suffer traumatic injury caused by the surfboard hitting them in the neck and rupturing an intervertebral disk

● Damage to spinal nerve roots in the sacral area from a trauma-induced fracture dislocation causes neurologic deficits specific to the nerve roots involved; damage can be unilateral or bilateral and motor and sensory loss may be apparent

● Damage to the spinal cord at the level of T4 to T6 or above can lead to autonomic dysreflexia, an emergency clinical condition characterized by an exaggerated autonomic response (life-threatening hypertension) to a stimulus; the triggering stimulus can be bladder distention, bowel distention, a hot or cold stimulus, or a skin stimulus (such as from tight clothing, a pressure ulcer, or an ingrown toenail)

— Impulses from a full bladder or other stimuli are sent by way of the spinothalamic tracts and posterior columns toward the brain but are blocked at the level of injury

— As these impulses travel up the spinal cord, they stimulate a sympathetic reflex in the gray horns of the thoracolumbar spinal cord; normally, these reflexes are inhibited by impulses from the brain

— Because the initial impulses to the brain are blocked at the level of injury, no inhibitory signals are sent to counter the sympathetic reflexes, resulting in a tremendous sympathetic response

— Symptoms of this sympathetic response include diaphoresis and flushing above the level of injury, with chills and severe vasoconstriction below the level of injury; paroxysmal hypertension, bradycardia, headache, and nausea also are present

— Autonomic dysreflexia is treated by removing the cause (for example, emptying the bladder or bowel) and administering antihypertensive drugs; the best treatment involves identifying the patient as susceptible to autonomic dysreflexia and preventing the syndrome through elimination of drafts, good skin and nail care, and regular bowel and bladder regimens

■ Diagnostic tests
  ◆ A series of spinal X-rays is done to check for fractures, dislocations, and degenerative changes of the vertebral column
  ◆ CT demonstrates bony pathology; myelography shows cord compression
  ◆ MRI shows soft tissue injury
  ◆ Angiography may be done with gunshot or stab wounds to assess vascular injuries
■ Medical management
  ◆ Treat the acute symptoms, and stabilize the injury
  ◆ Methylprednisolone begun within 8 hours of injury with a loading dose given I.V. and a drip following for 23 hours
  ◆ Use surgical interventions, if indicated, to repair fractures or decrease pressure on the spinal cord
  ◆ Crystalloid and colloid fluid replacement I.V. to maintain normal blood pressure as well as vasopressors
  ◆ Atropine to treat bradycardia
■ Nursing management
  ◆ Assess motor function and sensory abilities to detect changes from baseline values
  ◆ Prevent further damage by immobilizing the area, using special beds and equipment, as needed
  ◆ Assess for hypotension, bradycardia, and vasovagal reflex, which may result in cardiac arrest; be prepared to institute emergency measures
  ◆ Prevent hypothermia through temperature regulation (warming blankets) to prevent bradycardia
  ◆ Oxygenate before and after suctioning to prevent hypoxia and vasovagal reactions
  ◆ Avoid placing I.V. lines in paralytic limbs
  ◆ Keep in mind that immobilization places the patient at risk for hypoventilation, pneumonia, and pulmonary embolism; to prevent these complications, encourage coughing, deep breathing, and incentive spirometry; use proper technique in suctioning; apply heat physiotherapy; and measure vital capacity and tidal volume. Physical immobility from paralysis and spasticity can also result in muscle wasting, atony, and contractions
  ◆ Prevent skin breakdown and deep vein thrombosis with proper positioning, frequent turning, therapeutic range-of-motion (ROM) exercises, and antiembolism stockings
  ◆ Provide supportive care and treat complications resulting from the injury
    ▶ Arrhythmias, especially tachycardia and bradycardia, are common in patients with spinal cord injuries
    ▶ Respiratory disturbances also are common and associated with the level of injury
  ◆ Fluid volume deficit may result from gastric dilation (vomiting), hemorrhage, or gastric ulceration; administer antacids, histamine-2 antagonists, gastric lavage, and fluids as prescribed

◆ Urine retention may occur due to anatomic bladder or areflexia and can result in stone formation, renal deterioration, or urinary tract infection

▶ Indwelling catheters and monitoring urine cultures are necessary; when the patient's condition stabilizes, intermittent catheterization or self-catheterization programs may be initiated

◆ The patient and family members will need assistance coping with the emotional repercussions of these devastating injuries; patient issues typically involve disrupted self-concept and feelings of powerlessness; family coping may be ineffectual, given the situational crisis and long-term burden of care; consultative support is often required

❖ **Brain tumors (space-occupying lesions)**
■ Description
◆ Tumors of the brain act as space-occupying lesions and are life-threatening because they destroy brain tissue and nerve structures and also cause increased ICP
◆ Signs and symptoms are the result of compression, invasion, or destruction of brain tissue
◆ Complications include cerebral edema, intracranial hypertension, seizures, focal neurologic deficits, hydrocephalus, and hormonal changes
◆ Histologic features classify tumors and grade of malignancy on a scale from grade I to grade IV (malignant)
◆ Survival of the patient depends on histologic type, grade, location, and size; the patient's age; clinical status before surgery; and duration of symptoms
◆ Gliomas are nonencapsulated infiltrates that arise from neuroglial cells, displacing brain tissue; they comprise 40% to 50% of intracranial tumors

▶ Astrocytoma may occur in the brain or spinal cord; usually grade I or II with a survival rate of 50% to 85%
▶ Oligodendrogliomas are rare, slow-growing, calcified tumors originating in the oligodendrocytes
   • They occur in the cerebral hemispheres
   • Grade I, well-differentiated tumors carry a 5-year survival rate up to 85%; grade IV are 17%
◆ Other types include glioblastoma multiforme (often fatal), brain stem glioma, ependymoma, medulloblastoma, and pineal region tumors
▶ Extra-axial tumors arise from supporting structures of the central or peripheral nervous system; they include meningioma (vascular, firm, encapsulated, slow growing and benign) and acoustic neuroma (schwannoma, which are slow growing and benign)
▶ Developmental tumors include hemangioblastomas (slow growing and vascular), craniopharyngioma, and chordoma (invades bone)
◆ Pituitary tumors make up 10% to 15% of primary brain tumors and may be nonsecreting (chromophobe adenoma) or secreting (prolactin, growth hormone, or corticotropin secreting tumors)

◆ Metastatic tumors are the most common brain tumor, often originating from breast or lung tissue; lesions may be single or multiple, encapsulated or diffuse, and they affect the meninges or brain tissue; most patients die from their primary cancer

■ Clinical signs and symptoms

◆ Headache, seizures, mental changes, and drowsiness are the most common symptoms

◆ Other symptoms may include visual changes, vomiting, and dizziness

◆ Further nursing assessment will depict findings secondary to the location of the tumor, rate of growth, and degree of invasion of the brain tissue (frontal lobe, parietal, temporal, occipital, pituitary, and hypothalmic region, ventricular and periventricular, cerebellar, brain stem)

■ Diagnostic findings

◆ Visual field and funduscopic examination reveals papilledema, visual field defects

◆ CT scan and MRI reveal size and location of tumor

◆ Skull films reveal deviation of calcified pineal gland, erosion of bone or calcified areas

◆ Cerebral angiography reveals vascularity of tumor and vessels supplying it

◆ Endocrine studies are very helpful in pituitary and hypothalmic tumors

◆ CBF and radionucleotide studies can further differentiate the tumor

■ Medical management

◆ Surgery often is indicated, depending on the tumor's size, type, and extent

◆ Medical management for increased ICP and altered CPP depends on the severity of symptoms

◆ Supportive treatment as indicated

■ Nursing management

◆ Support of CPP, airway, and circulatory status, as condition indicates

◆ Monitor fluid status, oxygenation, nutrition, metabolic needs, and infection prevention

◆Protect the patient from seizure-related injury

◆ Nursing management related to location and extent of tumor

◆ Support the family and patient in coping with the illness

❖ Cerebral embolic events

■ Description

◆ Stroke is caused by occlusive vascular disease resulting from thrombotic or embolic events; these block CBF enough to cause cerebral ischemia or infarction. Stroke may also be caused by hemorrhage (25% of strokes) into the parenchyma, or hypertensive intracranial hemorrhage of the basal ganglia, cerebellum, or brain stem

◆ The clinical signs and symptoms of patients experiencing a hemorrhagic or embolic stroke depend on the cerebral area involved

■ Clinical signs and symptoms

◆ The patient may have a history of transient ischemic attacks, resulting in short-lived neurologic deficits, or reversible ischemic neurologic deficit, in which the deficit lasts more than 24 hours but leaves little or no deficits

◆ The main presenting symptoms are the sudden onset of signs and symptoms related to the area involved

▶ Right cerebral hemisphere injury may result in:
  • Left homonymous hemianopia (blindness in the left half of both visual fields)
  • Left hemiparesis or hemiplegia
  • Sensory agnosia manifested as astereognosis (can't recognize objects placed in hand with eyes closed), astratognosia (inability to identify position of body parts), tactile inattention, anosognosia (unaware of neurologic deficit), constructional apraxia (doesn't completely draw the left half of objects), dressing apraxia (inability to dress self properly), neglect (inattention to objects in the left visual field and left auditory stimuli), deviation of the head and eyes to the right

▶ Left cerebral hemisphere injury may result in:
  • Right homonymous hemianopia
  • Right hemiparesis or hemiplegia
  • Sensory agnosia: astereognosis, astratognosia, finger agnosia, right-left disorientation
  • Aphasia: expressive, receptive, or global impairment of speech or communication
    – In expressive (Broca's) aphasia, speech and writing are impaired, but verbal comprehension and reading ability usually remain intact; this type of aphasia results from damage to the posteroinferior frontal lobe
    – In receptive (Wernicke's) aphasia, verbal comprehension and reading are impaired, but speech is usually intact; this type of aphasia results from damage to the posterosuperior temporal lobe
    – In global aphasia, both expressive and receptive abilities are impaired; global aphasia results from damage to the frontotemporal lobe
  • Deviation of head and eyes to the left

■ Diagnostic tests

◆ A brain scan or CT scan may be performed (with best views 24 hours or more after the occluded event); ischemia and infarction are indicated by areas of decreased absorption; hemorrhage, as increased absorption

◆ Cerebral angiography may show vessels in spasm, aneurysm, AVMs, or displaced or stretched vessels

◆ MRI may be used to determine the location of the insult and possibly the causative agent

◆ Other studies include CBF (xenon isotope and PET) to support the diagnosis

■ Medical management
  ◆ Assess patient for fibrinolytic therapy immediately upon arrival (See *Suspected stroke algorithm*, page 202)
  ◆ Treat acute symptoms through supportive care
  ◆ Prescribe physical, occupational, and speech therapy to help the patient regain lost abilities
  ◆ Prevent recurring embolic events with anticoagulant therapy
■ Nursing management
  ◆ Assess for worsening neurologic impairment
  ◆ Orient the patient, and place personal objects within reach in the unaffected visual field; keep side rails up and call light within reach
  ◆ Use communication techniques appropriate for the patient's deficits
  ◆ Use caution when moving the patient to avoid dislocation of flaccid extremities
  ◆ Position the patient carefully to prevent pressure on affected areas and avoid skin breakdown
  ◆ Provide emotional support to the patient and family
  ◆ Teach the patient to scan affected fields or side and to gradually tend to that side

❖ **Intracranial hemorrhage**
  ■ Description
    ◆ Cerebral hematomas are classified by the space into which the bleeding occurs
      ▶ Epidural hematomas are formed by bleeding into the space between the skull and the dura
      ▶ Subdural hematomas are formed by bleeding into the space below the dura
      ▶ Intracerebral hematomas are formed by bleeding into the tissues of the brain
    ◆ Epidural hematomas are usually caused by arterial bleeding
      ▶ They're most commonly caused by a blow to the temporal area, which results in a skull fracture and shearing of the middle meningeal artery
      ▶ Because the bleeding is coming from an artery, not a vein, deterioration is rapid; this accounts for a high mortality rate of approximately 30%
    ◆ Subdural hematomas usually are caused by shearing of the cortical veins that bridge the dura and arachnoid membrane
      ▶ They typically result from acceleration-deceleration and rotational forces impinging the surface of the skull, causing cerebral contusion
      ▶ The skull may remain intact
    ◆ Hematoma formation caused by subdural hematomas may be classified as acute, subacute, or chronic
      ▶ Acute subdural hematomas cause clinical symptoms immediately or within the first 24 to 48 hours posttrauma
      ▶ Subacute subdural hematomas develop 3 to 20 days posttrauma

Suspected stroke algorithm

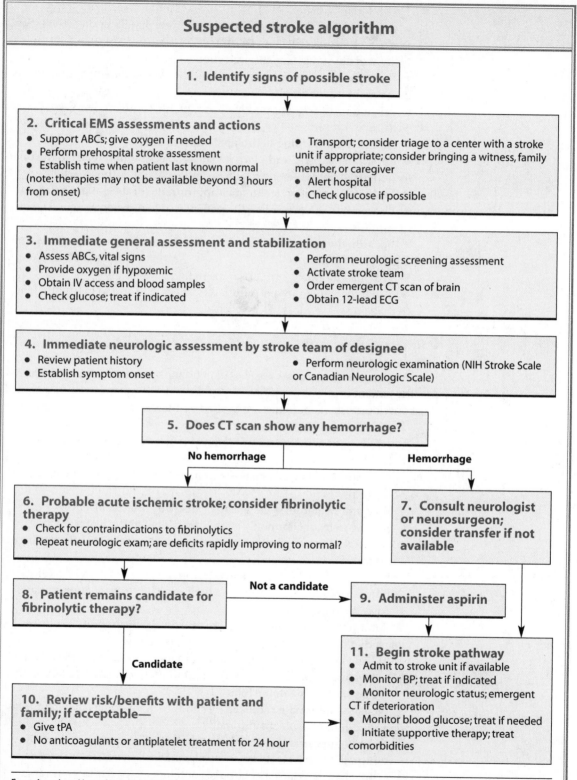

1. Identify signs of possible stroke

2. Critical EMS assessments and actions
- Support ABCs; give oxygen if needed
- Perform prehospital stroke assessment
- Establish time when patient last known normal (note: therapies may not be available beyond 3 hours from onset)
- Transport; consider triage to a center with a stroke unit if appropriate; consider bringing a witness, family member, or caregiver
- Alert hospital
- Check glucose if possible

3. Immediate general assessment and stabilization
- Assess ABCs, vital signs
- Provide oxygen if hypoxemic
- Obtain IV access and blood samples
- Check glucose; treat if indicated
- Perform neurologic screening assessment
- Activate stroke team
- Order emergent CT scan of brain
- Obtain 12-lead ECG

4. Immediate neurologic assessment by stroke team of designee
- Review patient history
- Establish symptom onset
- Perform neurologic examination (NIH Stroke Scale or Canadian Neurologic Scale)

5. Does CT scan show any hemorrhage?

No hemorrhage   Hemorrhage

6. Probable acute ischemic stroke; consider fibrinolytic therapy
- Check for contraindications to fibrinolytics
- Repeat neurologic exam; are deficits rapidly improving to normal?

7. Consult neurologist or neurosurgeon; consider transfer if not available

8. Patient remains candidate for fibrinolytic therapy?

Not a candidate

9. Administer aspirin

Candidate

10. Review risk/benefits with patient and family; if acceptable—
- Give tPA
- No anticoagulants or antiplatelet treatment for 24 hour

11. Begin stroke pathway
- Admit to stroke unit if available
- Monitor BP; treat if indicated
- Monitor neurologic status; emergent CT if deterioration
- Monitor blood glucose; treat if needed
- Initiate supportive therapy; treat comorbidities

From American Heart Association:"Guidelines for Cardiopulmonary Resuscitation and Emergency Cardiovascular Care," Circulation IV:112, December 2005. Used with permission.

▶ Chronic subdural hematomas are seen more than 20 days post-trauma
  • In chronic subdural hematomas, fibroblasts accumulate around and encapsulate the hematoma
  • As the red blood cells of the clot hemolyze, blood proteins disintegrate, and the encapsulated area has a higher osmotic concentration than the surrounding tissues
  • The osmotic gradient induces an influx of water into the capsule, causing it to swell

◆ Intracerebral hematomas may be caused by trauma, tumors, blood dyscrasias, anticoagulant therapy, or hypertension; 90% of cases result from congenital aneurysm, and 10% result from infection, trauma, or idiopathic causes; whatever the cause, the result is pooling of blood within cerebral tissues
  ▶ If the hematoma results from trauma, the usual cause is a missile injury or severe acceleration-deceleration force that causes laceration of deep cerebral tissues
  ▶ When caused by hypertension, the hematoma is called a hemorrhagic stroke
  ▶ The vessels usually involved are those of the circle of Willis, located at the base of the brain

■ Clinical signs and symptoms
◆ Epidural hematoma: brief loss of consciousness at the time of injury; the patient awakens and is lucid for several hours, then lapses into unconsciousness with rapid deterioration in neurologic status
◆ Subdural hematoma: decreased LOC and lateralizing signs
  ▶ Patients with acute and subacute subdural hematoma may exhibit a decreased sensorium that progresses to unconsciousness
    • In acute subdural hematoma, the patient commonly becomes unconscious immediately after the traumatic event and never regains consciousness
    • In subacute subdural hematoma, hematoma formation occurs at a slower rate; symptoms appear more slowly but are nonetheless acute when they do develop
  ▶ Chronic subdural hematoma: decreased LOC with a history of changes in behavior but not necessarily a history of recent trauma
    • Patients with chronic subdural hematoma are usually the elderly or alcoholics and have decreased cerebral volume as a result of atrophy
    • The initial hemorrhage isn't enough to cause significant clinical symptoms; it's the resultant swelling, which applies pressure to the surrounding cerebral tissues, that's symptomatic
    • Symptoms are generally insidious (for example, headache, absent-mindedness, and lethargy) and may be misdiagnosed as Alzheimer's disease or ascribed to the aging process or cerebral atrophy
◆ Intracerebral hematoma: possibly signs of increased ICP; symptoms vary according to the rate of bleeding and area of the brain in which it occurs

- Diagnostic tests
  - ◆ The diagnosis for epidural, subdural, and intracerebral hematomas is generally based on the patient's clinical presentation and medical history and CT scan results
  - ◆ Skull and cervical spine X-rays may help identify associated fracture
  - ◆ Lumbar puncture is contraindicated by the presence of increased ICP
- Medical management
  - ◆ Intervene accordingly, based on the location and extent of bleeding
  - ◆ Take immediate action for acute symptoms
    - ▶ Acute intervention generally entails immediate surgical intervention (for epidural hematoma) to remove the clot, cauterize the vessels, and prevent rapid neurologic deterioration
    - ▶ Osmotic diuretics shouldn't be administered before surgery, as the bleeding is stopped initially by the tamponade effect of the clot's expansion against the skull; administering osmotic diuretics would decrease swelling, allowing bleeding from the vessel to continue
    - ▶ Surgery may be deferred when there's a very small amount of bleeding, the patient remains neurologically stable, and there's no midline shifting of the cerebral structures
- Nursing management
  - ◆ Continuously assess for changes in neurologic status
  - ◆ Maintain the patient's airway if inadequate oxygenation and ventilation are present
  - ◆ Keep the cervical spine immobilized until injury has been ruled out
  - ◆ If the patient undergoes surgery, ensure that the head of the bed is elevated postoperatively to facilitate venous drainage

❖ **Neurologic infectious diseases**
- Brain abscesses
  - ◆ Description
    - ▶ Abscesses are pockets of infection in the brain tissues
    - ▶ They're most commonly caused by an infectious agent that has originated from an infected site elsewhere in the body, which is then carried in the bloodstream to the brain; examples of infections that can lead to brain abscesses include bacterial endocarditis, lung or skin abscesses, and ear, sinus, or tooth abscesses
    - ▶ The most common sites for abscesses to settle in the brain are the epidural and subdural spaces or the cerebrum
  - ◆ Clinical signs and symptoms
    - ▶ Fever and lethargy
    - ▶ Focal neurologic deficits, speech and motor deficits, and seizures
  - ◆ Diagnostic tests
    - ▶ The diagnosis is made by using a CT scan and lumbar puncture
    - ▶ Aspiration of the abscess, with culture and sensitivity testing, identifies the organism and helps determine appropriate medications
  - ◆ Medical management
    - ▶ Administer I.V. and intrathecal antibiotics

◗ Use surgical excision and drainage of the abscess to drain as much purulent fluid as possible

◆ Nursing management

◗ Use the same interventions as for a patient with meningitis (see pages 206 and 207)

◗ If the patient undergoes surgery, ensure that the head of the bed is elevated 30 degrees postoperatively to facilitate venous drainage

■ Encephalitis

◆ Description

◗ Encephalitis is an inflammation of the brain tissues, usually caused by a virus, fungus, bacterium (particularly *Rickettsia*), or parasite

◗ Acute encephalitis is typically caused by a virus

• Known infective viruses include herpes simplex, equine, and arbovirus

• Equine virus and arboviruses are transmitted by ticks and mosquitoes

◆ Clinical signs and symptoms

◗ Headache, fever, nausea, and vomiting

◗ Nuchal rigidity, positive Kernig's sign, positive Brudzinski's sign, photophobia, altered LOC, and seizures

◆ Diagnostic tests

◗ Diagnosis is generally determined by lumbar puncture

◗ In viral encephalitis, the CSF sample is cloudy and shows elevated protein level, normal glucose level, and the presence of WBCs

◆ Medical management

◗ Control the symptoms, using steroids (except in cases of herpes virus) and antiviral medications

◗ Administer antibiotic and antifungal medications after the causative organism has been identified

◗ Control increased ICP with osmotic diuretics (such as mannitol)

◆ Nursing management

◗ Continuously assess for changes in LOC and temperature

◗ Monitor for increasing ICP and possible causes

◗ Maintain an environment of subdued stimulation to decrease the risk of seizures

◗ Suppress elevated temperatures, which can cause increased ICP, with antipyretics and hypothermic blankets or tepid soaks

• The measures used to decrease temperature shouldn't induce shivering

• Shivering raises the metabolic rate and may increase ICP

■ Guillain-Barré syndrome

◆ Description

◗ Guillain-Barré syndrome is an inflammatory process of the nervous system characterized by demyelination of peripheral nerves; it results in progressive, symmetrical, ascending paralysis

◗ The exact cause is unknown, but the syndrome usually is preceded by a suspected viral infection accompanied by fever 1 to 3 weeks before the onset of acute bilateral muscle weakness in the lower extremities; autodigestion of the myelin sheath continues to ascend with development of flaccid paralysis within 48 to 72 hours

- ◆ Clinical signs and symptoms
  - ❱ The patient may present with progressive, ascending weakness with mild to moderate sensory changes (especially tingling and muscle pain)
  - ❱ Cranial nerve (IX, X, and XII) impairment, as evidenced by difficulties in speech, swallowing, and mastication
  - ❱ Inability to wrinkle the forehead or close the eyelids
  - ❱ Impaired facial expressions and disconjugate eye movements, indicating impairment of cranial nerves II, IV, V, VI, and VII
  - ❱ Impairment of the muscles of respiration, as the paralysis continues to ascend, and the cervical nerve roots are affected; respiratory failure occurs and supportive treatment is required to prevent death
  - ❱ Ascending bilateral muscle weakness, flaccid paralysis with pain, but no decrease in LOC
  - ❱ ANS dysfunction with fluctuation in blood pressure and heart rate
- ◆ Diagnostic tests
  - ❱ The hallmark of Guillain-Barré syndrome is the presence of albuminocytological dissociation (high protein count in the CSF); protein level peaks 10 to 20 days post onset
  - ❱ EMG and nerve conduction studies may be abnormal 1 to 2 weeks after onset
  - ❱ Sometimes lumbar puncture, MRI scan, and CT scan are used to diagnose this syndrome
- ◆ Medical management
  - ❱ Provide supportive care while myelin is regenerated; symptoms usually begin to subside within 2 weeks, with recovery in 2 years
  - ❱ Plasmapheresis to eliminate the protein causing the autoimmune demyelination
- ◆ Nursing management
  - ❱ Implement appropriate airway management techniques
  - ❱ Observe for signs of phlebitis; passive ROM exercises, antiembolism stockings, and anticoagulant therapy may be indicated
  - ❱ Maintain adequate hydration and nutrition
  - ❱ Monitor for complications of plasmapheresis (hypotension, hypoprothrombinemia with bleeding, arrhythmias, hypocalcemia), and treat symptoms promptly, as indicated
  - ❱ Promote comfort measures for relaxation, distraction, and pain control
  - ❱ Monitor vital signs, especially blood pressure and heart rate, as frequently as condition permits; administer medications to treat cardiovascular compromise (atropine, beta-blockers, vasoactive medications), as indicated
  - ❱ Prevent hazards of physical mobility
  - ❱ Assist with coping
- ■ Meningitis
  - ◆ Description

▶ Meningitis is an inflammatory process of the meninges and CSF within the subarachnoid space

▶ The infective agent can be introduced by way of the sinuses, ear canal, or bloodstream or through a penetrating head wound

   • In 80% to 90% of cases, meningitis is caused by streptococcal pneumonia, *Haemophilus influenzae*, or *Neisseria*

      • It can be caused by a viral or bacterial infection; mumps virus, tuberculosis, and fungal agents may also cause meningitis

◆ Clinical signs and symptoms

▶ Headache, fever, nausea, and vomiting

▶ Nuchal rigidity, positive Kernig's sign, positive Brudzinski's sign, photophobia, altered LOC, and seizures

▶ Neurologic abnormalities will reflect the cranial nerve involved

▶ Complications include Waterhouse-Friderichsen syndrome (adrenal hemorrhage) with resulting hemorrhage and shock, disseminated intravascular coagulation, encephalitis, hydrocephalus, and cerebral edema

◆ Diagnostic tests

▶ Diagnosis is generally determined by lumbar puncture, with results dependent on the type of organism

▶ The CSF is cloudy or xanthochromic (yellow) and shows elevated pressure, elevated protein level, decreased glucose level (bacterial), and the presence of WBCs

▶ CT may show hydrocephalus and diffuse enhancement in severe cases

◆ Medical management

▶ Control symptoms; patients with meningococcal meningitis must be isolated

▶ Administer antibiotics specific to the bacterial or fungal causative agent; antibiotics aren't given for viral or aseptic meningitis

◆ Nursing management

▶ Continuously assess for changes in LOC and temperature

▶ Monitor for increasing ICP and possible causes

▶ Maintain an environment of subdued stimulation to decrease the risk of seizures, promote comfort, and reduce pain

▶ Suppress elevated temperatures, which can cause increased ICP, with antipyretics and hypothermic blankets or tepid soaks

   • The measures used to decrease temperature shouldn't induce shivering

   • Shivering raises the metabolic rate and may increase ICP

■ Myasthenia gravis

◆ Description

▶ Myasthenia gravis is a chronic autoimmune disorder characterized by muscle fatigue that improves with rest but is exacerbated by activity

▶ The disorder is caused by an autoimmune response that destroys the acetylcholine receptor sites at the neuromuscular junction

◆ Clinical signs and symptoms

- ▶ Skeletal muscle weakness that increases with repetitive exercise and is accompanied by cranial nerve VII deficits
- ▶ Respiratory muscle impairment, which is usually the reason patients are treated in the intensive care unit
- ◆ Diagnostic tests
  - ▶ The Tensilon test is used to determine whether the patient is experiencing myasthenic or cholinergic crisis
    - • Tensilon (edrophonium chloride) is an anticholinesterase agent that, when given I.V. or I.M., dramatically revitalizes skeletal muscle function in a patient in myasthenic crisis; this recuperation lasts only a few minutes
    - • When Tensilon is given to a patient in cholinergic crisis, symptoms are exacerbated; although the exacerbation of symptoms lasts only a minute, respiratory support must be available
    - • Antibodies to acetylcholine receptors are found in the serum of 90% of patients with myasthenia gravis
  - ▶ EMG is used to measure the electrical activity of muscle cells
- ◆ Medical management
  - ▶ Administer anticholinesterase agents (such as pyridostigmine bromide [Mestinon]) to block the hydrolysis of acetylcholine at the neuromuscular junction
  - ▶ Consider surgical excision of the thymus or plasmapheresis to decrease the autoimmune response
  - ▶ Administer corticosteroids and other immunosuppressant drugs, if indicated
  - ▶ A patient in myasthenic crisis (inadequate anticholinesterase) presents a clinical picture much like that of a patient in cholinergic crisis (overdose of anticholinesterase); however, a patient in myasthenic crisis experiences increased blood pressure and tachycardia, whereas a patient in cholinergic crisis experiences GI symptoms (such as nausea, vomiting, salivation, and abdominal cramps), decreased blood pressure, bradycardia, and blurred vision
    - • Treatments for these crises are diametric opposites; therefore, it's of utmost importance to distinguish between the two types of crisis
    - • Neostigmine bromide (Prostigmin) is usually the drug of choice for myasthenic crisis; atropine, a cholinergic blocker, is the drug of choice for cholinergic crisis
- ◆ Nursing management
  - ▶ Administer medications, as prescribed, and according to the dosing schedule
  - ▶ Observe the patient closely for evidence of respiratory failure
  - ▶ Continuously assess muscle strength
- ■ West Nile encephalitis
  - ◆ Description
    - ▶ West Nile encephalitis is caused by a virus that may lead to encephalopathy, meningitis, or even death
    - ▶ The number of cases increases in warmer weather and in warmer climates

▶ The infection is transmitted from birds to humans with mosquitoes as the bridge vectors

▶ The greater risk is to those over 50 years of age and those with compromised immune systems

● The mortality rate is 3% to 15%

◆ Clinical signs and symptoms

▶ Headache, low-grade fever, myalgia, rash, swollen lymph glands, nausea, vomiting

▶ Severe infection may include high fevers, neck stiffness, stupor, and disorientation

▶ Complications include coma, tremors, paralysis, cranial nerve disruption, and myocarditis

◆ Diagnostic tests

▶ The enzyme-linked immunosorbent assay is the test of choice for a definitive diagnosis

● The specimen should be either serum or CSF collected at the time of the acute illness

▶ CBC will show normal or elevated leukocytes and anemia

◆ Medical management

▶ Control symptoms; administer I.V. fluids, control fever, provide respiratory support if needed

▶ High doses of ribavirin and interferon alfa-2b have some activity against the virus

◆ Nursing management

▶ Administer I.V. fluids to prevent dehydration; strictly monitor intake and output

▶ Continually assess neurological status for changes

▶ Continue to assess patient's cardiac status during acute phase of illness; watch for signs and symptoms of decreased cardiac output, such as tachycardia, hypotension, and confusion

▶ Administer medications to help with fever, nausea, and pain

▶ Suspected cases of West Nile encephalitis must be reported to the state Department of Health

▶ Provide oxygen therapy and respiratory support as needed

❖ **Seizure disorders**

■ Description

◆ Seizures are sudden paroxysmal discharges of a group of neurons that interfere with normal mental and behavioral activities

◆ Seizures may be triggered by toxic states, electrolyte imbalances, tumors, anoxia, inflammation of CNS tissue, increased ICP, trauma, hyperpyrexia, multiple sclerosis, Huntington's disease, Alzheimer's disease, or idiopathic causes

◆ Seizure activity is thought to be associated with an imbalance between the excitatory and inhibitory synaptic influences on the postsynaptic neurons; when this imbalance occurs, an area of excessive depolarization results, causing an abnormal pattern of electrical activity or a paroxysmal depolarization shift

◆ There are three theories of causation of this imbalance: alteration in the cellular sodium pump, acetylcholine-cholinesterase imbalance, and alteration in the conversion of glutamic acid to gamma-aminobutyric acid (GABA)

▶ The cellular sodium pump preserves the normal resting membrane potential by moving potassium out of the cell and sodium into the cell during depolarization; this active transport mechanism relies on sufficient amounts of oxygen and glucose

● When deprived of sufficient oxygen and glucose, the transport mechanism fails, and sodium is allowed to diffuse into the cell abnormally

● The resting membrane potential of the cell is lowered, making it more vulnerable to paroxysms of electrical activity

▶ Synaptic impulse transmission relies on the excitatory transmitter acetylcholine; the resting membrane potential is decreased in the presence of increased levels of acetylcholine

● Decreased levels of cholinesterase, an inhibitory neurotransmitter, decrease postsynaptic inhibition

● Increased levels of acetylcholine and decreased levels of cholinesterase make neuronal synaptic membranes more susceptible to repetitive electrical discharges

▶ The coenzyme pyridoxine is essential for the conversion of glutamic acid to the synaptic inhibitor GABA; inadequate amounts of pyridoxine result in decreased levels of GABA and loss of inhibition

◆ Seizures are classified as partial (focal) or generalized

▶ Partial seizures involve a localized or focal area of the brain

▶ Generalized seizures involve the entire brain and are associated with bilateral neuronal discharges

■ Clinical signs and symptoms

◆ Partial seizures usually don't impair consciousness and involve either motor or sensory symptoms

▶ For example, a Jacksonian seizure involves the clonic activity of a muscle that progresses to adjoining muscles

▶ The successive progression of the seizure reflects the wave of neuronal discharge activity in the brain

▶ Clinically, the patient experiences decreased LOC, impaired mentation and sensation, and amnesia

◆ Generalized seizures affect consciousness and, concurrently, motor and sensory functions

▶ Absence (petit mal) seizures cause transient loss of consciousness without tumultuous muscle motion and last for a few seconds

● Absence seizures may be accompanied by a vacant, blinking stare during the state of decreased consciousness

● Absence seizures are seen most frequently in children

▶ Generalized tonic-clonic (grand mal) seizures manifest initially as a preictal or aura phase consisting of vision disturbances or irritability

● Loss of consciousness is followed by stiffening of skeletal muscles (tonic phase) with progression to jerking movements (clonic phase)

- Breathing stops during the tonic phase; the clonic phase is characterized by hyperventilation
  - Autonomic dysfunction is demonstrated by the loss of bowel and bladder control
  - The postictal phase is characterized by flaccidity, with progressive return to consciousness and subsequent amnesia
- ❙ Myoclonic seizures cause brief, sudden contractions that generally involve the upper extremities
- ❙ Akinetic seizures cause brief, sudden episodes with loss of muscle control
- ❙ Status epilepticus is a clinical emergency, distinguished by continually recurring generalized tonic-clonic seizures that don't allow for recovery at the end of the postictal phase; principal concerns with status epilepticus are anoxia, arrhythmias, and acidosis

■ Diagnostic tests
  - ◆ The use of radiologic tests depends on the causative pathology
  - ◆ An EEG is used to identify the area of seizure focus
  - ◆ Laboratory tests are performed to look for abnormalities that may result in seizures (hypoglycemia, hypoxemia), toxicology, low anticonvulsant levels, and associated disorders (lead poisoning, sickle cell anemia, leukemia)

■ Medical management
  - ◆ Correct the causative pathology if the patient isn't in status epilepticus
  - ◆ For status epilepticus, administer lorazepam (Ativan) and diazepam (Valium) to interrupt the seizure activity, and maintain the airway (intubation may be necessary)
    - ❙ Because diazepam can't prevent a recurrence of seizures, phenytoin (Dilantin), phenobarbital, pentobarbital, or general anesthetic agents may be administered
    - ❙ Once the seizure activity has been stemmed, correction of the primary cause can be addressed
    - ❙ Temporal lobectomy or corpus callosotomy may be done in recurrent seizures

■ Nursing management
  - ◆ Maintain airway and oxygenation
  - ◆ Assess the seizure, noting the body parts involved, duration, the type and quality of movement, changes in neurologic status, and any precipitating events
  - ◆ Provide supportive care, and institute measures to prevent injury during the seizure
  - ◆ Administer seizure medication and monitor effect
  - ◆ Monitor for complications, such as blood pressure disturbances, arrhythmias, and hyperthermia

Review questions

1. An 18-year-old male motor vehicle accident victim is experiencing confusion and problems with reasoning. He most likely has a closed head injury involving the:

○ **A.** parietal lobe.

○ **B.** frontal lobe.

○ **C.** occipital lobe.

○ **D.** temporal lobe.

Correct answer: B The frontal lobe is responsible for high-level functioning, such as reasoning and abstract thinking.

2. To identify the type and extent of injury to the head-injured patient, the nurse can expect him to undergo:

○ **A.** CT.

○ **B.** MRI.

○ **C.** EEG.

○ **D.** single photon emission tomography.

Correct answer: A CT is a useful diagnostic tool to identify bleeding within the brain.

3. A patient suddenly becomes unresponsive as you are speaking to him, and he develops trembling of all extremities. Your priority is to:

○ **A.** notify the doctor immediately.

○ **B.** administer diazepam I.V.

○ **C.** establish an airway.

○ **D.** perform a rapid neurologic examination.

Correct answer: C Initially, the patient's airway, breathing, and circulation are the priority, followed by seizure assessment and treatment.

4. A 50-year-old patient has a bleeding aneurysm within the circle of Willis area as evidenced on a CT. After surgical clipping, medical management would include:

○ **A.** calcium channel blockers, anticonvulsants, and analgesics.

○ **B.** diuretics, positive inotropic agents, and nonsteroidal anti-inflammatory drugs.

○ **C.** vasodilators, antiplatelet agents, and antibiotics.

○ **D.** dopamine, antihypertensives, and fluids.

Correct answer: A Calcium channel blockers help regulate heart rate and blood pressure, anticonvulsants control seizure activity, and analgesics provide pain relief.

5. A patient isn't expected to survive a massive aneurysmal bleed, despite aggressive efforts by the staff, and brain death is suspected. The medical staff is beginning to test the patient for brain death criteria. The nurse should:

○ **A.** call for pastoral care support for the family.

○ **B.** approach the family regarding organ donation.

○ **C.** allow the family unlimited visiting.

○ **D.** notify the nursing supervisor of the situation.

Correct answer: B The priority is to determine the family's feelings and understanding of the situation. In most states, the law requires approaching the family regarding organ donation.

CHAPTER 7

Gastrointestinal disorders

❖ Anatomy
- ■ Mouth
  - ◆ The mouth consists of the lips, cheeks, teeth, gums, tongue, palate, and salivary glands; the tongue is a mass of striated and skeletal muscles covered by mucous membranes
  - ◆ The salivary glands (submandibular, parotid, and sublingual) secrete 1,000 to 1,500 ml of saliva per day
  - ◆ The mouth is connected to the esophagus by the pharynx; the walls of the pharynx are composed of fibrous tissues surrounded by muscle fibers
  - ◆ Motor impulses for swallowing are transmitted via cranial nerves V, IX, X, and XII in the pharyngeal area
- ■ Esophagus
  - ◆ Located behind the trachea, the esophagus is 10" to 12" (25.4 to 30.5 cm) long and passes through the thoracic and abdominal cavities
  - ◆ The top one-third of the esophagus is striated muscle; the bottom two-thirds is smooth muscle
  - ◆ The superior end of the esophagus is opened and closed by the hypopharyngeal sphincter; the distal end is opened and closed by the lower esophageal sphincter
  - ◆ Peristaltic waves move food through the esophagus to the stomach
- ■ Stomach
  - ◆ The stomach is located in the epigastric umbilical and left hypochondriac areas of the abdomen
  - ◆ It's divided into the fundus, or upper part; the greater curvature, which lies below the fundus; the body, which makes up the largest portion of the stomach; the pyloric part, near the outlet to the intestines; and the lesser curvature, which lies between the pyloric sphincter and the esophagus
  - ◆ The stomach consists of an outer layer of longitudinal muscle fibers, a middle layer of circular fibers, and an inner layer of transverse fibers
  - ◆ The gastric mucosa, which contains large numbers of gastric, cardiac, and pyloric glands, lines the interior of the stomach; secretion of gastric enzymes is necessary for digestion; the gastric hormones gastrin and histamine are also secreted to aid digestion
  - ◆ The submucosal layer of the stomach is composed of blood vessels, lymph vessels, and connective and fibrous tissues
  - ◆ Rugae (folds) on the interior of the stomach allow for distention

- Small intestine
  - ◆ The small intestine is a tubular structure that extends from the pyloric sphincter to the cecum
  - ◆ It's divided into three sections: the duodenum, which makes up the first several inches; the jejunum, which is about 8' (2.4 m) long and extends from the ileocecal valve; and the ileum, which is about 12' (3.6 m) long
  - ◆ The lumen contains small, fingerlike projections called villi, which vastly increase the surface area of the small intestine
  - ◆ The small intestine also contains several glands, including Lieberkühn's crypts, which are found between the villi and produce mucus; absorptive and secreting cells; Brunner's glands; and Peyer's patches, which play a role in the immune system
  - ◆ The primary function of the small intestine is nutrient absorption
- Large intestine
  - ◆ Also called the colon, the large intestine extends from the ileum to the anus
  - ◆ About 5' to 6' (1.5 to 1.8 m) long and 2½" (6.3 cm) in diameter, the large intestine is divided into three segments: the cecum, the colon (ascending, transverse, and descending), and the rectum
  - ◆ The large intestine contains no villi
  - ◆ The major function is absorption of water and elimination of food residue (feces)
- Innervation of the GI system
  - ◆ The GI tract has its own intrinsic nervous system, which is under the control of the autonomic nervous system; the autonomic nervous system can change the effects of the GI system at any point
  - ◆ Cranial nerve X (vagus nerve) is the primary nerve for the parasympathetic nervous system; sympathetic nervous fibers parallel the major blood vessels of the entire GI tract
    - ❱ Parasympathetic stimulation increases the activity of the GI tract
    - ❱ Sympathetic stimulation decreases, or may even halt, the activity of the GI tract
- Accessory organs of the GI system
  - ◆ Salivary glands
    - ❱ There are three salivary glands: the parotid gland, submandibular gland, and sublingual gland
    - ❱ Each salivary gland occurs in pairs
  - ◆ Pancreas
    - ❱ The pancreas is both an endocrine and a digestive system organ
    - ❱ This fish-shaped, lobulated gland lies behind the stomach
      - • The head and neck of the pancreas lie in the C-shaped curve of the duodenum
      - • The body lies behind the duodenum
      - • The tail is a thin, narrow segment below the spleen
    - ❱ The duct of Wirsung is the main pancreatic duct and runs the entire length of the organ
    - ❱ Small pancreatic sacs called acinar cells manufacture the juices used in digestion

▶ The ampulla of Vater is the short segment of the pancreas, located just before the common bile duct

▶ Pancreatic function is controlled by the phases of digestion and the vagus nerve of the parasympathetic system

▶ The duct of Wirsung and the bile duct merge at the ampulla of Vater and enter the duodenum

◆ Gallbladder

▶ The gallbladder can store up to 50 ml of bile, which is released when fatty food is present in the small intestine

▶ The gallbladder has four parts

• The fundus is the distal portion of the body and forms a blind sac

• The body connects the fundus to the infundibulum

• The infundibulum connects the body to the neck of the gallbladder

• The cystic duct merges with the duct system of the liver to form the common bile duct

◆ Liver

▶ The largest single organ in the body, the liver weighs 3 to 4 lb (1.4 to 1.8 kg)

▶ The liver is located in the right upper quadrant of the abdomen, lying against the right inferior diaphragm

▶ It's divided into a right and left lobe by the falciform ligament

• The right lobe is larger than the left

• The falciform ligament attaches the liver to the abdominal wall

▶ The hepatic lobule is the functioning unit of the liver

• Each lobule has its own hepatic artery, portal vein, and bile duct; these structures constitute the portal triad

• Sinusoids are intralobular cavities between columns of epithelial cells, lined with Kupffer's cells

❖ **Physiology**

■ Mouth

◆ Food that enters the mouth is mechanically altered by mastication

◆ To help break down starch, food is mixed with saliva

■ Esophagus

◆ When a bolus of food enters the esophagus, the hypopharyngeal sphincter opens

◆ Gravity and peristaltic wave motion advance the bolus of food down the esophagus

◆ When the lower esophageal sphincter opens, the food passes into the stomach

■ Stomach

◆ When the upper portion of the stomach receives the food bolus, the gastric glands are stimulated to secrete lipase, pepsin, intrinsic factor, mucus, hydrochloric acid, and gastrin

◆ The food bolus is churned until it becomes a semiliquid mass called chyme

◆ Gastric motility—the ability of the stomach to churn the food—is affected by the quantity and pH of the contents, the degree of mixing, peristalsis, and the ability of the duodenum to accept the food mass

Where nutrients are absorbed in the GI tract	
Location	**Nutrient**
Duodenum-jejunum	Triglycerides, fatty acids, amino acids, simple sugars (glucose, fructose, galactose), fat-soluble vitamins (A, D, E, and K), water soluble vitamins (C, B complex, niacin), folic acid, calcium, electrolytes, and water
Ileum	Bile salts, vitamin B_{12}, chloride, and water
Colon	Potassium and water

- ◆ The stomach empties at a rate proportional to the volume of its contents and distends to hold a large quantity of food
- ■ Small intestine
  - ◆ The principal function of the small intestine is to absorb nutrients from the chyme (see *Where nutrients are absorbed in the GI tract*)
    - ▶ The chyme leaving the stomach isn't sufficiently broken down to be absorbed
    - ▶ The pancreas, liver, and gallbladder contribute to the continued breakdown of chyme
  - ◆ Food is absorbed in the small intestine through hydrolysis, nonionic movement, passive diffusion, facilitated diffusion, and active transport
  - ◆ The small intestine uses mixing contractions to mix the food with digestive juices and propulsive contractions to move the food through the system
    - ▶ The myenteric reflex occurs when distention of the small intestine activates the nerves to continue the contraction sequence
    - ▶ The gastroileal reflex regulates the movement of chyme from the small intestine to the large intestine
  - ◆ The ileocecal valve at the terminal ileum prevents the chyme from returning to the ileum from the large intestine
- ■ Large intestine
  - ◆ The large intestine absorbs water and some electrolytes and retains the chyme for elimination of waste products
    - ▶ The chyme moves slowly through the large intestine to allow for water reabsorption
    - ▶ Normally, the large intestine removes 80% to 90% of the water from the chyme
    - ▶ The bacteria found in the large intestine (primarily *Escherichia coli*) helps digest cellulose and synthesize vitamins and other nutrients
  - ◆ Haustral contractions are weak peristaltic contractions that move the chyme through the large intestine
- ■ Pancreas
  - ◆ The acinar glands secrete water, salt, amylase, and lipolytic and proteolytic enzymes as well as nuclease and deoxyribonuclease
  - ◆ Amylase digests carbohydrates

▶ The lipolytic enzymes lipase and phospholipase break down fats of all types

▶ The proteolytic enzyme trypsin breaks down protein

▶ The enzymes nuclease and deoxyribonuclease break down the nucleotides in deoxyribonucleic acid and ribonucleic acid

◆ The cells lining the acinar glands contain large amounts of carbonic anhydrase and make the pancreatic secretions strong bases

◆ Pancreatic secretion is triggered by the presence of undigested food in the small intestine

■ Gallbladder

◆ The gallbladder stores and concentrates bile

▶ Bile salts react with water, leaving a fat-soluble end product to mix with cholesterol and lecithin

▶ Bile pigments and bilirubin result from the breakdown of hemoglobin

▶ Vagal stimulation increases bile secretions through the sphincter of Oddi

◆ During normal digestion, the gallbladder contracts in response to the hormone cholecystokinin when food is present in the small intestine

■ Liver

◆ The liver synthesizes and transports bile and bile salts for fat digestion

◆ The hepatic cells synthesize bile, which flows through a series of ducts to the common hepatic duct and the gallbladder

❖ Gastrointestinal assessment

■ Noninvasive assessment techniques

◆ Inspect the abdomen from above and from the side

▶ Note any distention of the abdomen; check for symmetry, skin texture, color, scarring, lesions, rashes, and moles

▶ Note the location and condition of the umbilicus; assess abdominal movements, breathing, and pulse

▶ Normally, the abdomen should be flat with no scars and the umbilicus at midline

◆ Lift the head and observe the abdominal muscles

◆ Auscultate all four quadrants, noting normal and abnormal sounds

◆ Percuss all four quadrants, noting the presence of fluid, air, or masses; tympany is the normal sound in the abdomen above the gastric bubble. Dullness may be percussed over the liver, spleen, or stool-filled colon

◆ Percuss the liver

▶ Percussing the liver helps determine its size and location; first percuss from the umbilicus up the right abdomen for a change in sound from tympany to dullness, and mark this site; next, percuss downward from above the nipple on the right midclavicular line for a change in sound from resonance to dullness, and mark this site

▶ Measure the space between the two sites for approximate liver size; the normal liver is 2½″ to 4¾″ (6 to 12 cm); note the liver's position

◆ Percuss the spleen in the left lateral area between the 6th and 10th ribs

◆ Lightly palpate (indent the skin ½″ [1.3 cm]) all four quadrants to assess for tenderness, guarding, and masses

◆ Deeply palpate the abdomen (indent the skin 2″ to 3″ [5 to 7.6 cm]) to identify tenderness and masses in deeper tissues and rebound tenderness
◆ Palpate the liver, spleen, and kidneys; normally, most abdominal organs are *not* palpable
◆ Assess for inguinal lymph nodes
■ Diagnostic tests and procedures
◆ Magnetic resonance imaging (MRI) is used to evaluate sources of GI bleeding, fistulas, or abscesses; MRI is also used to evaluate vascular structure or diagnose tumors in the GI tract
◆ Ultrasonagraphy helps define fluid, masses, stones, cysts, or other abnormalities of the GI organs; special equipment adaptations allow ultrasound use in endoscopic procedures to quantify masses or assess levels of infiltration to the surrounding tissue
◆ Computed tomography (CT) of the abdomen is used to visualize all GI organs; CT can help diagnose tumors, evaluate vasculature, and locate perforations or other disorders
◆ Scintigraphy uses radioactive isotopes to reveal displaced anatomical structures, changes in organ size, or presence of focal lesions or tumors
◆ Esophagogastroduodenoscopy (EGD) uses a flexible fiber-optic endoscope to directly visualize the esophageal and gastric mucosa, pylorus, and duodenum; EGD can be extended to include the pancreas and gallbladder
◆ Proctoscopy and sigmoidoscopy use a rigid or flexible fiber-optic sigmoidoscope to directly visualize the mucosa of the colon's distal segment and rectum
◆ Colonoscopy uses a flexible fiber-optic colonoscope to directly visualize colonic mucosa up to the ileocecal valve
◆ Endoscopic retrograde cholangiopancreatography (ERCP) involves insertion of a flexible fiber-optic scope through the stomach into the duodenum; the scope has a side-viewing port that allows a cannula to enter the ampulla of Vater to observe the biliary duct system; radiopaque dye is injected into the biliary tree to observe for abnormalities, such as bile stones or strictures. Therapeutic techniques can be performed during ERCP, including gallstone removal or sphincterotomy (widening of the ampulla)
◆ Barium enema (lower GI series) introduces liquid barium into the colon to visualize its movement, position, and filling of the various segments
◆ Barium swallow (upper GI series) involves ingestion of liquid barium to visualize the position, shape, and activity of the esophagus, stomach, duodenum, and jejunum
◆ Cholecystography involves ingestion of a contrast medium, followed by fatty meal consumption; X-rays of the dye-filled gallbladder are then taken to assess gallbladder function and detect gallstones
◆ Cholangiography uses an I.V. contrast medium to visualize the hepatic, cystic, and common bile ducts for patency
◆ Gastric analysis with histamine or Histalog tests a sample of gastric contents for the presence of hydrochloric acid after I.M. or subcutaneous histamine administration

◆ Hydrogen breath tests diagnose intestinal bacteria overgrowth, lactose (and other carbohydrate) malabsorption, and fat absorption

◆ Fecal occult blood tests detect the presence of blood in the stool, using a stool sample from the rectum

◆ Fecal studies are used to observe for malabsorption, pathogens, occult blood, and protein loss

◆ *Helicobacter pylori* studies—done with serum, gastric biopsy, or breath test—detect the presence of helicobacteria in the GI tract that predispose the patient to peptic ulcer disease

◆ 24-hour pH monitoring (pneumogram) directly detects gastroesophageal reflux or may be used to evaluate noncardiac chest pain

■ Key laboratory values

◆ Amylase (normal value: 26 to 102 units/L)

▶ An elevated amylase level results from acute pancreatitis, duodenal ulcer, cancer of the head of the pancreas, and pancreatic pseudocysts

▶ A decreased amylase level is seen in chronic pancreatitis, pancreatic fibrosis and atrophy, cirrhosis of the liver, and acute alcoholism

◆ Bilirubin (normal value: total, 0.1 to 1.0 mg/dl; direct, less than 0.5 mg/dl; indirect, 1.1 mg/dl)

▶ An elevated bilirubin level results from biliary obstruction, hepatocellular damage, pernicious anemia, hemolytic anemia, and hemolytic disease of the neonate

▶ A decreased bilirubin level occurs in certain malnutrition states

◆ Cholesterol (normal values: total ≤ 200 mg/dl; LDL ≤ 100 mg/dl; HDL ≥ 40 mg/dl)

▶ An elevated cholesterol level results from hyperlipidemia, obstructive jaundice, diabetes, and hypothyroidism

▶ A decreased cholesterol level occurs with pernicious anemia, hemolytic jaundice, hyperthyroidism, severe infections, and terminal diseases

◆ Iron (normal value: 50 to 170 mcg/dl)

▶ An elevated level occurs with pernicious anemia, aplastic anemia, hemolytic anemia, hepatitis, and hemochromatosis

▶ A decreased level occurs with iron deficiency anemia

◆ Leucine aminopeptidase (normal value: 75 to 200 units/ml)

▶ An elevated value occurs with liver and biliary tract disease, pancreatic disease, metastatic cancer of the liver or pancreas, and biliary obstruction

▶ A decreased value isn't associated with any disease states

◆ Lipase (normal value: less than 160 units/L)

▶ An elevated level occurs with acute or chronic pancreatitis, biliary obstruction, cirrhosis, hepatitis, and peptic ulcer

▶ A decreased level occurs with fibrotic disease of the pancreas

◆ Pepsinogen (normal value: 200 to 425 units/ml)

▶ An elevated level isn't associated with any disease states

▶ A decreased level occurs with conditions involving decreased gastric acidity, pernicious anemia, and achlorhydria

◆ Protein (normal value: total, 7.0 to 7.5 g/dl)

▶ An elevated level occurs with hemoconcentration and shock states

◗ A decreased level occurs with malnutrition or hemorrhage
◆ Aspartate aminotransferase (normal value: 12 to 31 units/L)
  ◗ An increased level occurs with liver disease, myocardial infarction, and skeletal muscle disease
  ◗ A decreased level isn't associated with any disease states
◆ Alanine aminotransferase (normal value: 8 to 50 international units/L)
  ◗ A highly elevated level occurs with liver disease
  ◗ A decreased level isn't associated with any disease states
◆ Gastric analysis
  ◗ The normal value for free hydrochloric acid is 0 to 30 mEq/L; for total acidity, 15 to 45 mEq/L; and for combined acid, 10 to 15 mEq/L
  ◗ All values are increased in peptic ulcer disease; all values are decreased in pernicious anemia, gastric carcinoma, gastritis, and aging

❖ **Acute GI hemorrhage**
■ Description
  ◆ Common causes of GI hemorrhage include duodenal ulcer, gastric ulcer, erosive gastritis, varices, esophagitis, Mallory-Weiss syndrome, and bowel infarction
■ Medical management
  ◆ Administer colloids, crystalloids, and whole blood or packed cells to maintain blood pressure
  ◆ Administer vitamin K, calcium, or platelets to reduce bleeding
  ◆ Initiate vasopressin or sclerotherapy to reduce variant bleeding
  ◆ Initiate pharmacological agents to decrease gastric acid secretion and diminish acid effects on gastric mucosa, including proton pump inhibitors, histamine blockers, and antacids
  ◆ Endoscopy is the treatment of choice for ulcers and varices with profuse blood loss; sclerotherapy or band ligation of bleeding varices may be done through the endoscope
  ◆ Transjugular intrahepatic portosystemic shunt is an interventional radiology technique that creates a parenchymal tract from the hepatic to portal vein; this relieves pressure from variceal bleeding, lowering portal pressure
  ◆ Insert an esophageal tube to control bleeding from esophageal varices (see *Comparing esophageal tubes*, page 222)
  ◆ Surgery may be indicated if bleeding is life-threatening
■ Nursing management
  ◆ Monitor vital signs (blood pressure, heart rate and rhythm, respiratory rate, and temperature) every 5 minutes until the patient is stable; frequent monitoring of vital signs allows early detection of abnormalities and prompt initiation of treatment to prevent further complications
  ◆ Monitor cardiac output and hemodynamic pressures, including central venous pressure (CVP), right arterial pressure, pulmonary artery wedge pressure (PAWP), and pulmonary artery pressure (PAP); these parameters are critical indicators of cardiac function, reflecting left ventricular function, fluid status, and arterial perfusion of vital organs
  ◆ Monitor hemoglobin level and hematocrit for indication of further hemorrhage; decreased levels are seen 4 to 6 hours after a bleeding episode;

Comparing esophageal tubes

Three types of esophageal tubes are the Linton tube, the Minnesota esophagogastric tamponade tube, and the Sengstaken-Blakemore tube.

Linton tube

The Linton tube, a three-lumen, single-balloon device, has ports for esophageal and gastric aspiration. Because the tube doesn't have an esophageal balloon, it isn't used to control bleeding for esophageal varices.

Large-capacity gastric balloon
Esophageal aspiration lumen
Gastric aspiration lumen
Gastric balloon-inflation lumen

Minnesota esophagogastric tamponade tube

The Minnesota esophagogastric tamponade tube has four lumens and two balloons. It has pressure-monitoring ports for both balloons.

Gastric balloon
Esophageal balloon
Gastric balloon-inflation lumen
Gastric balloon pressure-monitoring port
Gastric aspiration lumen
Esophageal aspiration lumen
Esophageal balloon pressure-monitoring port
Esophageal balloon-inflation lumen

Sengstaken-Blakemore tube

The Sengstaken-Blakemore tube, a three-lumen device with esophageal and gastric balloons, has a gastric aspiration port that allows drainage from below the gastric balloon and is also used to instill medication.

Gastric balloon
Esophageal balloon
Gastric balloon-inflation lumen
Gastric aspiration lumen
Esophageal balloon-inflation lumen

values are also decreased by hemodilution and crystalloid fluid replacement

◆ Monitor blood urea nitrogen (BUN), serum electrolyte, creatinine, and ammonia levels

▶ Sodium and potassium levels are transiently decreased following volume restoration and increased after a bleeding episode; the body responds to bleeding by conserving sodium and water to maintain volume

▶ The potassium level increases over time as transfusions free potassium, releasing it into serum; the breakdown of red blood cells (RBCs) in the intestines frees additional potassium

▶ The calcium level decreases after massive transfusions of stored blood; citrate in the stored blood binds circulating calcium

▶ BUN and creatinine levels increase after a bleeding episode, as the breakdown of blood into intestinal products overwhelms the kidneys' capacity to excrete them; hypovolemia and shock lead to decreased glomerular filtration

▶ The ammonia level increases, as liver dysfunction impairs clearance of the intestinal products of blood breakdown; encephalopathy results

◆ Monitor arterial blood gas (ABG) values, and remember that respiratory alkalosis can develop early; decreased perfusion of the lungs during shock stimulates hyperventilation, and lactic acid buildup leads to metabolic acidosis

◆ Frequently assess for chest congestion, as evidenced by crackles and wheezes, dyspnea, shortness of breath, orthopnea, and cough with pink, frothy sputum; patients with GI hemorrhage are at high risk for impaired gas exchange related to hemoglobin deficit and for pulmonary edema due to fluid overload

◆ Assess urine output and specific gravity hourly; a high urine specific gravity and output less than 30 ml per hour indicates renal failure secondary to decreased circulating volume or compensatory vasoconstriction

◆ Monitor the patient for signs of respiratory distress or back pain, which may indicate esophageal rupture or tracheal occlusion caused by the esophageal tube balloon

◆ Maintain traction on the Sengstaken-Blakemore tube; keep the gastric and esophageal balloons at the correct pressures, with periodic deflation and inflation as prescribed; traction of inflated balloons against varices maintains tamponade of bleeding mucosal surfaces; periodic deflation and inflation of the balloons prevents tissue necrosis

◆ Maintain patent gastric aspiration and oropharyngeal ports; because these tubes aren't vented, intermittent suction must be applied to maintain patency

◆ Keep the head of the bed elevated to maximize lung ventilation

◆ Administer supplemental oxygen, as prescribed, to maintain or reestablish normal oxygenation status

◆ Monitor for signs of continued bleeding by checking gastric aspirate and stools, which may appear black, sticky, or dark red (melena) if they contain blood; prompt recognition of further bleeding episodes allows early intervention to stem the bleeding and prevent hypovolemic shock

◆ Assess the patient's level of consciousness (LOC) and neuromuscular function and response; these signs and symptoms may result from elevated serum ammonia secondary to increased protein load from GI bleeding

◆ If symptoms of encephalopathy develop, orient the patient to time, place, and person as necessary to decrease anxiety and fear; increased anxiety level and fear could directly affect the central nervous system (CNS) and influence hemodynamic stability

◆ Explain all procedures before initiating to help decrease the patient's anxiety

◆ Encourage the patient to verbalize his feelings; this supports development of adaptive coping skills

❖ **Hepatic failure and hepatic coma**
- Description
  - ◆ The liver is vital to most bodily processes; even mild disorders of the biliary system can cause life-threatening alterations in bodily functions
    - ◆ Cirrhosis causes liver cells to degenerate
      - ▶ As the affected liver cells degenerate, nodule formation and scar tissue result; this leads to a resistance to hepatoportal blood flow and hepatoportal hypertension
      - ▶ Ultimately, cirrhosis causes decreased functioning of the liver, hepatic encephalopathy, and hepatic coma
    - ◆ Fulminant hepatitis is a severe, often fatal, form of hepatitis in which liver cells fail to regenerate, leading to necrotic progression
    - ◆ Hepatic failure results from severe hepatic necrosis, accompanied by loss of the liver's synthetic and excretory functions; it eventually leads to multiple organ dysfunction syndrome
    - ◆ Causes of hepatic failure include viral hepatitis (see *Types of viral hepatitis*), alcoholism, and drug overdose
- Clinical signs and symptoms
  - ◆ Asterixis and hyperactive reflexes
  - ◆ Slurred speech
  - ◆ Generalized seizures
  - ◆ Tachycardia, arrhythmias, and fever
  - ◆ Peripheral edema, ascites
  - ◆ Rapid, shallow respirations with fetor hepaticus
  - ◆ Jaundice and mucosal bleeding
  - ◆ Hepatomegaly and tenderness in the right upper quadrant of the abdomen
  - ◆ Dark amber urine and decreased urine output
  - ◆ Laboratory results may reveal coagulopathy (prothrombin time [PT] greater than 13 seconds, activated partial thromboplastin time greater than 40 seconds), elevated white blood cell (WBC) count, hypoglycemia, and elevated serum ammonia; laboratory findings vary depending on etiology
- Medical management
  - ◆ Administer oxygen, as indicated
  - ◆ Neomycin to clean the gut and lactulose to decrease serum ammonia levels
  - ◆ Restrict dietary sodium to 200 to 500 mg per day

Types of viral hepatitis

Use this table to compare the features of various types of viral hepatitis characterized to date. Other types are emerging.

Feature	Hepatitis A	Hepatitis B	Hepatitis C	Hepatitis D	Hepatitis E	Hepatitis G
Incubation	15 to 45 days	30 to 180 days	15 to 160 days	14 to 64 days	14 to 60 days	2 to 6 weeks
Onset	Acute	Insidious	Insidious	Acute	Acute	Presumed insidious
Age-group commonly affected	Children, young adults	Any age	More common in adults	Any age	Ages 20 to 40	Any age, primarily adults
Transmission	Fecal-oral, sexual (especially oral-anal contact), nonpercutaneous (sexual, maternal-neonatal), percutaneous (rare)	Blood-borne; parenteral route, sexual, maternal-neonatal; virus is shed in all body fluids	Blood-borne; parenteral route	Parenteral route; most people infected with hepatitis D are also infected with hepatitis B	Primarily fecal-oral	Blood-borne; similar to Hepatitis B and C
Severity	Mild	Commonly severe	Moderate	Can be severe and lead to fulminant hepatitis	Highly virulent with common progression to fulminant hepatitis and hepatic failure, especially in pregnant patients	Moderate
Prognosis	Generally good	Worsens with age and debility	Moderate	Fair, worsens in chronic cases; can lead to chronic hepatitis D and chronic liver disease	Good unless pregnant	Generally good; no current treatment recommendations
Progression to chronicity	None	Occasional	10% to 50% of cases	Occasional	None	Not known; no association with chronic liver disease

◆ Restrict fluid intake to about 1,500 ml per day; space the fluid intake throughout a 24-hour period, with the greatest volume during the day and the least at night

◆ Administer diuretics in combination with an aldosterone antagonist, such as spironolactone
◆ Administer dextran or albumin
■ Nursing management
◆ Monitor vital signs (blood pressure, heart rate and rhythm, respiratory rate, and temperature) every 5 to 15 minutes until stable, then every 15 to 30 minutes
  ▶ In the patient with hepatic failure, blood pressure eventually decreases due to fluid transudation and the release of vasoactive substances from the damaged liver
◆ Monitor CVP every hour
  ▶ Elevated CVP may be a sign of fluid overload, which can directly affect cardiac output
  ▶ Decreased CVP may be a sign of low circulatory volume and leakage of fluid into the third space
◆ Monitor for signs of cardiovascular changes, such as flushed skin, hypertension, bounding pulses, and enhanced precordial impulse
  ▶ Cardiovascular symptoms may occur initially due to the patient's hyperdynamic state
  ▶ Arrhythmias can be caused by electrolyte changes; bradycardia may be noted with severe hyperbilirubinemia
◆ Monitor ABG and arterial oxygen saturation values
  ▶ Patients with hepatic failure are at risk for respiratory problems related to encephalopathy and altered LOC
  ▶ Additionally, pleural effusion can compress lung tissue, as ascitic fluid leaks into the pleural space; if this occurs, the patient may become hypoxemic
◆ Monitor the patient's complete blood count and PT; assess for signs of impaired coagulation, including bruising, nosebleeds, and petechiae
  ▶ Clotting factors are deficient in patients with hepatic failure, which could lead to disseminated intravascular coagulation
  ▶ Decreased hemoglobin level and hematocrit indicate recent bleeding episodes and the liver's inability to store hematopoietic factors, including iron, folic acid, and vitamin B_{12}
  ▶ Decreased WBC and platelet counts are associated with splenomegaly; an elevated WBC count indicates infection
◆ Monitor sodium, potassium, calcium, and magnesium levels
  ▶ Initially, sodium and water retention occur in intravascular spaces due to decreased metabolism of antidiuretic hormone (ADH)
    • As the liver becomes congested and hepatoportal vein pressure increases, fluid seeps into the peritoneal cavity, causing decreased plasma volume
    • This results in release of ADH and aldosterone, with activation of the renin-angiotensin-aldosterone system
    • As a result, sodium and water retention occur, with the eventual development of dilutional hyponatremia
  ▶ Hypokalemia may result from diarrhea, aldosterone secretion, and the use of diuretics

Stages of hepatic encephalopathy

Hepatic encephalopathy progresses as the serum ammonia level increases and as the liver continues to fail; it's divided into four stages. Identification of the signs and symptoms of a particular stage can help the nurse determine the extent of encephalopathy and, consequently, hepatic failure.

Stage	Signs
Stage I—Prodromal stage	Disorientation; tremors of the extremities; personality changes (usually becoming hostile, uncooperative, and belligerent); slurred speech; forgetfulness
Stage II—Impending stage	Tremors progressing to asterixis, lethargy, abberant behavior, apraxia
Stage III—Stuporous stage	Hyperventilation with stupor; patient noisy and abusive when stimulated
Stage IV—Comatose stage	Hyperactive reflexes; positive Babinski's sign; coma; musty, sweet breath odor

▶ Hypocalcemia results from decreased dietary intake and decreased absorption of vitamin D

▶ Hypomagnesemia is caused by the liver's inability to store magnesium

▶ Hypoglycemia can occur when the impaired liver can't metabolize glycogen; monitor blood glucose levels frequently, as indicated

◆ Assess serum albumin and total protein levels; these decrease due to impaired protein synthesis

◆ Check the results of liver function tests, and monitor bilirubin and ammonia levels

▶ Aspartate aminotransferase, alanine aminotransferase, alkaline phosphatase, and lactate dehydrogenase levels increase as a result of damage to hepatocellular or biliary tissue in liver failure

▶ The bilirubin level increases as a result of liver dysfunction, leading to jaundice

▶ The ammonia level increases due to impaired hepatic synthesis of urea

◆ Monitor for signs of hepatic encephalopathy by assessing the patient's general appearance, behavior, orientation, and speech patterns; signs of hepatic encephalopathy worsen as a result of the high ammonia level caused by liver dysfunction (see *Stages of hepatic encephalopathy*)

◆ Monitor GI status by assessing for nausea, vomiting, increased abdominal pain, and decreased or absent bowel sounds

▶ Increased intra-abdominal pressure caused by ascites compresses the GI tract and reduces its capacity to hold food

▶ Venous congestion in the GI tract can lead to nausea

▶ Pain can result from continued venous engorgement of internal organs and ascites

◆ Check for increased abdominal girth, rapid weight loss or gain, asterixis, tremors, confusion, and signs of bleeding

▶ Increased abdominal girth indicates worsening portal hypertension

◗ Rapid weight loss or gain is a sign of negative nitrogen balance; weight gain may also result from fluid retention

◗ Asterixis (irregular flapping of forcibly dorsiflexed and outstretched hands) indicates worsening hepatic encephalopathy

◗ Tremors result from impaired neurotransmission, caused by failure of the liver to detoxify enzymes that act as false neurotransmitters

◗ Confusion results from cerebral hypoxia due to high serum ammonia levels (a result of the liver's inability to convert ammonia to urea)

◗ Bleeding is a sign of decreased PT and clotting factor deficiency

◆ Provide periods of uninterrupted rest

◗ Physical activity depletes the body of the energy required to heal the damaged liver

◗ Adequate rest may prevent a relapse

◆ Give vitamin K, as prescribed; vitamin K is required for the synthesis of blood coagulation factors II (prothrombin), VII (proconvertin), IX (plasma thromboplastin component or Christmas factor), and X (Stuart factor or Stuart-Prower factor)

◆ Avoid injections if possible, and apply pressure to all puncture sites for 5 minutes; the patient is at increased risk for bleeding and hemorrhage due to deficiency of vitamin K-dependent clotting factors

◆ Tell the patient to avoid straining or coughing, which may precipitate bleeding of esophageal varices or hemorrhoids (secondary to portal hypertension)

◆ Examine all vomitus and stools for the presence of blood; occult bleeding can be life-threatening because of the patient's volume deficit

◆ Maintain a safe environment to prevent injuries that could trigger a hemorrhage, such as injuries from falls

◆ Provide mouth care; administer antiemetics, such as trimethobenzamide (Tigan) or dimenhydrinate (Dramamine), before meals as prescribed

◗ Accumulation of food particles in the mouth contributes to foul odors and taste, which diminish appetite

◗ Use of prophylactic antiemetics reduces the likelihood of anorexia

◆ Administer high-calorie (1,600 to 2,500 calories per day) carbohydrate nutrients with supplemental vitamins via nasogastric (NG) tube or I.V. line; when encephalopathy subsides, introduce protein sources, beginning at a rate of 20 g per day

◗ In the patient with liver dysfunction, catabolism creates a nutritional deficit that must be counteracted with a high caloric intake

● Proteins must not be given to patients with hepatic encephalopathy because the diseased liver can't metabolize protein

● Protein intolerance can become chronic, depending on the severity and chronicity of the liver dysfunction

◗ To prevent aspiration in patients with hepatic encephalopathy or coma, administer nutrition with a small-bore tube (such as a Dobhoff tube); for patients experiencing persistent vomiting, administer I.V. (see *Enteral feeding routes*)

◆ Administer I.V. fluids and electrolytes, as prescribed

Enteral feeding routes

The table below shows various enteral feeding routes and the indications for their use.

Access	Indications
Nasogastric or orogastric	• Short-term • No esophageal reflux • Gag reflex intact • Normal gastric and duodenum emptying
Nasoduodenal or nasojejunal	• Short-term • Esophageal reflux • High risk of pulmonary aspiration • Delayed gastric emptying
Esophageal or pharyngostomy	• Long-term • Head or neck tumors • Nasopharyngeal access contraindicated
Gastrostomy	• Long-term • Swallowing dysfunction • Nasoenteric access contraindicated • Normal gastric and duodenum emptying • Esophageal stricture or neoplasm
Jejunostomy	• Long-term • Esophageal reflux • High risk of pulmonary aspiration • Impaired gastric emptying • Failure to access upper GI tract • Postoperative feeding in trauma, malnourishment, or upper GI surgery

▶ Hepatic failure can cause decreased renal blood flow and reduced glomerular filtration, resulting in renal failure; renal failure in the presence of hepatic failure is called hepatorenal syndrome

▶ Fluids and electrolytes maintain circulating plasma volume and hemodynamic stability

◆ Administer lactulose, as prescribed

▶ Lactulose passes unchanged into the large intestine, where it's metabolized by bacteria, producing lactic acids and carbon dioxide

▶ This metabolic process decreases the pH to about 5.5, which favors the conversion of ammonia to ammonium ions and subsequent excretion in the stool

▶ The laxative action of lactulose further enhances evacuation of ammonia-rich stools

▶ Neomycin therapy may be ordered if lactulose alone doesn't reduce ammonia levels

◆ Administer enemas as prescribed to remove ammonia from the intestine

◆ Use a special mattress that reduces pressure on the skin, turn the patient frequently, and keep the skin clean and moisturized with lotion to prevent skin breakdown

◆ Monitor for adverse effects of medications, and avoid administering opioid analgesics, sedatives, and tranquilizers; in patients with liver dysfunction, metabolism of these drugs is decreased, thereby increasing the risk of drug toxicity

❖ Acute pancreatitis
■ Description
◆ Acute pancreatitis is an inflammation of pancreatic tissues
◆ It's caused by the premature activation and release of proteolytic enzymes, which autodigest the organ itself
◆ The enzyme trypsin is thought to play a role in the pathology of pancreatitis
◆ The inflammatory response within the pancreas can be hemorrhagic, with tissue necrosis extending to the vascular compartment, or nonhemorrhagic, with acute interstitial or acute edematous inflammation caused by the escape of digestive enzymes into surrounding tissue
◆ The inflammatory and autodigestive process leads to tissue necrosis; precipitation of calcium, with resultant hypocalcemia; release of necrotic toxins, which serve as precursors to sepsis; leakage of large volumes of albumin-rich pancreatic exudates into the peritoneum; and, ultimately, shock and death
■ Clinical signs and symptoms
◆ Severe epigastric pain
◆ Nausea and vomiting
◆ Hypotension and tachycardia
◆ Distended abdomen with distant bowel sounds and guarding on palpation (peritonitis)
◆ Turner's sign (bruising at the flanks) and Cullen's sign (bluish discoloration at the umbilicus) are late signs of pancreatitis, indicating retroperitoneal bleeding
◆ Laboratory tests show increased amylase and lipase levels, increased WBC count, and decreased potassium; abdominal CT is the definitive diagnostic tool for acute pancreatitis; ultrasonography and endoscopic retrograde cholangiopancreatography may also be used in diagnosis
■ Medical management
◆ The patient should have nothing by mouth to reduce stimulation of gastric secretions
◆ Insert an NG tube for drainage or suction
◆ Administer I.V. meperidine, and assess its effectiveness in pain relief
◆ Administer antacids to decrease inflammation
◆ Keep the patient on nothing-by-mouth status, and maintain NG tube drainage until bowel sounds return and abdominal pain subsides
◆ While the patient is on nothing-by-mouth status, administer I.V. fluid solutions; add potassium chloride, calcium, multivitamin supplements, thiamine, and folic acid to maintain nutritional status
◆ Consult with a nutritional support team or dietitian on the patient's nutritional status and nutrition repletion program; total parenteral nutri-

tion can prevent stimulation of gastric enzymes and provide nutritional and electrolyte balance (see *Types of parenteral nutrition,* pages 232 and 233)

◆ Institute alternate feeding methods if nothing-by-mouth status must be prolonged

■ Nursing management

◆ Monitor vital signs (blood pressure, heart rate and rhythm, respiratory rate, and temperature) every 5 to 15 minutes until the patient is stable, then every 30 to 60 minutes; frequent monitoring of vital signs permits early recognition of abnormalities and prompt initiation of treatment to prevent further complications

◆ Monitor hemodynamic parameters (CVP, PAP, PAWP, and cardiac output) as ordered; the patient's hemodynamic status provides an indication of the effectiveness of interventions

◆ Monitor for signs and symptoms of hypovolemia and shock, including increased pulse rate; normal or slightly decreased blood pressure; urine output less than 30 ml per hour; restlessness, agitation, and change in mentation; increasing respiratory rate; diminished peripheral pulses; cool, pale, or cyanotic skin; increased thirst; and decreased hemoglobin level and hematocrit

▶ Hypovolemia, a major cause of death secondary to pancreatitis, may have several origins, including decreased oral intake, nothing-by-mouth status, and excess fluid loss through NG tube drainage or vomiting

▶ In addition, pancreatic enzymes destroy vessel walls, resulting in bleeding; plasma shifts (secondary to increased vascular permeability due to the inflammatory response) also contribute to hypovolemia

▶ The compensatory response to decreased circulatory volume involves efforts to raise blood oxygen levels, heart and respiratory rates increase, and circulation to the extremities is reduced, resulting in decreased peripheral pulses and cool skin

▶ Diminished oxygen to the brain causes changes in mentation

▶ Decreased circulation to the kidneys leads to decreased urine output

◆ Monitor fluid status by assessing parenteral and oral intake, urine output, and fluid loss resulting from NG tube drainage or vomiting

▶ Fluid shifts, NG suctioning, and nothing-by-mouth status can disrupt fluid balance in a patient with acute pancreatitis; stress may cause sodium and water retention

▶ Early detection of a fluid deficit allows prompt intervention to prevent hypovolemic shock

◆ Collaborate with the physician to replace fluid losses at a rate sufficient to maintain urine output greater than 0.5 ml/kg/hour; this promotes optimal tissue perfusion

◆ Monitor for signs and symptoms of hypocalcemia, including mentation changes, numbness and tingling of fingers and toes, muscle cramps, seizures, and electrocardiogram (ECG) changes. Check for Chvostek's sign (facial twitching when the cheek is tapped) and Trousseau's sign (hand spasm when a blood pressure cuff is inflated over the arm for 3 minutes)

Types of parenteral nutrition

Type	Solution components per liter	Uses
Total parenteral nutrition by central venous (CV) catheter or peripherally inserted central catheter into the superior vena cava through the infraclavicular vein (most common), supraclavicular vein, internal jugular vein, or antecubital fossa	• $D_{15}W$ to $D_{25}W$ (1 L dextrose 25% = 850 nonprotein calories) • Crystalline amino acids 2.5% to 8.5% • Electrolytes, vitamins, trace elements, and insulin, as ordered • Lipid emulsion 10% to 20% (usually infused as a separate solution)	• When needed for 2 weeks or more • For a patient with large calorie and nutrient needs • Provides calories, restores nitrogen balance, and replaces essential vitamins, electrolytes, minerals, and trace elements • Promotes tissue synthesis, wound healing, and normal metabolic function • Allows bowel rest and healing; reduces activity in the gallbladder, pancreas, and small intestine • Improves tolerance of surgery
Peripheral parenteral nutrition by peripheral catheter	• D_5W to $D_{10}W$ • Crystalline amino acids 2.5% to 5% • Electrolytes, minerals, vitamins, and trace elements, as ordered • Lipid emulsion 10% or 20% (1 L dextrose 10% and amino acids 3.5% infused at the same time as 1 L of lipid emulsion = 1,440 nonprotein calories) • Heparin or hydrocortisone, as ordered	• When needed for 2 weeks or less • Provides up to 2,000 calories/day • Maintains adequate nutritional status in a patient who can tolerate relatively high fluid volume, one who usually resumes bowel function and oral feedings after a few days, and one susceptible to infections associated with the CV catheter

▶ Hypocalcemia may result from the kidneys' inability to metabolize vitamin D, which is needed for calcium absorption

▶ Retention of phosphorus causes a reciprocal drop in serum calcium level

▶ A low serum calcium level produces increased neural excitability (tetany), which leads to muscle spasms and CNS irritability (manifested as seizures); it also causes cardiac muscle hyperactivity, as evidenced by ECG changes (monitor QT interval)

▶ Calcium binds with free fats, which are excreted because of a lack of lipase and phospholipase—enzymes needed for digestion

◆ If hypocalcemia occurs, administer calcium via bolus infusion, as prescribed; consult with a dietitian on a high-calcium, low-phosphorus diet; monitor for hyperphosphatemia and hypomagnesemia; and observe for ECG changes

◆ Monitor for signs and symptoms of sepsis; monitor temperature, vital signs, and WBC count

◆ Monitor glucose levels in blood and urine; injury to pancreatic beta cells decreases insulin production, but injury to pancreatic alpha cells increases glucagon production

◆ Monitor for signs and symptoms of hyperglycemia, including polyuria and polydipsia

Special considerations

Basic solution
- Nutritionally complete
- Requires minor surgical procedure for CV line insertion
- Highly hypertonic solution
- May cause pneumothorax (typically during catheter insertion), phlebitis, thrombus formation, air embolus, infection, sepsis, and metabolic complications (glucose intolerance, electrolyte imbalance, essential fatty acid deficiency)
- Must be delivered in a vein with high blood flow rate because glucose content may be increased beyond the level a peripheral vein can handle (commonly six times more concentrated than blood)

I.V. lipid emulsion
- May not be used effectively in a severely stressed patient (especially a patient with burns)
- May interfere with immune mechanisms; in a patient suffering from respiratory compromise, reduces carbon dioxide buildup
- Given by way of CV line

Basic solution
- Nutritionally complete for a short time
- Can't be used in a nutritionally depleted patient
- Can't be used in a volume-restricted patient
- Doesn't cause weight gain
- Avoids insertion and care of the CV line, but requires adequate venous access site; must be changed every 72 hours
- May cause phlebitis and increases risk of metabolic complications
- Less chance of metabolic complications than with CV line
- To avoid venous sclerosis, must contain no more than 10% dextrose, so patient must tolerate large fluid volume to meet nutritional needs

I.V. lipid emulsion
- As effective as dextrose for calorie source
- Diminishes phlebitis if infused at the same time as basic nutrient solution
- Irritates vein in long-term use
- Reduces carbon dioxide buildup when pulmonary compromise is present

◗ Without insulin, cells can't utilize glucose
◗ As a result, protein and fats are metabolized, leading to the production of ketones
◆ Monitor for later manifestations of ketoacidosis, such as serum glucose level greater than 300 mg/dl, positive serum and urine ketones, acetone breath, headache, Kussmaul's respirations, anorexia, nausea, vomiting, tachycardia, decreased blood pressure, polyuria, polydipsia, and decreased serum sodium, potassium, and phosphate levels
◗ Excessive ketone bodies cause headaches, nausea, vomiting, and abdominal pain
◗ The respiratory rate and depth increase in an attempt to increase carbon dioxide excretion to reduce acidosis
◗ Glucose inhibits water reabsorption in the renal glomerulus, leading to osmotic diuresis with severe loss of water, sodium, potassium, and phosphate
◆ If ketoacidosis occurs, initiate appropriate treatment protocols: administer normal or half-normal saline solution I.V., begin an I.V. infusion of dextrose 5% when the serum glucose level is between 250 and 300 mg/dl, add insulin (about 6 to 10 units per hour) to I.V. fluids, administer I.V. potassium and phosphate supplements, and administer bicarbonate I.V., as prescribed; these interventions restore the insulin-glucagon ratio and

treat circulatory collapse, ketoacidosis, and electrolyte imbalance in a patient with severe acidosis

◆ Monitor serum potassium, sodium, and phosphate levels

▶ Acidosis causes hyperkalemia and hyponatremia

▶ Insulin therapy promotes the return of potassium and phosphate to the cells, causing serum hypokalemia and hypophosphatemia

◆ Monitor BUN and serum albumin, protein, and cholesterol levels and hemoglobin and hematocrit

▶ The presence of insufficient pancreatic enzymes in the GI tract results in insufficient protein catabolism and decreased protein absorption, producing decreased levels of BUN, serum albumin, cholesterol, and transferrin

▶ A decreased transferrin level causes inadequate iron absorption and transport, resulting in decreased hemoglobin level and hematocrit

◆ Monitor serum amylase, lipase, calcium, bilirubin, and alkaline phosphatase levels; urine amylase level; and WBC count

▶ Elevated levels of serum amylase, serum lipase, and urine amylase are signs of pancreatic cell injury

▶ Serum calcium level decreases as fatty acids combine with calcium during fat necrosis

▶ The serum bilirubin and alkaline phosphatase levels and WBC count are increased by hepatobiliary involvement, obstructive processes, and the inflammatory response

◆ Monitor for signs and symptoms of alcohol withdrawal: tremors, diaphoresis, anorexia, nausea, vomiting, increased heart and respiratory rates, agitation, visual or auditory hallucinations, and alcohol withdrawal delirium

▶ Chronic alcohol abuse may cause pancreatitis, and the signs and symptoms of alcohol withdrawal may be apparent even when the patient denies alcoholism

▶ Signs of alcohol withdrawal can begin 24 hours after the last drink and may continue for 1 to 2 weeks; monitor for withdrawal symptoms and seizures, and administer medications as prescribed

◆ Monitor arterial oxygen saturation to detect hypoxia and hypoxemia

◆ Monitor for signs and symptoms of hypovolemic shock; if hypovolemic shock occurs, place the patient in the supine position with his legs elevated (unless contraindicated)

◆ Monitor neurologic status every hour; fluctuating glucose level, acidosis, and fluid shifts can affect neurologic functioning

◆ Monitor cardiac function and circulatory status by assessing skin color, capillary refill time, peripheral pulses, and serum potassium level

▶ Severe dehydration can reduce cardiac output and cause compensatory vasoconstriction

▶ Arrhythmias can be caused by potassium imbalances

◆ Monitor for signs of paralytic ileus, which may manifest as localized, sharp, or intermittent pain

▶ Paralytic ileus results from impaired peristaltic activity of the bowel, caused by ischemia from hypovolemia

▶ It also can be related to the use of opioid analgesics, which affect peristaltic action

◆ Assess for physical signs of acute pain, such as increased heart and respiratory rates, elevated blood pressure, restlessness, facial grimacing, and guarding; some patients are reluctant to admit pain, and the assessment of these signs and symptoms may be the only method to determine pain level

◆ Assess verbal complaints of abdominal pain, and determine its specific location and intensity; acute pancreatitis can cause severe and diffuse pain

◆ Work with the patient to determine the most effective methods of pain management

◆ Intervene to reduce accumulated gas, which may be painful; encourage frequent position changes, administer nonnarcotic analgesics, advance the diet slowly, avoid large meals, and restrict dietary fat intake

◆ Ensure that the NG tube is properly secured, apply a water-soluble lubricant around the nares, and turn the patient every 2 hours; these interventions help reduce the discomfort associated with NG tube placement

◆ Monitor the frequency, consistency, odor, and amount of stools

▶ Decreased secretion of pancreatic enzymes impairs protein and fat digestion; these undigested fats are excreted in the stool

▶ Steatorrhea (large amounts of fat in the stool) indicates impaired digestion

◆ Assess the patient's nutritional status with weight on admission and daily thereafter, monitor hourly intake, and inspect for signs of malnutrition, including fragile and lackluster hair, sunken eyes with pale conjunctivae, dry and swollen oral mucous membranes, and smooth or coated tongue

▶ Pancreatitis can negatively affect nutrition due to decreased intake and impaired digestion

▶ Changes in weight provide an indication of nitrogen balance; weight loss reflects a negative nitrogen balance and breakdown of muscle mass (catabolism), whereas weight gain reflects a positive nitrogen balance and buildup of muscle mass (anabolism)

◆ Evaluate the adequacy of the patient's diet in meeting nutritional requirements; when the patient can tolerate the NG tube clamped for several hours, small amounts of clear liquids may be given; the diet is generally advanced to a bland, high protein and carbohydrate diet; antacids and pancreatic replacement enzymes may be given when food is introduced

◆ Assess the patient's complaints of nausea, vomiting, stomatitis, gastritis, and flatus; these symptoms can adversely affect eating patterns

◆ Position the patient on his side with his knees flexed to reduce pressure and tension on the abdominal muscles

◆ Place the patient in semi-Fowler's position to allow for maximum expansion of the diaphragm; this helps decrease ventilatory effort and increase ventilation

◆ Restrict the patient to bed rest, and provide a quiet environment; keeping him rested and in bed decreases the metabolic rate, GI stimulation, and GI secretion, thereby reducing abdominal pain

◆ Provide reassurance, simple explanations, and emotional support to help reduce the patient's anxiety; a high level of anxiety increases the metabolic demand for oxygen

◆ Explain all procedures before proceeding to decrease the patient's anxiety

❖ **Gastroesophageal reflux**
  ■ Description
    ◆ Backflow of gastric or duodenal contents into the esophagus, past the lower esophageal sphincter (LES)
      ❱ Normal pressure of the LES usually prevents gastric contents from entering the esophagus
      ❱ When pressure in the stomach exceeds the LES pressure, or the LES is deficient, reflux can occur
    ◆ Several factors predispose a patient to reflux
      ❱ Pyloric surgery (alteration or removal of the pylorus), which allows reflux of bile or pancreatic juice
      ❱ NG intubation for longer than 4 days
      ❱ Any agent that may lower the pressure of the LES: food, alcohol, cigarettes, anticholinergics, morphine, diazepam, calcium-channel blockers
      ❱ The presence of a hiatal hernia with an incompetent sphincter
      ❱ Any condition or position that may increase intra-abdominal pressure
    ◆ Reflux esophagitis may occur from the continual presence of acid in the esophagus
      ❱ Sedentary or bedridden patients are at risk for aspiration of the gastric contents
  ■ Clinical signs and symptoms
    ◆ Some patients may not have symptoms
    ◆ Patients frequently complain of heartburn and regurgitation
      ❱ Symptoms frequently occur 1 to 2 hours after eating and worsen with exercise, lying down, or when bending over
      ❱ Patients report relief from symptoms after using an antacid or sitting upright
    ◆ Hypersecretion of saliva causes sudden fluid accumulation in the throat
    ◆ A dull substernal ache upon swallowing is associated with long-term reflux and esophageal spasm, stricture, or esophagitis
    ◆ Bright red or dark brown blood may be seen in vomitus
    ◆ Chronic pain that radiates to the neck, jaw, and arm mimics angina; often from an esophageal spasm
  ■ Diagnostic tests
    ◆ Esophageal acidity is the most sensitive and accurate test. It monitors the acid level in the esophagus for 12 to 36 hours

◆ Esophageal manometry is used to evaluate the resting pressure of the LES and to determine sphincter competence

◆ An acid perfusion test confirms the esophagitis

◆ Esophagoscopy and a biopsy will allow visualization of the esophagus; this is used to evaluate the extent of the disease and to determine if there are any pathologic changes in the mucosa

■ Medical management

◆ Histamine-2 receptor blocker provides symptom relief

◆ Proton-pump inhibitors treat erosive esophagitis

◆ Surgery (fundoplication, vagotomy or pyloroplasty) may be needed for patients with refractory symptoms or serious complications

■ Nursing management

◆ Elevate the head of the bed at all times, if possible. If patient is intubated and receiving enteral feedings, turn off the feeding when patient is supine

◆ Provide care to the patient after surgery, if indicated

◆ Teach the patient about the causes of reflux and the lifestyle changes that can be made

◆ Give medications as ordered

◆ Consult with a dietitian to develop a diet that will help minimize reflux symptoms

❖ **Bowel infarction, obstruction, and perforation**

■ Description

◆ Bowel infarction results from decreased blood flow to the bowel, which causes vasoconstriction and vasospasm

▶ Vasoconstriction and vasospasm can lead to ischemic bowel, tissue necrosis, gangrenous changes, peritonitis, and local abscess

▶ Bowel infarction is associated with mural thrombosis during the postmyocardial infarction period, decreased cardiac output, arteriosclerosis, cirrhosis, emboli, dislodged plaques, and hypercoagulability

◆ Bowel obstruction occurs when the normal flow of intestinal contents is impeded by a disturbance in the neural stimulation of bowel peristalsis or by other factors (such as inflammation, edema, Crohn's disease, and tumors)

◆ Chronic inflammation and thinning of the bowel mucosa can predispose the bowel to perforation

■ Clinical signs and symptoms

◆ Nausea, vomiting, weight loss, and severe abdominal pain

◆ Hypotension, tachycardia, low-grade fever, and signs of hypovolemia

◆ High-pitched, hyperactive bowel sounds early in the process, then diminished sounds late in the disease

◆ Distended and tender abdomen

◆ Laboratory test results show mild leukocytosis and low hemoglobin and hematocrit

■ Medical management

◆ Insert an NG tube or decompression tube to drain secretions and relieve pressure

◆ Obtain a series of abdominal X-rays to help locate the obstruction

◆ CT or MRI can determine the obstruction's location; monitor for signs of bowel strangulation or peritonitis

◆ Order fluid replacement therapy to prevent hypovolemia and replace electrolytes such as potassium as indicated by laboratory values

◆ Recommend surgery, if indicated, when the cause is diagnosed

■ Nursing management

◆ Monitor vital signs (blood pressure, heart rate and rhythm, respiratory rate, and temperature) every 15 minutes until the patient is stable, then every hour

▶ Increases in blood pressure and heart and respiratory rates can result from the release of catecholamines in response to pain and anxiety

▶ Changes in vital signs also may indicate the presence of infection or changes in fluid volume within the bowel

▶ In a patient with bowel obstruction, body temperature seldom rises above 100° F (37.7° C); higher temperatures—with or without guarding and tenderness—and a sustained elevation in pulse rate suggest strangulated obstruction or peritonitis

▶ Assess the effectiveness of NG decompression by measuring abdominal girth and auscultating for resumption of peristalsis

◆ Assess for nonverbal signs of pain, including grimacing, furrowed brow, tachycardia, shallow or rapid respirations, flushing, restlessness, diaphoresis, and facial pallor

▶ Nonverbal signs of pain may indicate a level of pain that the patient can tolerate without medication; however, it's more likely that the pain is simply not recognized as such (or as manageable with medication) by the patient

▶ Nonverbal signs of pain should be confirmed with the patient to ensure that the pain exists before deciding on the most appropriate course of action

◆ Assess verbal complaints of pain by having the patient identify the location and type of pain, whether it's relieved by the passage of stools, and what measures bring relief; ask the patient to rate the pain on a scale of 1 to 10, with 1 indicating no pain and 10 indicating the greatest pain possible, then compare the level of pain before and after analgesic medication is given

◆ Administer I.V. meperidine, as prescribed, and assess its effectiveness in relieving pain; for pain relief in patients with bowel disease, meperidine is preferred to morphine because morphine may decrease peristaltic activity

◆ Have the patient lie on one side with his knees flexed; this position promotes comfort by reducing pressure and tension on the abdomen

◆ Work with the patient to determine the most effective methods of pain management

◆ If the patient has bowel obstruction secondary to Crohn's disease, assess his understanding of the illness; this chronic disease requires strict adherence to the prescribed medical regimen to prevent or reduce exacerbations

◆ Assess for signs and symptoms of infection; a patient with bowel obstruction or perforation associated with Crohn's disease may have a lowered natural resistance as a result of malnutrition, anemia, alterations in the immune system, or long-term corticosteroid treatment

◆ Assess for signs and symptoms of dehydration, including decreased skin turgor, dry mucous membranes, thirst, weight loss greater than 0.5 kg per day, low blood pressure, weak and rapid pulse rate, and output less than intake with a urine specific gravity greater than 1.030

▶ Excessive loss of fluid and electrolytes may result from vomiting

▶ Impaired absorption of fluid and electrolytes is associated with inflammation and ulceration of the small intestine, as seen in Crohn's disease

▶ A prolonged, inadequate oral intake may be associated with pain, nausea, fatigue, fear of precipitating an attack of abdominal pain, or prescribed dietary restrictions

◆ Monitor potassium level and check for signs and symptoms of hypokalemia, including muscle weakness and cramping, paresthesia, nausea, vomiting, hypoactive or absent bowel sounds, and drowsiness; hypokalemia may result from the loss of potassium-rich intestinal secretions

◆ Monitor magnesium and calcium levels, and assess for signs and symptoms of hypocalcemia, including changes in mental status; arrhythmias; positive Chvostek's sign; positive Trousseau's sign; muscle cramps; tetany; seizures; and numbness and tingling in the fingers, toes, and circumoral area

▶ Absorption of calcium and magnesium is impaired in patients with Crohn's disease

▶ This impairment occurs because of the lack of absorption of vitamin D and fat from the inflamed small intestine; excess fats then bind calcium and magnesium and are excreted in the stool

◆ Assess for signs and symptoms of metabolic acidosis, such as drowsiness, disorientation, stupor, rapid and deep respirations, headache, nausea, and vomiting; obstruction at the end of the small intestine causes loss of bases with fluids and increases the risk of developing metabolic acidosis

◆ Assess the patient's pattern of bowel elimination, noting frequency, characteristics, and amount of stool; note whether blood, fat, mucus, or pus is present in the stool; identification of the bowel pattern ensures timely intervention when a change from the normal pattern occurs

◆ Assess the patient's nutritional status, including total protein and albumin levels; intolerance of certain foods; intake of caffeine-containing drinks and alcohol; appetite; usual weight and recent weight loss; and presence of nausea, weakness, or fatigue

▶ Hypoproteinemia can result from loss of protein through the damaged intestinal epithelium

▶ Weakness results from weight loss caused by decreased nutrient intake and decreased absorption; cachexia may also occur

◆ Monitor for signs and symptoms of intestinal obstruction, including wavelike abdominal pain, abdominal distention, vomiting, change in bowel sounds (initially hyperactive, progressing to absent), and impaction

▶ Inflammation, edema, decreased peristalsis, and tumors may cause bowel obstruction

▶ As a result, intestinal contents are propelled toward the mouth instead of the rectum

◆ Monitor for signs and symptoms of fistulas, fissures, and abscesses; these signs and symptoms include purulent drainage, fecal drainage from the vagina, increased abdominal pain, burning rectal pain after defecation, signs of sepsis (fever and increased WBC count), cyanotic skin tags, and perianal induration, swelling, and redness

▶ The inflammation and ulceration caused by Crohn's disease can penetrate the intestinal wall and form an abscess or fistula in other parts of the intestine or skin

▶ Abscesses and fistulas can cause cramping, pain, and fever and may interfere with digestion

▶ Sepsis may arise from seeding of the bloodstream with bacteria from fistula tracts or abscess cavities

◆ Monitor for signs and symptoms of GI bleeding, including decreased hemoglobin and hematocrit, fatigue, irritability, pallor, tachycardia, dyspnea, anorexia, and increased circumference of the abdomen; chronic inflammation of the bowel can erode vessels, resulting in bleeding

◆ Monitor for signs of anemia, including decreased hemoglobin, decreased RBC count, and vitamin B_{12} and folic acid deficiency

▶ Anemia can result from GI bleeding, bone marrow suppression (which is associated with chronic inflammatory disease), and inadequate intake or impaired absorption of vitamin B_{12}, folic acid, and iron

◆ Administer antibiotics and corticosteroids, as prescribed

▶ Antibiotics decrease the bacteria count in the bowel and are administered prophylactically in anticipation of rupture or perforation and surgical intervention

▶ Corticosteroids are administered to patients with inflammatory bowel disease to prevent or reduce the inflammatory process

◆ Maintain the patency of the NG tube for drainage or suction, as prescribed

▶ Maintaining suction on the NG tube allows for decompression of the GI system

▶ Decompression decreases gastric secretions and peristaltic activity above the bowel obstruction, which could contribute to the patient's pain

◆ Restrict the patient to bed rest in a quiet environment; this measure helps reduce GI stimulation and secretion, decreasing abdominal pain

◆ Turn the patient every 2 hours, and encourage range-of-motion exercises, as tolerated; even though the patient is restricted to bed rest, these movements are necessary to stimulate peristaltic activity

◆ Assist with the insertion of a Miller-Abbot, Levin, or salem sump tube; these tubes, which extend into the small intestine, contain radiopaque weights at the end of a lumen that act as a bolus of food to stimulate peristalsis

◆ Maintain sterile technique during all invasive procedures to prevent contamination and nosocomial infections; long-term corticosteroid use predisposes the patient to infection because it reduces the immune system response

◆ Encourage a fluid intake of 2,500 ml per day when the patient is taking fluids to help soften stool and prevent dehydration

◆ Administer I.V. vitamin supplements, particularly when anorexia and nausea are present, until the obstruction is resolved; then advance to a low-residue, high-protein, high-calorie diet

▶ Supplemental vitamins are necessary while the patient is on nothing-by-mouth status to prevent malnourishment and maintain immune system functioning

▶ Iron supplements may be necessary to prevent or treat anemia

▶ A low-residue diet promotes bowel rest and is less irritating to the mucosal lining

▶ A diet high in protein and calories replaces nutrients lost through the intestinal wall by way of exudation or bleeding; calories are needed for energy to conserve the protein, which is essential for healing

◆ Arrange a dietary consultation to plan an adequate nutritional regimen; total parenteral nutrition may be needed

◆ Place the patient in Fowler's position, if tolerated; maintain oxygen therapy, as prescribed; encourage deep-breathing exercises, nose-breathing, and avoidance of air swallowing

▶ Abdominal distention creates pressure on the diaphragm, inhibiting chest expansion; Fowler's position releases pressure on the diaphragm

▶ Breathing exercises allow maximum expansion of the lungs and help prevent further abdominal distention

▶ Supplemental oxygen maintains optimal tissue perfusion

◆ Encourage the patient to turn, if possible, and deep-breathe every 2 hours; imposed bed rest and immobility cause pooling of secretions in the lungs, which could lead to infection

◆ Organize nursing tasks so that the patient has uninterrupted periods of rest; overactivity can increase fatigue and oxygen use

❖ **Acute abdominal trauma**
■ Description
◆ Abdominal trauma is defined as any injury that occurs from the nipple line to midthigh; it's seldom limited to a single organ
◆ Abdominal trauma is classified as blunt or penetrating
▶ Blunt trauma commonly results from motor vehicle accidents, assaults, falls, and sports injuries
▶ Penetrating trauma may be caused by motor vehicle accidents, assaults, and knife or gunshot wounds
◆ Because a patient with bowel trauma may have other abdominal injuries, the priority should be on the risk of hemorrhage and peritonitis associated with abdominal trauma, rather than pathological changes in a specific organ
■ Clinical signs and symptoms
◆ Slightly distended abdomen with multiple ecchymotic areas

◆ Decreased bowel sounds
◆ Acute upper thoracic and abdominal pain
◆ Tenderness on palpation
◆ Hypotension and tachycardia
◆ Decreased urine output
◆ Cold, clammy skin
◆ Laboratory tests showing decreased hemoglobin and hematocrit, as well as abnormal liver enzyme, BUN, and creatinine values; the abnormal values depend on the organs affected by the injury
◆ Blood in the stool

■ Medical management
◆ Insert a central I.V. line, and begin fluid replacement
◆ Insert an NG lavage tube
◆ Administer supplemental oxygen
◆ Review abdominal X-rays, CT scans, ultrasonography, and MRI scans to assess the extent of injury
◆ Recommend surgery, if indicated

■ Nursing management
◆ Continuously monitor vital signs (blood pressure, heart rate and rhythm, respiratory rate, and temperature); in patients with multisystemic trauma, close monitoring of vital signs permits identification of overt or covert changes in the patient's status
◆ Continuously assess arterial oxygen saturation level, which reflects oxygen perfusion of tissues, using pulse oximetry
◆ Frequently assess breath sounds and respiratory effort; patients who have experienced blunt abdominal trauma must be closely observed for complications
◆ Perform a patient assessment (including airway-breathing-circulation with cervical spine precautions and hemorrhage control); monitor the patient every 15 minutes until stable, and then every hour; frequent monitoring permits identification of overt or covert changes in status
◆ Perform an abbreviated neurologic examination, using the Glasgow Coma Scale and assessing pupillary responses, every 15 minutes until the patient is stable, and then every hour; changes in neurologic status may indicate cerebral ischemic conditions
◆ Perform capillary refill checks when vital signs are assessed; continue to monitor urine output, noting the color, amount, consistency, and specific gravity; these assessments reflect the adequacy of tissue perfusion
◆ Establish a patent airway, using a chin-lift or jaw-thrust maneuver without hyperextending the neck; a patent airway provides the initial route for adequate oxygen intake
◆ Check the abdomen for ecchymoses; assess for Cullen's sign (ecchymosis around the umbilicus) and Turner's sign (ecchymosis in either flank)
  ▶ Ecchymosis may indicate internal bleeding
  ▶ Cullen's sign may indicate retroperitoneal bleeding into the abdominal wall
  ▶ Turner's sign indicates retroperitoneal bleeding

◆ Assess for Kehr's sign (left shoulder pain); this sign—a classic finding in patients with splenic rupture—is caused by the presence of blood below the diaphragm that irritates the phrenic nerve

◆ Auscultate the abdomen for bowel sounds; absent or diminished bowel sounds may result from the presence of blood, bacteria, or a chemical irritant in the abdominal cavity

◆ Auscultate the abdomen for bruits, which indicate renal artery injury

◆ Percuss the abdomen, noting any resonance over the right flank with the patient lying on his left side (Ballance's sign); percuss for resonance over the liver and for areas of dullness over hollow organs that normally contain gas, such as the stomach, large intestine, and small intestine

  ▶ Ballance's sign indicates a ruptured spleen

  ▶ Normal percussion over the liver elicits a dull sound; resonance, which is caused by free air, is pathological

  ▶ Dullness over hollow organs may indicate the presence of blood or fluid

◆ Lightly palpate the abdomen to identify areas of tenderness, rebound tenderness, guarding, rigidity, and spasm

◆ Check for rectal bleeding; assess urine output every hour, and monitor for protein or blood in the urine; check the amount of gastric drainage from an NG tube every hour, monitoring for bleeding

  ▶ Close observation of the patient is necessary in the initial postinjury phase to identify overt or covert signs of bleeding

  ▶ Signs of bleeding may necessitate an exploratory laparotomy to repair abdominal injuries

◆ Assess verbal complaints of pain, including its severity, location, and intensity; a complete and continuing assessment of the patient's pain permits the most effective pain management interventions and provides information about the extent of tissue, nerve, or vessel damage caused by blunt trauma

◆ Provide high-flow oxygen at 6 to 10 L per minute, using a mask, cannula, or oral or nasal adjuncts; oxygen delivery in the proper amount with the appropriate method helps maintain adequate tissue oxygenation

◆ Use mechanical ventilation, as needed, to maintain forced inspiratory oxygen at 100%; patients with an obstructed airway may require ventilatory support by means of endotracheal or nasotracheal intubation, cricothyrotomy, or tracheotomy

◆ Monitor serial ABG values, as prescribed; ABG measurements accurately reflect gas exchange requirements in injured patients with decreased tissue perfusion

◆ Monitor breath sounds every 15 minutes until the patient is stable, and then every hour; observe for tracheal shifting to the contralateral side; although the initial respiratory assessment may be negative, tension pneumothorax may develop as a result of blunt trauma to the chest

◆ Place the patient in a supine position with his legs elevated, unless contraindicated because of hypertension; the best position for a hypotensive patient is in a supine position with his legs elevated because this prevents blood from pooling in the lower extremities and allows maximum perfusion of vital organs

▶ A modified Trendelenburg's position initially facilitates venous return and augments blood pressure

▶ Continued use of the Trendelenburg position overstimulates baroceptors in the carotid arteries and aortic arch; this decreases blood pressure, producing rebound hypotension

◆ Continue to assess for signs of occult bleeding (such as a rigid abdomen); review results of guaiac stool tests; early detection of occult bleeding via continued reassessment may reveal initially missed injuries or a significant change in the patient's status

◆ To replace lost fluid volume, maintain large-bore I.V. infusions with crystalloids, colloids, and blood, as prescribed

▶ Crystalloids are replaced at a rate of 3 ml for each milliliter of blood loss

▶ Blood is replaced in a 1:1 ratio, that is, at a rate of 1 ml for each milliliter of blood loss

◆ Consider using a pneumatic antishock garment to enhance peripheral resistance, achieve arterial tamponade, promote shunting of blood to vital organs, and splint fractures to decrease blood loss; if used, monitor the patient's response

◆ Monitor serial hematocrit and WBC count as well as chemistry and enzyme laboratory test results

▶ The initial hemoglobin level and hematocrit don't reflect true blood loss—the values appear higher than they actually are because of hemoconcentration resulting from volume loss; serial hemoglobin and hematocrit measurements can identify true blood loss

▶ An elevated WBC count may indicate a ruptured spleen

▶ Elevated serum amylase concentrations may signal injury to the pancreas or bowel

◆ Obtain a baseline 12-lead ECG and perform continuous ECG monitoring

◆ Consider implementing hemodynamic monitoring to detect the status of cardiopulmonary function and measure cardiac output

◆ Position the patient to alleviate pain or reduce discomfort; medication for pain may not be administered in the immediate posttraumatic phase because it may mask physical symptoms of injury

◆ Administer pain medication, as prescribed, and monitor the patient's response

◆ Communicate frequently with the patient and family to establish a trusting relationship; encourage the patient and family to verbalize feelings, and involve them in the treatment plan

◆ Explain all procedures before proceeding to help decrease the patient's anxiety

◆ Refer the patient to support services, as needed, including social services, pastoral care, and psychological counseling; these services can be valuable during acute and rehabilitative treatment phases

Review questions

1. The nurse is assessing a 22-year-old male patient who was thrown head-first off his bicycle when he ran into a parked car. Which of the following signs would indicate splenic rupture?

○ **A.** Cullen's sign

○ **B.** Turner's sign

○ **C.** Kehr's sign

○ **D.** Chvostek's sign

Correct answer: C Kehr's sign—left shoulder pain—is a classic finding in the patient with splenic rupture. It's caused by the presence of blood below the diaphragm that irritates the phrenic nerve.

2. After suffering an acute GI hemorrhage, a 75-year-old patient is resuscitated in the emergency department with I.V. crystalloids and packed cells. His vital signs are as follows: blood pressure, 90/40 mm Hg; pulse rate, 160 beats/minute; respiratory rate, 32 breaths/minute; CVP, 4. In the intensive care unit (ICU) 1 hour later, his vital signs are as follows: blood pressure, 130/72 mm Hg; pulse rate, 122 beats/minute; respiratory rate, 36 breaths/minute, CVP, 12. The patient appears short of breath and has a slight cough. The nurse suspects:

○ **A.** respiratory alkalosis.

○ **B.** encephalopathy.

○ **C.** cardiac failure.

○ **D.** pulmonary edema.

Correct answer: D Patients with GI hemorrhage are at high risk for impaired gas exchange related to hemoglobin deficit and for pulmonary edema resulting from fluid overload. The patient should be assessed for chest congestion (crackles, wheezes, dyspnea, orthopnea, and cough with pink frothy sputum) to confirm the nurse's suspicion.

3. A patient with hepatic failure in the ICU is confused about time, place, and person. For safety, the nurse should initially:

○ **A.** reorient the patient.

○ **B.** increase the frequency of patient observation.

○ **C.** restrain the patient.

○ **D.** administer a mild sedative.

Correct answer: A Initially, the nurse should reorient the patient to time, place, and person by helping him recall admission to the ICU. Familiar objects, clocks, and calendars can help increase the patient's sense of orientation.

4. A 56-year-old patient with pancreatitis develops fine tremors, agitation, and tachycardia 48 hours after ICU admission. These signs may indicate:

○ **A.** alcohol withdrawal.

○ **B.** adverse reaction to medications.

○ **C.** ICU psychosis.

○ **D.** generalized tonic-clonic seizure.

Correct answer: A Chronic alcohol abuse can cause signs of alcohol withdrawal beginning 24 hours after the last drink and continuing for 1 to 2 weeks. Signs include tremors, diaphoresis, anorexia, nausea, vomiting, increased heart rate and respirations, agitation, visual or auditory hallucinations, and delirium.

5. A patient is experiencing changes in mentation, numbness and tingling of the fingers and toes, muscle cramps, and ECG changes. The patient should be evaluated for:

○ **A.** hypoglycemia.

○ **B.** hypocalcemia.

○ **C.** hypovolemia.

○ **D.** hyperglycemia.

Correct answer: B Hypocalcemia produces increased neural excitability, which leads to muscle spasms, CNS irritability (such as seizures), and cardiac muscle hyperactivity (evidenced by ECG changes).

Renal disorders

❖ **Anatomy**
  ■ Kidneys
    ◆ The kidneys are small, paired organs located in the retroperitoneal connective tissue of the posterior abdominal wall, with one kidney situated on each side of the vertebral column in the flank or lumbar areas; an adrenal gland sits atop each kidney
    ◆ In the supine position, the kidneys extend from the T12 to L3 level, with the right kidney usually slightly lower than the left, due to the liver being located just above the right kidney
      ▶ A single kidney of an adult male weighs 4.4 to 6.0 oz (125 to 170 g); an adult female's weighs 4.0 to 5.5 oz (114 to 155 g)
      ▶ Each kidney is 1″ to 1¼″ (2.5 to 3.8 cm) thick, 4¼″ to 4¾″ (11 to 12 cm) long, and 2″ to 3″ (5 to 7.5 cm) wide
    ◆ The kidneys appear slightly bean-shaped, with their long axis lying approximately vertical; they present anterior and posterior surfaces, medial and lateral margins, and superior and inferior poles
    ◆ On the medial surface of each kidney is the hilus, through which the renal pelvis, renal artery, renal vein, lymphatics, and nerve plexus pass into the renal sinus
    ◆ Each kidney is surrounded by a tough, fibrous tissue called the renal capsule, which restricts distention
    ◆ Associated renal structures include the ureters (fibromuscular tubes that propel urine from the renal pelvis to the bladder), urinary bladder (pouch for holding 400 to 500 ml of urine), and urethra (tube through which urine passes for excretion)
  ■ Kidney cross section
    ◆ The renal cortex is a pale, outer region that contains all the glomeruli, proximal and distal convoluted tubules, and adjacent parts of the loop of Henle; it's the site of aerobic metabolism and formation of ammonia and glucose
    ◆ The medulla is a darker, inner region that contains collecting ducts and loops of Henle grouped into 8 to 18 renal pyramids; it's the site of anaerobic and glycolytic metabolism needed for active transport
      ▶ The base of each renal pyramid extends toward the renal pelvis to form a papilla; the tip of the papilla has 10 to 25 small openings that serve as the renal collecting ducts (Bellini's ducts)
      ▶ The cortex, which is about ⅜″ (1 cm) thick, forms a cap over each renal pyramid and lies between each pyramid to form renal columns

◆ The calyces are cuplike structures that enclose the renal pyramids
▶ The minor calyx receives urine from the collecting tubules; several minor calyces join to form a major calyx
▶ The major calyx directs urine from the renal sinus to the renal pelvis; the major calyces join to form the renal pelvis, which then directs urine to the ureter
▶ The walls of the calyces, renal pelvis, and ureters contain smooth muscle, which helps propel urine to the bladder by the hydrostatic (gravitational) flow and rhythmic contractions (peristalsis)

■ Microscopic renal structures
◆ The nephron is the structural and functional unit of the kidney; it contains the renal corpuscle and the renal tubule
▶ The renal corpuscle consists of Bowman's capsule and the glomerulus, which lies inside Bowman's capsule
 • Bowman's capsule contains specialized tubules that support the glomerulus
 • The glomerulus is a capillary bed that's permeable to virtually all plasma components, including water, electrolytes, nutrients, and waste, but relatively impermeable to large negatively charged protein molecules and cells (glomerular barrier)
▶ The renal tubule is divided into the proximal convoluted tubule, loop of Henle, distal convoluted tubule, and collecting duct
◆ At birth, each human kidney contains approximately 1 million nephrons in different stages of development; nephrons mature after birth, but new nephrons aren't formed
◆ If nephrons are damaged or destroyed, the remaining functional nephrons compensate by hypertrophy and by filtering a higher solute load

■ Renal blood flow
◆ The kidneys receive 20% to 25% of cardiac output via the renal arteries at rest when mean arterial pressure is 80 to 170 mm Hg via autoregulation; during physical or emotional stress, the kidneys may receive only 2% to 4% of cardiac output
◆ The abdominal aorta gives rise to the renal artery, which enters the hilus of each kidney and usually divides into anterior and posterior branches
▶ Segmental or lobar arteries from the anterior branch supply the anterior side of the kidney; this supply fans out in the cortex and branches to form afferent arterioles that enter the tuft of glomerular capillaries
▶ Efferent arterioles leave the glomerular capillary bed to form a peritubular capillary network; this network becomes progressively larger and leaves the kidney via the hilum to join with the inferior vena cava
◆ Each kidney normally is supplied by one artery and one vein, but nearly one-third of all human kidneys have multiple vessels that usually occur on the right side (seldom on the left)
◆ The juxtaglomerular apparatus is a specialized structure made up of juxtaglomerular cells (smooth-muscle cells that contain inactive renin) and macula densa cells (a portion of the distal tubule that lies close to the afferent arterioles)

▶ The juxtaglomerular apparatus works by monitoring arterial blood pressure and serum sodium level

▶ It can be triggered by low arterial blood pressure in the afferent and efferent arterioles, low sodium content within the distal tubule, or increased sympathetic stimulation of the kidneys; when the triggers are activated, renin is secreted to increase blood pressure and sodium reabsorption from the distal convoluted tubule increases

■ Lymphatic system

◆ Interstitial fluid leaves the kidneys via the lymphatic system

◆ The renal lymphatic system drains into the aortic and para-aortic nodes of the lumbar lymphatic chain and then into the thoracic duct

■ Innervation

◆ Nerve fibers from the celiac plexus form a renal plexus around the renal artery; this plexus is joined by the lower splanchnic nerve or the renal branch of the lesser splanchnic nerve

◆ These sympathetic, afferent nerve fibers conduct pain impulses and control blood flow to the kidney by means of dilation or constriction of supplying vessels

❖ Physiology

■ Formation of urine

◆ Normal urine volume averages 1 to 2 L daily

◆ Urine composition varies slightly among individuals, but all urine contains urea (waste product of protein and amino acid metabolism); uric acid (waste product of purine metabolism by the liver); creatinine (waste product of muscle [protein] metabolism); ions (potassium, sodium, calcium, and chloride); hormones and their breakdown products (for example, chorionic gonadotropin); and vitamins (particularly the water-soluble B-complex vitamins and vitamin C)

▶ Certain medications, such as penicillin and aspirin, are excreted in the urine

▶ The presence of glucose, albumin, red blood cells (RBCs), or calculi in the urine is an abnormal finding

◆ The amount of glomerular ultrafiltration is determined by pressure gradients

▶ The glomerular capillary hydrostatic pressure normally is 55 mm Hg (or one-half the mean arterial pressure), which encourages filtration

▶ A glomerular colloid osmotic pressure less than 25 mm Hg and Bowman's capsule pressure less than 10 mm Hg oppose the glomerular hydrostatic pressure to discourage glomerular filtration (see *Values for normal glomerular ultrafiltration,* page 250)

◆ The glomerular filtration rate (GFR) is the volume of fluid filtered into the Bowman's capsule per unit time and depends on renal plasma flow

▶ It is calculated as follows: GFR $= (U_x \times V) P_x$, where x refers to the substance freely filtered by the glomerulus and not secreted or absorbed by the tubules, U_x is the urine concentration of x, V is the urine flow rate, and P_x refers to the plasma concentration of x

▶ Normal GFR is 125 ml per minute, or 180 L per day, of which about 99% is returned to the blood via tubular transport processes

Values for normal glomerular ultrafiltration

The net filtration pressure is determined by subtracting the colloid osmotic pressure and the Bowman's capsule pressure from the glomerular hydrostatic pressure.

Measurement	Normal value
Glomerular hydrostatic pressure	55 mm Hg
Colloid osmotic pressure	25 mm Hg
Bowman's capsule pressure	10 mm Hg
Net filtration pressure	20 mm Hg

▶ The GFR doesn't vary enough to affect urine volume, except in certain pathologic conditions
◆ The tubular functions of reabsorption and secretion occur through active and passive processes; these processes are directly affected by mean arterial pressure, electrochemical gradients, and hormones
   ▶ In the active process, ion transport occurs against a gradient, thus requiring energy; it also employs membrane protein pumps with a maximum rate of tubular activity
   ▶ In the passive process, diffusion occurs across a concentration gradient, requiring no energy
◆ The proximal convoluted tubule (PCT) is the site for reabsorption of glucose, amino acids, phosphates, uric acid, and potassium from the tubular filtrate, which enter the blood through the peritubular capillaries
   ▶ Reabsorption of these substances occurs mainly through an active process in the tubular epithelium
   ▶ The PCT also actively reabsorbs sodium (this particular process is stimulated by aldosterone) and passively reabsorbs approximately 80% of water by osmosis
   ▶ It also reabsorbs and secretes bicarbonate and hydrogen to help regulate the acid-base balance
◆ The loop of Henle is divided into an ascending segment (thick limb) and a descending segment (thin limb); the ascending loop of Henle contains an active sodium pump and is impermeable to water, whereas the descending loop of Henle is permeable to water only
   ▶ The primary function of the loop of Henle is the concentration or dilution of urine
   ▶ The loop of Henle performs this function by maintaining a hypertonic interstitial fluid gradient through the removal of sodium chloride that increases the osmotic force and promotes reabsorption of water in the collecting tubules (concentration of urine)
◆ The distal convoluted tubule is the site for reabsorption of water, sodium chloride, and sodium bicarbonate and the secretion of hydrogen, potassium, ammonia, and other blood-borne substances

◗ Antidiuretic hormone (ADH) synthesized by the hypothalamus and secreted by the posterior pituitary gland controls the amount of water and urea reabsorbed from the distal tubule

◗ The hormone aldosterone controls the reabsorption of electrolytes, especially sodium, from the tubular lumen

◆ The collecting duct system consists of the initial collecting tubule, the cortical collecting duct, and the inner and outer medullary segments; the collecting duct system, which is controlled by ADH, is the site of the final osmotic reabsorption of water before urine enters the renal pelvis; the absence of ADH results in excess water excretion in the urine

■ Excretion of metabolic waste products

◆ The primary function of the kidneys is the excretion of more than 200 metabolic waste products

◆ The effectiveness of the kidneys in excreting metabolic waste is measured by the levels of blood urea nitrogen (BUN) and creatinine

◗ Creatinine, which plays a role in muscle (protein) metabolism, is the most sensitive laboratory determinant of kidney function; creatinine normally is excreted at a rate equal to the GFR

◗ Urea is a protein metabolite; its excretion is influenced by urine flow, low blood volume, fever, infection, trauma, drug use, and diet

● Elevated BUN without a concomitant increase in creatinine is a sign of decreased renal perfusion and volume depletion

● Elevated BUN with a concomitant increase in creatinine is an indicator of renal disease

■ Regulation of body water

◆ The principal role of the thirst mechanism is to maintain normal hydration status

◗ The thirst mechanism is located in the anterior hypothalamus

◗ The subjective feeling of thirst is triggered when there is a deficit in the extracellular volume and a higher plasma osmolarity; angiotensin stimulates thirst by directly affecting the brain; the renin-angiotensin system is an important regulator of water balance when extracellular volume is decreased

◆ Secretion of ADH by the posterior pituitary gland is stimulated by increased serum osmolarity and decreased extracellular fluid (ECF) volume

◗ ADH acts on the distal tubule and collecting duct, causing more water to be reabsorbed from the tubular filtrate and returned to the blood

◗ ADH has an antidiuretic effect, resulting in sodium reasborption by the sodium-potassium-adenosine triphosphate pump, under the influence of aldosterone

◆ Aldosterone is a mineralocorticoid secreted by the adrenal cortex; its primary effect is to increase renal tubular sodium reabsorption and cause selective renal potassium excretion

◆ The renal countercurrent mechanism can adjust urine osmolarity for concentration or dilution; this mechanism is a continuous process that occurs in the juxtamedullary nephrons, descending loop of Henle, and vasa recta

❖ **Renal regulation of the acid-base balance**
  ◆ The kidneys minimize variations in fluid balance through the retention and excretion of hydrogen; fluid balance is also regulated by the lungs, blood, serum bicarbonate (HCO_3^-) level, and plasma protein level
  ◆ Excretion of hydrogen ions occurs after acid is buffered by ammonia or phosphate, so that the blood pH level won't drop
  ◆ Reabsorption of HCO_3^- begins in the proximal tubule and is completed in the distal tubule; HCO_3^- is reabsorbed, along with sodium, when the bicarbonate level in the filtrate is above 28 mEq/L
    ▶ CO_3^- is completely reabsorbed in the glomerulus until the level in the filtrate is less than or equal to 28 mEq/L; phosphate is then secreted to react with hydrogen
    ▶ HCO_3^- is synthesized in the distal tubule
      • Carbonic acid (H_2CO_3) results from the hydration of carbon dioxide (CO_2) by way of carbonic anhydrase
      • CO_2 is a product of cellular metabolism
      • New HCO_3^- is formed as CO_2 reacts with water and the resulting carbonic acid dissociates, as shown in the following equation: $H_2O + CO_2 \rightarrow H_2CO_3 \rightarrow H^+ + HCO_3^-$
■ Regulation of blood pressure
  ◆ Normal plasma volume must be maintained for blood pressure control
    ▶ Decreased plasma volume reduces arterial blood pressure, leading to vasoconstriction that eventually impairs oxygenation
    ▶ Increased plasma volume raises blood pressure by increasing cardiac preload and cardiac output
  ◆ Vasoconstriction of the circulatory system is controlled by the renin-angiotensin-aldosterone system
    ▶ As the GFR decreases, renin is secreted from juxtaglomerular apparatus into the afferent arterioles
    ▶ Renin then acts on renin substrate to split vasoactive angiotensin
    ▶ Pulmonary capillary cells convert angiotensin I into angiotensin II, which is a potent vasoconstrictor acting directly upon the tunica media; as arterial pressure increases, renal perfusion and glomerular filtration increase
    ▶ Fluid response is balanced by angiotensin II, which stimulates aldosterone to increase sodium reabsorption
  ◆ Constriction of the renal arterioles increases ECF volume, thereby increasing blood pressure
  ◆ Dilation of the renal vascular system is stimulated by prostaglandins
    ▶ Prostaglandins are found in most cells, especially those of the kidneys, brain, and gonads
    ▶ Prostaglandins inhibit the distal tubule response to ADH; this results in sodium and water excretion and decreased circulating volume
■ Synthesis and maturation of RBCs
  ◆ The kidneys control the production of RBCs by producing erythropoietin (EPO), a hematopoietic growth factor that acts as a hormone; 90% of circulating EPO originates from the kidney; 10% is from extrarenal sources
  ◆ EPO stimulates bone marrow release and RBC maturation

Components of the medical history in a patient with renal disease

Obtaining a thorough history is important in assessing the cause of renal disease and in determining subsequent treatment. The outline below details what to look for when performing a health history interview and a physical assessment.

A. Previous evidence of renal disease
  1. Previous elevated blood urea nitrogen or creatinine level
  2. History of albuminuria (foamy urine), hematuria (dark urine), edema, or urinary tract infections (UTIs)
  3. Incidence of renal disease during previous medical examinations
  4. History of hypertension
  5. Symptoms of lower UTI (urinary frequency, burning, hesitancy, urgency)
  6. Oliguria, polyuria, nocturia
  7. History of infections (throat, skin)
  8. Family history of renal disease (polycystic kidney disease, Alport's disease [hearing loss])
B. History of systemic diseases
  1. Diabetes mellitus
  2. Collagen vascular diseases (systemic lupus erythematosus, periarteritis, Sjögren's disease, Wegener's granulomatosis, Henoch-Schönlein purpura)
  3. Cancer (myeloma, breast, lung, colon, lymphoma)
  4. Essential hypertension
  5. Sickle cell disease
  6. Primary or secondary amyloidosis
  7. Goodpasture's syndrome
  8. Renal calculi
  9. Hereditary nephritis

C. History of drug exposure
  1. Nonsteroidal anti-inflammatory drugs
  2. Penicillins
  3. Aminoglycosides
  4. Chemotherapeutic drugs
  5. Abuse of opioid drugs
  6. Recent use of drugs associated with temporary renal failure (such as angiotensin-converting enzyme inhibitors)
  7. Exposure to heavy metals (lead, gold, cadmium), cleaning products, pesticides, or mercury
D. History of factors contributing to prerenal or postrenal azotemia
  1. Heart failure
  2. Diuretic use
  3. Nausea, vomiting, diarrhea, high fever, bleeding
  4. Sodium-restricted diet
  5. Cirrhosis of the liver or hepatitis
  6. Lower UTIs
  7. Pelvic disease
  8. Recent illnesses (infections, surgeries) or severe injuries (endotoxins, severe hypotension, or skeletal muscle distractions that result in kidney damage)
  9. Exposure to radioactive dyes
E. Uremic symptoms
  1. Nausea, vomiting, anorexia
  2. Weight loss
  3. Pruritus
  4. Weakness, fatigue
  5. Lethargy, drowsiness, stupor, convulsions, coma
  6. Bleeding abnormalities
  7. Uremic peritonitis
  8. Pleuritis

▶ EPO is probably produced in the kidney's peritubular interstitial cells

❖ **Renal assessment**
  ■ Noninvasive assessment techniques
    ◆ In a patient with renal disease, the medical history is often the most important element in making the diagnosis (see *Components of the medical history in a patient with renal disease*)
    ◆ The physical examination includes an assessment of vital signs, fluid volume status, and signs of systemic disease, uremia, or obstruction
      ▶ Vital sign assessment
        • Blood pressure, noting pulse pressure and a positive paradoxical pulse
        • Heart rate and rhythm

- Low temperature with erythrocyte sedimentation rate decline due to immunosuppression
- Respirations
▶ Signs of altered volume status
  - Depletion: changes in orthostatic blood pressure and pulse rate as well as decreased skin turgor, resulting in tenting and decreased weight
  - Overload: jugular venous distention, crackles, ascites, pulmonary edema, heart failure, shortness of breath, liver congestion and enlargement, pitting edema, and increased weight
▶ Possible signs of systemic disease
  - Skin: malar rash or butterfly-shaped rash over the nose and cheeks (systemic lupus erythematosus [SLE]), purpura (vasculitis, Henoch-Schönlein purpura), macular rash (acute interstitial nephritis), and scleroderma
  - Head, ears, eyes, nose, and throat: alopecia (SLE), uveitis (sarcoidosis or vasculitis), papilledema (malignant hypertension), diabetic retinopathy, hypertension, throat infection, and hearing loss (Alport's syndrome)
  - Pulmonary system: consolidation (glomerulonephritis secondary to pneumonia)
  - Heart: murmurs (endocarditis), pericardial friction rub
  - Abdomen: bruits (renal artery stenosis), costovertebral angle tenderness
  - Extremities: livedo reticularis (vasculitis), blue extremities (embolic events), Janeway's lesions, Osler's nodes, and angiokeratomas
▶ Signs of uremia
  - Skin: uremic frost and ecchymosis
  - Heart: pericardial friction rub and paradoxical pulse (tamponade)
  - Extremities: asterixis, Trousseau's sign, and Chvostek's sign
  - Lungs: Kussmaul's respirations (metabolic acidosis)
◆ Signs of obstruction
  - Percussible bladder
  - Enlarged prostate
  - Phimosis
■ Noninvasive imaging techniques
  ◆ Ultrasonography is used to determine the size and symmetry of the kidneys and to pinpoint the location of cysts, fluid collection, and calculi; imaging before and after voiding is helpful in making the diagnosis
  ◆ Renal radionuclide scan (renogram) is used to assess glomerular filtration, renal plasma flow, arterial occlusion, and obstruction of outflow
  ◆ Renal arteriography is used to assess renal arterial vasculature; the testing dye is nephrotoxic, and all patients receiving it should be monitored closely
  ◆ Computed tomography (CT) is used to identify tumors and lymphoceles
  ◆ Magnetic resonance imaging (MRI) detects morphological changes, especially in renal transplantation
  ◆ Cystoscopy can detect bladder or urethral problems

◆ Retrograde pyelography, retrograde urethrography, and voiding cystourethrography are specialized X-rays that show specific renal deficits
◆ Excretory urography is used less often since the advent of ultrasonography, but it remains useful for detecting papillary necrosis and abnormalities of the renal calyces and collecting ducts

■ Invasive assessment techniques
◆ A kidney biopsy is the most direct method of determining the histological cause of intrinsic parenchymal disease; contraindications include serious bleeding disorders, morbid obesity, and severe hypertension
◆ Biopsies can be open (surgical) or closed (percutaneous method)

■ Key laboratory values
◆ Blood
  ▶ Serum abnormalities are found in acute renal failure (ARF) or chronic renal failure (CRF)
  ▶ BUN level (normal value: 10 to 20 mg/dl) may be elevated (also elevated with volume depletion)
  ▶ Creatinine level (normal value: 0.7 to 1.4 mg/dl) may be elevated
  ▶ Ratio of BUN level to creatinine level (normal value is 10:1)
    ● If decreased (less than 10:1), may indicate liver disease, protein restriction, or excess fluid intake
    ● If increased (greater than 10:1), may indicate volume depletion, low "effective" blood volume, catabolism, or excess protein intake
  ▶ Potassium level (normal value: 3.5 to 5.5 mg/dl) may be elevated
◆ Urine
  ▶ Normal urine specific gravity ranges from 1.010 to 1.030
    ● A specific gravity less than 1.010 is consistent with a defect in the kidneys' ability to concentrate urine and may be caused by diabetes insipidus
    ● A specific gravity greater than 1.030 indicates severe dehydration, which may result from proteinuria
  ▶ Normal urine pH ranges from 4.5 to 8.0
  ▶ Normal creatinine clearance, an excellent clinical indicator of renal function, is 100 to 110 ml per minute
  ▶ Glucose in the urine is an abnormal finding and may be related to diabetes
  ▶ Acetone in the urine is seen in diabetic ketoacidosis
  ▶ Protein in the urine indicates nephrotic syndrome
◆ Urine electrolyte profile
  ▶ A 24-hour urine examination (in which all urine voided during a 24-hour period is saved) is used to determine the urine electrolyte profile and can be used to differentiate between prerenal and postrenal causes of renal failure; prerenal causes are indicated by decreased renal perfusion, but postrenal causes generally stem from obstruction
  ▶ Urine sodium concentration (normal value: 40 to 220 mEq/L/24 hours) indicates water and salt balance and differentiates oliguria associated with ARF from other prerenal causes
  ▶ BUN (normal value: 9 to 16 g/24 hours); an increase in BUN indicates impaired renal function
◆ Culture and sensitivity tests

▶ These tests may reveal the presence of hyaline, blood, granular, fatty, or renal tubular casts in the urine

- RBC casts are a sign of active glomerulonephritis
- The presence of white blood cells (WBCs) and casts indicate renal infection
- Granular casts can indicate acute tubular necrosis, interstitial nephritis, acute or chronic glomerulonephritis, chronic renal disease, or proteinuric states
- Fatty casts may indicate nephrotic syndrome or proteinuric states
- Renal tubular casts may indicate renal failure

▶ These tests are also used to check urine for the presence of bacteria, WBCs, RBCs, crystals, and eosinophils

❖ **Acute renal failure**
  ■ Description
    ◆ ARF is a syndrome that can be broadly defined as rapid (hours to a few days) deterioration of renal function, resulting in the accumulation of nitrogenous wastes and fluid and electrolyte imbalance
    ◆ ARF typically occurs when the GFR is decreased by 50% or more; six major syndromes are associated with decreased GFR
      ▶ *Prerenal azotemia* results from renal hypoperfusion (ischemia) that's immediately reversed by the return of blood flow and doesn't damage the renal structures
        - The renal response to prerenal azotemia is multiphasic
        - Decreased renal blood flow from the cortex to the medulla leads to decreased afferent glomerular arterial pressure, which decreases the GFR and causes fluid reabsorption in the tubules
        - Prerenal causes of ARF include:
          − Dehydration
          − Sepsis/shock
          − Hypovolemic shock
          − Vena cava obstruction
          − Trauma with bleeding
          − Sequestration (burns, peritonitis)
          − Hypovolemia (diuretics)
          − Cardiovascular failure (heart failure, vascular pooling, tamponade, arrhythmia)
          − Hemorrhage
          − GI losses (diarrhea, vomiting)
          − Extreme acidosis
          − Anaphylaxis/shock
          − Renal artery stenosis or thrombosis
      ▶ *Acute (intrinsic) renal failure* (also called acute tubular necrosis) is caused by renal hypoperfusion or a nephrotoxin; it can't be immediately reversed, and it causes some damage to tubular cells; recovery time varies from days to weeks
        - Renal hypoperfusion may be caused by intravascular volume depletion (resulting from trauma, burns, or hemorrhage), decreased cardiac output (caused by severe heart failure, pulmonary hyperten-

sion, or positive-pressure mechanical ventilation), or an increase in the renal-systemic vascular resistance ratio

— Renal vasoconstriction, which may cause ARF if it occurs for an extended period, results from the use of amphotericin B or alpha-adrenergic agents (for example, norepinephrine) or from hypercalcemia

— Systemic vasodilation results from decreased afterload, use of antihypertensive medications, anaphylactic shock, sepsis, drug overdose, or liver failure; it decreases blood pressure, causing decreased renal blood flow and ARF

● Nephrotoxic ARF is usually reversible if identified early

— Exogenous nephrotoxins can cause tubule destruction, papillary necrosis, and acute interstitial nephritis

— Common nephrotoxins include aminoglycosides and other antibiotics, radiologic contrast agents, anesthetics (methoxyfluorane), chemotherapeutic agents, heavy metals, hemoglobinuria (from hemolysis), organic solvents (carbon tetrachloride), disseminated intravascular coagulation (DIC), and other drugs (cimetidine, cyclosporine, phenytoin, loop and thiazide diuretics, and nonsteroidal anti-inflammatory drugs)

▶ *Acute interstitial nephritis* is caused by interstitial inflammation

▶ *Acute glomerulonephritis* or *vasculitis* results from glomerular or vessel inflammation

▶ *Acute renovascular disease* is caused by obstruction of the renal artery or vein in a single kidney or by bilateral kidney disease

▶ *Obstructive uropathy* results from obstruction of the urinary collecting system

● Extraureteral obstruction may be caused by a tumor or an inflammatory aortic aneurysm

● Intraureteral obstruction may be caused by blood clots, calculi, or edema

● Bladder outlet obstruction can result from calculi, blood clots, prostatic hypertrophy, or bladder infection

● Urethral obstruction may be caused by a congenital valve defect, stricture, phimosis, or tumor

◆ In major trauma or systemic infections, breakdown of skeletal muscle cell membranes (rhabdomyolysis) may release muscle cell contents, such as myoglobin (normally found only within muscle cells), into the blood; myoglobin can cause obstruction if filtered into the tubules, possibly resulting in renal parenchymal disease (intrarenal failure). Common risk factors for rhabdomyolysis include:

▶ Direct physical trauma, malignant hyperthermia, or status epilepticus, which produces extensive damage to the muscle cell membrane (sarcolemma)

▶ Heat stroke or electrical shock, which produces thermal injury to the sarcolemma

▶ Systemic infections, particularly viral, which produce inflammation and may lead to ischemia as edema accumulates in muscle compartments bounded by fascia

◗ Alcohol or cocaine abuse, with overdose followed by prolonged immobility in which gravitational fluid shifts contribute to edema
◆ Loss of sarcolemma integrity allows myoglobin as well as other intracellular components (creatine kinase, uric acid, potassium, and phosphate) to enter the blood; with injury of 100 to 200 g of muscle, the binding capacity of plasma proteins is exceeded and free myoglobin is released into the urine, changing its color (pigmenturia, a dark reddish brown color); myoglobin nephrotoxicity occurs with a renal tubular pH of less than 5.6, which is common with dehydration and acidosis
◗ Concomitant with acute rhabdomyolysis is some degree of DIC, which usually resolves spontaneously within 2 weeks, but may require transfusion of clotting factors in fresh frozen plasma
◗ The patient is commonly acutely ill with fever, weakness, malaise, nausea, vomiting, and pain and swelling of the affected muscles; manifestations associated with ARF include oliguria, azotemia, electrolyte imbalances, and hypervolemia
■ Clinical signs and symptoms
◆ Pruritus (the most common symptom), poor skin turgor, anorexia, nausea, vomiting, weight loss (resulting from decreased food intake or increased catabolism) or weight gain (resulting from edema or ascites), and generalized weakness and fatigue
◆ Metallic taste, stomatitis, and GI hemorrhage
◆ Hypertension or hypotension, pericarditis, and cardiomyopathy
◆ Pulmonary edema, pleural effusion, and dyspnea
◆ Encephalopathy and stupor
◆ Osteodystrophy
■ Diagnostic tests
◆ Laboratory tests of blood and urine samples may show abnormal values
◆ Ultrasonography, to assess the size and symmetry of the kidneys
◆ Renal arteriography, to check the renal vasculature
◆ Kidney biopsy is the definitive diagnostic test for renal disorders
■ Medical management
◆ Initiate preventative strategies for known risk factors
◆ Individualize treatment for the patient's condition
◆ Determine if the patient is a candidate for dialysis, peritoneal dialysis, or continuous renal replacement therapies, which include slow continuous ultrafiltration, continuous arteriovenous hemodialysis or hemodiafiltration, continuous venovenous hemofiltration, and continuous venovenous hemodialysis or hemodiafiltration
◆ Prescribe medications, as indicated, to control blood pressure, metabolic disturbances, fluid balance, and anemia
◆ Restrict the patient's intake of sodium, phosphorus, potassium, protein, magnesium, and caffeine; fluid intake is usually restricted to 500 ml per day, plus the previous day's output
■ Nursing management
◆ Record the patient's weight on admission to determine the baseline hydration status; then weigh the patient daily at the same time
◗ Weight is an indicator of overhydration or dehydration

◗ Assessment of fluid intake and output must take into account insensible losses through the skin, lungs, and intestines (average of 700 to 800 ml per day) and the catabolic rate (average of 350 ml per day includes fluids derived from ingested food)

◆ Monitor vital signs every 1 to 4 hours, and assess for signs and symptoms of hypervolemia and hypovolemia

◆ Perform a review of all body systems, which should include heart and breath sounds to determine cardiac and pulmonary response to volume status and laboratory values to determine the treatment plan's effectiveness

◆ Restrict fluid intake, as prescribed; fluid intake is usually limited to 500 ml per day, plus the previous day's output

◆ Restrict the patient's intake of sodium, phosphorus, potassium, protein, magnesium, and caffeine; these substances are excreted by the kidneys and can accumulate in toxic levels when the kidneys aren't functioning properly

◆ Administer fluid challenges (normal saline solution or albumin), as prescribed, to help control hypotension secondary to volume depletion

◆ Encourage the patient to participate as much as possible in dietary and fluid management; patient compliance is the most important factor in the successful treatment of renal disease

◆ Monitor potassium, sodium, calcium, phosphate, and magnesium levels for indications of electrolyte imbalance

◆ Monitor for conditions that may produce electrolyte imbalance, such as vomiting, diarrhea, nasogastric tube suctioning, and tissue destruction resulting from trauma or burns

◆ Administer antihypertensive medications, as prescribed, and monitor their effects; hypertension is a common complication of renal failure

◆ Administer such medications as dopamine and digoxin, as prescribed, for renal hypoperfusion; by increasing cardiac output, these medications indirectly increase renal perfusion

◆ Monitor the effects of dialysis, and recommend changes in ideal body weight after consultation with dialysis unit personnel and a dietitian; long-term dialysis causes a breakdown in muscle mass or decreases in "dry" or "ideal" body weight, so most dialysis patients retain fluids, and their weight seems stable

❖ **Chronic renal failure**
■ Description
◆ CRF is a progressive and irreversible loss of renal function, usually developed over many years; nephron damage (nephropathy) results from fibrous scar tissue, toxic or ischemic tubular damage, tubular obstruction, interstitial edema, leukocyte infiltration, and focal tubular necrosis

◆ Renal parenchymal ischemia (vascular injury) leads to thickening, fibrosis, or focal lesions of the renal blood vessels, resulting in tubular atrophy, interstitial fibrosis, and functional disruption

◆ Subsequent renal insufficiency, which occurs when renal function reserve is exhausted and the GFR is reduced by 75%, is manifested by mild azotemia

◆ Polyuria and nocturia result from impaired tubular transport and concentration of urine (alteration of the medullary gradient with loss of concentrating ability)

◆ With a loss of more than 90% of functional nephrons, end-stage renal disease results, manifested by a GFR of consistently less than 10 ml per minute

◆ Nephrons may be damaged by toxic, inflammatory, ischemic, or degenerative processes; in the United States, CRF's most prevalent cause is diabetic nephropathy due to glycosylation of glomerular proteins and other factors; other causes include hypertension, primary disorders of the kidney, and systemic disorders (vasculitis, sickle cell disease, SLE, and acquired immunodeficiency syndrome); only a small number of ARF cases lead to CRF

■ Clinical signs and symptoms

◆ While onset is gradual and depends on the duration of renal failure and the patient's response to treatment, CRF produces clinical manifestations similar to ARF, including:

  ▶ Azotemia

  ▶ Fluid and electrolyte imbalance, metabolic acidosis

  ▶ Anemia, bleeding or clotting disorders

  ▶ Renal osteodystrophy (bone demineralization) due to decreased renal activation of vitamin D, with subsequent decreased absorption of dietary calcium; retention of phosphate, resulting in an increased urinary loss of calcium; and increased circulating parathyroid hormone (as a result of decreased urinary excretion of parathyroid hormone), resulting in demineralization of bones and teeth

◆ Malnutrition due to anorexia, malaise, and restricted dietary protein; leads to capillary fragility, decreased immune function, and impaired wound healing

  ▶ Grayish-yellow cast to skin due to retention of urinary pigments (urochromes); pruritus, probably due to release of inflammatory mediators by residual toxins in the skin; and a powdery, white coating on the skin (uremic frost) due to crystallization of uric acid and other substances in sweat

  ▶ Peripheral neuropathy due to toxic effects on sensitive nervous system cells, restless legs syndrome

  ▶ Weakness, decreased deep tendon reflexes

■ Medical management

◆ Restriction of protein intake to 0.6 to 0.8 g per day; low-phosphate diet

◆ Strict glycemic control in patients with diabetes with divided-dose insulin, oral hypoglycemic therapy, or dietary measures

◆ Drug therapy with angiotensin-converting enzyme inhibitors (for example, captopril) to interrupt the renin-angiotensin-aldosterone system to improve renal blood flow and protect against hypertensive nephropathy

◆ Drug therapy with diuretics to increase sodium and water excretion

◆ Drug therapy with recombinant erythropoietin (for example, Procrit) to treat anemia

◆ Calcium and vitamin D supplements to prevent or treat renal osteodystrophy

◆ Renal replacement therapy, if conservative therapy is insufficient, with hemodialysis or peritoneal dialysis

◆ Renal transplantation

■ Nursing management

◆ Nursing management in CRF is essentially the same as in ARF

❖ **Electrolyte imbalance**

■ Description

◆ Electrolyte imbalance results when an electrolyte value is outside of safe parameters

◆ In a patient with a renal disorder, sodium, potassium, calcium, phosphate, and magnesium levels must be monitored closely

▶ Sodium

- Hyponatremia (serum sodium concentration less than 135 mEq/L)
- Hypernatremia (serum sodium concentration greater than 145 mEq/L)

▶ Potassium

- Hypokalemia (serum potassium level less than 3.5 mEq/L)
- Hyperkalemia (serum potassium level greater than 5.5 mEq/L)

▶ Calcium

- Hypocalcemia (serum calcium level less than 8.5 mg/dl)
- Hypercalcemia (serum calcium level greater than 10.5 mg/dl)

▶ Phosphorus

- Hypophosphatemia (serum phosphate level less than 2.5 mg/dl)
- Hyperphosphatemia (serum phosphate level greater than 5 mg/dl)

▶ Magnesium

- Hypomagnesemia (serum magnesium level less than 1.4 mEq/L)
- Hypermagnesemia (serum magnesium level greater than 2.1 mEq/L)

■ Clinical signs and symptoms

◆ Hyponatremia

▶ The severity of symptoms is related to the degree and rate of sodium loss

▶ The most serious symptoms (ranging from apathy, lethargy, confusion, and delirium to seizures and coma) occur when the serum sodium level is less than 120 mEq/L, reflecting hyperosmality and central nervous system (CNS) dehydration

◆ Hypernatremia

▶ Neurologic deficits result from shrinking brain cells, which occur in proportion to the degree of hypernatremia

▶ Severe symptoms are seen when the serum sodium level is greater than 155 mEq/L

▶ The expected normal renal response to hypernatremia is the excretion of a minimal volume of maximally concentrated urine in response to ADH; a lack of ADH, neurohypophysial insufficiency (diabetes insipidus), hypercalcemia, osmotic diuretic therapy, or uncontrolled diabetes mellitus can cause polyuria and lead to hypernatremic dehydration

◆ Hypokalemia
  ▶ The most prominent symptoms are fatigue and muscle weakness, leading to flaccid paralysis and increased susceptibility to arrhythmias
  ▶ Severe hypokalemia can lead to cardiac arrest
◆ Hyperkalemia
  ▶ The initial complaint is usually numbness (paresthesias) of the extremities, nausea, vomiting, diarrhea, muscle cramps, weakness, irritability, and restlessness
  ▶ Electrocardiogram (ECG) changes indicate the condition's severity; peaked and elevated T waves, widening QRS complex, prolonged PR interval, and loss of P wave occur; sine wave formation may be seen
◆ Hypocalcemia
  ▶ Acute hypocalcemia must be distinguished from protein-bound calcium secondary to hypoalbuminemia and from surgical correction of primary hyperparathyroidism
  ▶ In true hypocalcemia, neuromuscular symptoms (paresthesia and tetany) predominate, and the ECG may show a prolonged QT interval
  ▶ Chvostek's sign (facial twitching in response to tapping on the facial nerve) and Trousseau's sign (carpal spasm after 3 minutes of inflation of a blood pressure cuff to above systolic pressure) indicate hypocalcemia
  ▶ Other findings include abdominal spasms and cramps, skeletal muscle cramps, laryngeal spasm, impaired memory, irritability, decreased cardiac output, or bleeding
◆ Hypercalcemia
  ▶ The most common symptoms of severe hypercalcemia are nausea, vomiting, confusion, somnolence, polyuria, and polydipsia; other signs include muscle weakness or atrophy, personality or behavioral changes, pathologic fractures, bone pain, excessive thirst, anorexia, constipation, hypertension, and ECG changes (shortened QT interval, atrioventricular block)
  ▶ Hypercalcemia places the patient at increased risk for metastatic calcification and renal calculi
◆ Hypophosphatemia
  ▶ Severe hypophosphatemia manifests as skeletal muscle weakness and cardiomyopathy; rhabdomyolysis and hemolysis have also been reported; other signs and symptoms include ataxia, paresthesias, confusion, coma, seizures, muscle weakness, joint stiffness, bone pain, anorexia, dysphagia, anemia, platelet dysfunction, and impaired immunity
  ▶ This condition is commonly seen in alcoholics, patients in the recovery phase of diabetic ketoacidosis, and those receiving total parenteral nutrition (TPN); it can also result from excessive use of phosphate binders
◆ Hyperphosphatemia
  ▶ Hyperphosphatemia is usually correlated with hypocalcemia, which stimulates the secretion of parathyroid hormone and resorption of calcium from bone

▶ Signs and symptoms include osteoporosis, bone pain, pathologic fractures, abdominal cramps, tachycardia, nausea, diarrhea, and increased deep tendon reflexes

◆ Hypermagnesemia

▶ Magnesium balance is necessary for functional integrity of the neuromuscular system

▶ The most common signs and symptoms are CNS depression, respiratory paralysis, lethargy, coma, bradycardia, and hypotension

◆ Hypomagnesemia

▶ Signs include tremors, tetany, seizures, positive Chvostek's or Trousseau's signs, tachycardia, hypertension, ventricular arrhythmias, and personality changes

■ Medical management

◆ Hyponatremia

▶ In the patient with hyponatremia, the goal is to treat the underlying cause, increase the sodium concentration to a safe level, and reduce free water intake

▶ A hypovolemic patient should receive I.V. isotonic saline solution and albumin if hypoalbuminemia is present

▶ If neurologic symptoms develop, the saline infusion rate should be increased at a rate of 1 to 2 mEq/L per hour

▶ In the patient with chronic hyponatremia (hyponatremia persisting for more than 48 hours), the saline infusion rate should be increased to a maximum of 0.6 mEq/L per hour

▶ If the patient has water excess, a hypertonic saline solution (such as 3% sodium chloride) should be infused at a rate of 50 mg sodium per hour; in the normovolemic patient, suggest water restriction or increased water excretion by loop diuretics in conjunction with increased sodium and potassium intake

◆ Hypernatremia

▶ The causative factors of hypernatremia must be determined before treatment can begin

▶ Water loss can be replaced with hypotonic sodium chloride solution and dextrose 5% in water if the patient has moderate volume depletion or with isotonic saline solution if the patient has severe volume depletion, until volume is restored; lower the serum sodium level no faster than 2 mEq/L per hour to prevent cerebral edema

◆ Hypokalemia

▶ The management of hypokalemia begins with treating the underlying cause, while monitoring for cardiac changes (U waves on ECG) (See *Electrolyte effects on the ECG,* page 264)

▶ Oral or I.V. potassium is administered to raise the potassium level to within normal range

▶ Provide a diet with potassium-rich foods (bananas, apricots, orange juice, and broccoli)

◆ Hyperkalemia

▶ As with hypokalemia, initial management of hyperkalemia begins with treating the underlying cause, while monitoring for cardiac changes (tall pointed T waves on ECG)

Electrolyte effects on the ECG

ECG effects of hypokalemia

As the serum potassium concentration drops, the T wave becomes flat, and a U wave appears (shaded area). The rhythm strip below shows typical ECG effects of hypokalemia.

ECG effects of hyperkalemia

The classic and most striking ECG feature of hyperkalemia is tall, peaked T waves. This rhythm strip shows a typical peaked T wave (shaded area).

ECG effects of hypocalcemia

Decreased serum concentrations of calcium prolong the QT interval, as shown (shaded area) in this rhythm strip.

ECG effects of hypercalcemia

Increased serum concentrations of calcium cause shortening of the QT interval (shaded area). The rhythm strip shown here illustrates this key ECG finding in hypercalcemia.

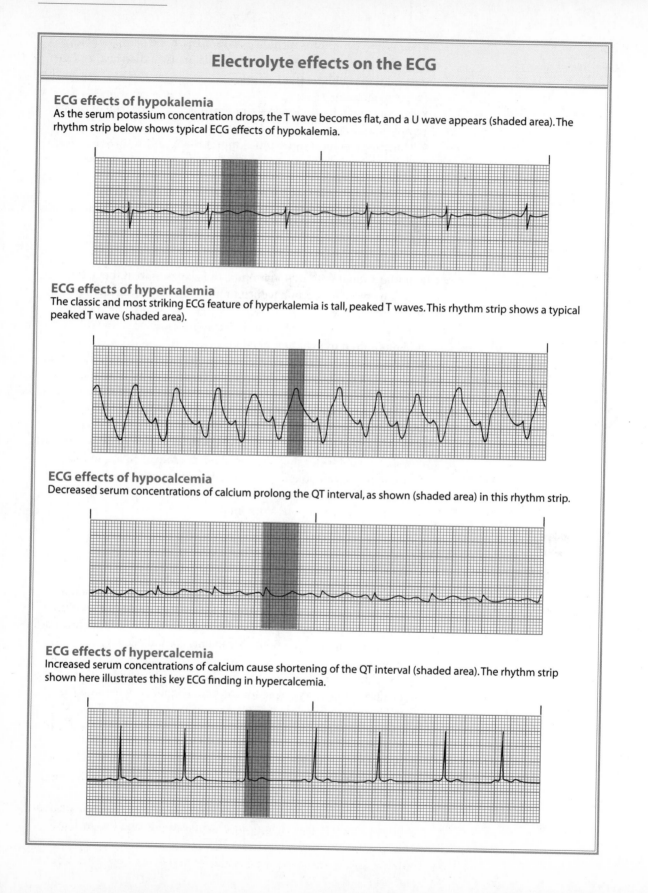

◗ When the potassium level is above 6 mEq/L, the patient should receive I.V. calcium gluconate to stabilize the myocardium

◗ Potassium can be shifted into the cells through the administration of I.V. sodium bicarbonate, hypertonic dextrose, and insulin

◗ Hemodialysis may be the quickest treatment for hyperkalemia, if dialysis access is intact

◗ Potassium can be removed less quickly through the use of potassium-binding resins (such as sodium polystyrene sulfonate [Kayexalate] or sorbitol) or diuretics

  • Kayexalate works by exchanging potassium for sodium in a 1:1 ratio in the bowel cell wall

  • Sorbitol induces diarrhea to remove potassium

◆ Hypocalcemia

◗ In patients with hypocalcemia, urgent treatment is usually required to relieve tetany and to prevent arrhythmias and seizures

◗ Administer I.V. calcium gluconate for short-term treatment of hypocalcemia; administer oral calcium carbonate for long-term therapy

◗ Monitor the ECG for lengthening QT intervals

◆ Hypercalcemia

◗ Along with treating the underlying cause, an isotonic sodium chloride infusion is used to control hypercalcemia through volume expansion and plasma calcium dilution

◗ Corticosteroids are administered to decrease calcium absorption in the intestines; if indicated, the patient may receive calcitonin therapy to regulate calcium level

◗ A low phosphate level may also need to be corrected in patients with hypercalcemia

◗ Monitor ECG for shortening QT interval

◆ Hypophosphatemia

◗ Hypophosphatemia can be managed orally or by administering I.V. phosphorus at a rate of 1 mmol/L/kg over 24 hours

◗ Hypophosphatemia secondary to TPN or acute respiratory alkalosis doesn't require replacement therapy

◗ Provide phosphate-rich foods (milk products); monitor for signs of infection (greater risk due to changes in white blood cell function)

◆ Hyperphosphatemia

◗ Hyperphosphatemia is treated with phosphate binders, such as aluminum hydroxide or aluminum carbonate, to decrease GI absorption of phosphorus

◗ Fluid intake or I.V. isotonic saline may be increased, if adequate renal function exists to promote renal phosphate excretion

◗ Administer hypertonic dextrose with regular insulin to temporarily drive phosphorus into the cell

◗ Dialysis for patients with compromised renal function

◗ Restrict dietary intake of phosphate-containing foods (such as milk and milk products)

◆ Hypomagnesemia

◗ In addition to treating the underlying cause of hypomagnesemia, management consists of magnesium-replacement therapy, with careful monitoring for subsequent signs and symptoms of hypermagnesemia

▶ Monitor vital signs during rapid infusions to detect respiratory or cardiac complications

▶ Provide dietary intake of magnesium-rich foods (for example, dairy products, green vegetables, meat, seafood, and cereals)

◆ Hypermagnesemia

▶ In addition to treating the underlying cause of hypermagnesemia, any magnesium-replacement therapy should be discontinued (for example, magnesium-containing antacids or laxatives or magnesium-rich dialysate)

▶ If indicated, I.V. calcium gluconate can be administered to counteract the neuromuscular and cardiac toxicities of hypermagnesemia

▶ Dialysis may be indicated for hypermagnesemic renal failure; a temporary cardiac pacemaker may be necessary with bradyarrhythmias

■ Nursing management

◆ Monitor the patient for various signs and symptoms of electrolyte imbalance; electrolyte abnormalities are potentially fatal if left untreated

◆ Observe for central pontine myelinolysis, which may result from excessively rapid correction of hyponatremia

◆ Dilute oral potassium supplements before administration; this step is necessary for proper absorption and to alleviate GI distress

◆ Infuse I.V. potassium supplements slowly to prevent hyperkalemia and, possibly, ventricular fibrillation

◆ Ensure that the patient is connected to a heart monitor during potassium replacement therapy; electrolyte replacement therapies can affect cardiac function

◆ Monitor for ECG changes, record the patient's intake and output, and check neurologic status frequently; these assessments are necessary to identify treatment complications

◆ Check whether the patient is receiving digoxin therapy; electrolyte abnormalities, especially abnormalities in the potassium level, increase the risk of digoxin toxicity

❖ Kidney transplantation

■ Description

◆ Patients with end-stage renal disease are candidates for kidney transplantation

◆ The transplanted kidney may be donated by a living relative or taken from a cadaver

◆ To prevent rejection of the transplanted organ, immunosuppressant medications are given

■ Contraindications

◆ Contraindications to kidney transplantation vary among transplant centers

◆ The three absolute contraindications are incurable cancer, refractory noncompliance, and patient refusal to provide informed consent

■ Medical management

◆ Determine whether the patient is a candidate for kidney transplantation

◆ Maintain potential recipients on dialysis before surgical kidney transplantation

■ Nursing management
  ◆ Determine the patient's level of knowledge about the transplant procedure and its implications; a patient-teaching plan that covers all aspects of transplantation is necessary for the procedure's success
  ◆ Before the transplant procedure, monitor the patient's vital signs; check when the patient last underwent dialysis; perform a physical assessment; assess for recent exposure to infection; review laboratory test results, including blood crossmatching and baseline values; ensure that a chest X-ray was taken; maintain the patient on nothing-by-mouth status; teach the patient how to turn, cough, and deep-breathe; and initiate immunosuppressant therapy
  ◆ After the transplant procedure, maintain adequate respiratory function and fluid volume status, monitor for signs and symptoms of rejection or infection, and assess renal transplant function
    ▶ Immunosuppressant medications leave the patient vulnerable to infection
    ▶ The typical initial signs and symptoms of rejection are decreased urine output, abdominal pain, and low-grade fever
  ◆ Help the patient manage emotional aspects of the procedure; after major surgery involving transplantation of an organ from another person, many patients have difficulty coping emotionally
  ◆ Before discharge, educate the patient about diet, fluid intake, medications, activity level, signs and symptoms of infection and rejection, and follow-up appointments

❖ **Continuous arteriovenous hemofiltration**
  ■ Description
    ◆ In continuous arteriovenous hemofiltration (CAVH), arterial blood is diverted through a small artificial kidney filter (see *CAVH setup*, page 268)
      ▶ An arterial port and a venous port are placed on opposite sides of the filter to connect the filter to a larger artery and a major vein
      ▶ Blood flows through the filter and back through the venous system
      ▶ Ultrafiltrate is removed by means of a drain port
    ◆ The patient's systolic blood pressure must be at least 80 mm Hg for CAVH to function properly
    ◆ CAVH is used to manage short-term renal problems in hemodynamically unstable patients who can't tolerate hemodialysis or peritoneal dialysis
  ■ Medical management
    ◆ Determine the patient's suitability for CAVH
    ◆ Obtain vascular access
    ◆ Determine the appropriate length of treatment
  ■ Nursing management
    ◆ Frequently monitor the filter site and connections for clots, leaks, and kinks; these common complications prevent the device from working properly
    ◆ Don't allow the patient to lie on the filter, which can kink the tubes or damage the filter

CAVH setup

The illustration below shows how to set up equipment for continuous arteriovenous hemofiltration (CAVH). The doctor inserts two large-bore, single-lumen catheters (depicted below). One catheter is inserted into an artery, most commonly the femoral artery. The other catheter is inserted into a vein, usually the femoral, subclavian, or internal jugular vein.

The patient's arterial blood pressure serves as a natural pump, driving blood through the arterial line. A hemofilter removes water and toxic solutes (ultrafiltrate) from the blood. Replacement fluid is infused into a port on the arterial side. This same port can be used to infuse heparin. The venous line carries the replacement fluid and purified blood to the patient.

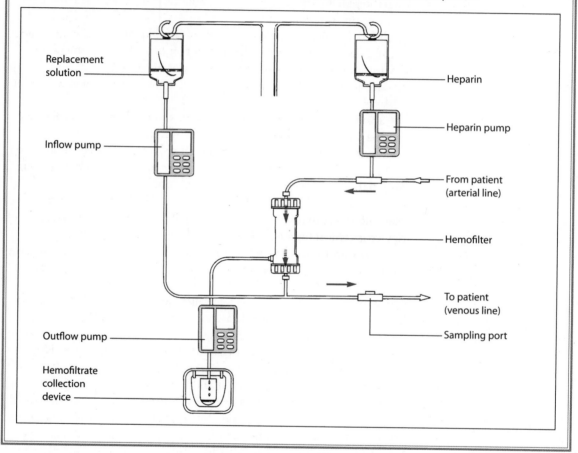

- Replacement solution
- Inflow pump
- Outflow pump
- Hemofiltrate collection device
- Heparin
- Heparin pump
- From patient (arterial line)
- Hemofilter
- To patient (venous line)
- Sampling port

◆ Use aseptic technique when handling this type of filter and tubes because infectious organisms can be easily introduced into the bloodstream

❖ **Hemodialysis**
- ■ Description
  - ◆ Hemodialysis is the removal of waste products or toxins from the blood by diffusion across a semipermeable membrane, while the blood is circulated outside the body
  - ◆ Hemodialysis is indicated for CRF and ARF resulting from trauma or infection; it's also used to rapidly remove toxic substances, including alcohol, barbiturates, and poisons
  - ◆ There are no absolute contraindications to hemodialysis

■ Medical management
  ◆ Determine the patient's suitability for hemodialysis
  ◆ Obtain vascular access by means of surgical insertion of a double-lumen subclavian catheter, atrioventricular fistula, or atrioventricular graft
  ◆ Determine the length of treatment, and select the dialysis machine pressure settings
■ Nursing management
  ◆ Educate the patient about hemodialysis and the associated vascular access procedures
  ◆ Before hemodialysis is started, monitor the patient's vital signs, including heart rate and rhythm; assess volume status by checking the patient's weight, neck vein distention, PAWP, central venous pressure (CVP), and intake and output; and review laboratory and X-ray reports
    ▶ These assessments are necessary to determine the dialysis machine settings
    ▶ They also provide baseline parameters for assessing postdialysis data
  ◆ Assist the physician with vascular access placement; this procedure may be done in the patient's room, but is usually performed in the operating room
  ◆ After vascular access is obtained, secure all connections and verify placement before beginning hemodialysis; patency of the vascular access device is critical for successful hemodialysis
  ◆ Follow anticoagulant protocols to prevent dialyzer clotting complications; patients with active bleeding or contraindications to heparin can be dialyzed on a heparin-free or citrate anticoagulant regimen
  ◆ Check activated clotting times to monitor the effects of heparin administration
    ▶ Activated clotting times should be determined 1 hour after dialysis is started and 30 minutes before dialysis is discontinued or if clots are seen
    ▶ Activated clotting times should be determined every 3½ to 4 minutes during dialysis in patients with subclavian catheters, Hemocaths, or external shunts
  ◆ Don't perform venipuncture, administer I.V. therapy or injections, or take a blood pressure reading with a cuff on the extremity with vascular access; all these activities can damage the vascular access and impede hemodialysis
  ◆ Instruct patients not to lie on the extremity having vascular access, wear tight clothing, or injure the extremity in any way
  ◆ Monitor access sites for bleeding, which is one of the most serious complications of vascular access

❖ **Peritoneal dialysis**
  ■ Description
    ◆ In peritoneal dialysis, the peritoneum surrounding the abdominal cavity serves as a dialyzing membrane
    ◆ Peritoneal dialysis is indicated for ARF, CRF, refractory heart failure, and intraperitoneal chemotherapy

◆ There are three forms of peritoneal dialysis: continuous ambulatory peritoneal dialysis, continuous cyclic peritoneal dialysis, and intermittent peritoneal dialysis

▶ *Continuous ambulatory peritoneal dialysis* is the treatment of choice; it involves exchanges over a 24-hour period, 7 days a week

▶ *Continuous cyclic peritoneal dialysis* uses a cycling machine that infuses and drains dialysate fluid while the patient sleeps at night; during the day, the patient doesn't have any dialysate fluid in the peritoneal cavity

▶ *Intermittent peritoneal dialysis (also called automated peritoneal dialysis)* can be performed manually or with a cycling machine; typically, it's done at night, and the dialysate from the last exchange remains in the peritoneal cavity during the day, then drained at the initiation of the next exchange

■ Contraindications

◆ An absolute contraindication to peritoneal dialysis is significant loss of peritoneal surface resulting from adhesions or recurrent peritonitis

◆ Relative contraindications include the presence of ostomies, extreme obesity, recent abdominal surgery or trauma, and tuberculous or fungal peritonitis

◆ Continuous ambulatory peritoneal dialysis and continuous cyclic peritoneal dialysis may be contraindicated when the patient has a condition exacerbated by intraperitoneal pressure, such as hernia, hemorrhoids, or lower back pain

■ Medical management

◆ Determine the patient's suitability for peritoneal dialysis

◆ Surgically insert an abdominal catheter

◆ Determine the solution concentration based on laboratory values

■ Nursing management

◆ Educate the patient about peritoneal dialysis, including peritoneal catheter placement, what to expect before and after the procedure, the importance of aseptic technique, use of local anesthetics, anticipated discomfort, and postprocedure activity; after the catheter is inserted, the patient is responsible for much of his own care and must thoroughly understand the dialysis procedure

◆ Assist the physician with catheter placement; a patient undergoing peritoneal dialysis typically has a trocar catheter surgically inserted into his peritoneum

◆ Before peritoneal dialysis is started, monitor the patient's vital signs, including heart rate and rhythm; assess volume status by checking the patient's weight, neck vein distention, PAWP, CVP, and intake and output; and review laboratory and X-ray reports; due to some degree of pre-existing renal failure, the patient must be closely monitored before dialysis begins

◆ Inspect the catheter and exit site for dialysate leaks and signs and symptoms of infection; these complications are commonly seen after the catheter is inserted

◆ Review how to use the manual or automated dialysis system, dialysate volume, dialysate dextrose concentration, and fill, dwell, and drain times with the patient

◆ Explain to the patient how medications are added to the dialysate, and ensure that he understands the parameters for adjusting dialysate dextrose concentrations and knows how to care for the catheter exit site; this information is crucial to prevent infection

◆ Teach the patient how to perform the peritoneal dialysis procedure; ascertain patency by draining the first dialysate solution and then allowing other infusions to fill, dwell (usually for 20 to 45 minutes), and drain

◆ Check the color and consistency of the drainage

▶ Normal drainage is clear and pale yellow

▶ Bleeding or bloody drainage isn't unusual during the first to fourth exchanges

▶ Cloudy fluid usually indicates peritonitis, which requires immediate treatment

◆ Teach the patient to monitor his vital signs and record total body intake and output (have him record the measured amount of fluid removed for each exchange, and record the negative and positive balance); make sure that patients with diabetes are aware that dialysate contains glucose and some absorption may occur; confirm that they know how to monitor their blood glucose level

◆ Teach the patient how to obtain outflow fluid samples for baseline culture and sensitivity tests

❖ Renal trauma

■ Description

◆ Injury to the kidney or lower urinary tract

◆ Blunt injuries are the most common cause of renal trauma and may be caused by motor vehicle accident, fall, sport-related impact, or assault

◆ Penetrating injuries are most often caused by gunshot or stab wounds

◆ The right kidney is more susceptible to injury due to its lower position

▶ Right kidney trauma is often seen with an injury to the liver

◆ Left kidney trauma is often seen with an injury to the spleen

◆ Renal traumas are divided into five classes

▶ Class I (renal contusion): The kidney is compressed between the vertebral column and the lower ribs; the kidney may have a subcapsular hematoma and minor cortical lacerations

▶ Class II (cortical laceration): Cortical laceration is often caused by a fracture of ribs 10 through 12 or one of the transverse processes of the vertebrae; the kidney has a damaged renal capsule and parenchyma and may also have damage to the collecting system

▶ Class III (caliceal laceration): In this injury, a large single laceration or several smaller ones extend into the collecting system

▶ Class IV (renal fracture or shattered kidney): The kidney has extensive lacerations at multiple sites, and the collecting system has damage

▶ Class V (vascular pedicle injury or renal artery thrombosis): A vascular pedicle injury is often caused by a penetrating injury involving a tear or laceration to the renal vasculature; a renal artery thrombosis is usually caused by a blunt injury and occurs when the intima is torn away, and blood is forced into the space; this results in a thrombosis that occludes the vessel

■ Clinical signs and symptoms
   ◆ The patient may have upper quadrant pain; persistent flank pain may indicate a renal artery thrombosis
      ▶ Renal colic pain radiates from the flank into the groin, thigh, or external genitals; this may indicate a passage of clots
   ◆ Hematuria, due to bleeding in the kidney, may be microscopic or gross
   ◆ The patient may have decreased or absent urine output
   ◆ The patient may have abdominal distention, flank swelling, a mass, or a hematoma in the flank area
   ◆ Entrance or exit wound may be seen if the causative injury was a penetrating trauma
   ◆ Bruit may be auscultated with a renal artery thrombosis
   ◆ Retroperitoneal bleeding may be indicated by back pain, signs of hemorrhage with no visible bleeding site noted, or Grey Turner's sign (ecchymosis over the flank)
   ◆ Many physical signs are hard to see because of the location of the kidneys beneath abdominal organs, bony structures, and back muscles
   ◆ If the bladder has ruptured, the absorption of urine will cause hyperkalemia, hypernatremia, uremia, and acidosis
■ Diagnostic tests
   ◆ BUN and creatinine are elevated
   ◆ If bleeding is present, the hemoglobin and hematocrit will be decreased
   ◆ A urinalysis will be positive for blood
   ◆ Chest X-ray will show fractured ribs on the affected side
   ◆ Kidney-ureter-bladder X-ray will evaluate the position, size, and structure of the renal system; it may show rib fracture, bowel displacement, or obliteration of renal shadow from bleeding
   ◆ An intravenous pyelogram will show the renal vasculature and functional tissue; it will identify renal pedicle injury, renal infarct, a hematoma, and the presence of lacerations or shattered kidney
   ◆ Renal ultrasound is not used for early identification of injury due to lack of precision
   ◆ CT of the kidneys will reveal lacerations, infarcts, hematomas, and urine extravasation; if contrast is used, arterial occlusion can also be detected; renal CT is the diagnostic tool of choice in renal trauma
   ◆ An MRI will give a clearer picture if needed before a surgical intervention
■ Medical management
   ◆ Administer analgesics as needed for pain
   ◆ Provide volume replacement with crystalloids, colloids, or blood products as indicated
   ◆ Surgical repair may be needed for extensive renal trauma, bladder injury, or injury to the ureters
   ◆ Administer antibiotics to prevent infection
■ Nursing management
   ◆ Keep patient on bed rest with limited activities
   ◆ Administer pain medication as needed

◆ Obtain intravenous access with a minimum of two large-gauge I.V. catheters; be prepared to administer fluid and blood products if patient begins to hemorrhage

◆ Send blood to laboratory for laboratory values, and send blood to blood bank for type and cross if needed

◆ Monitor lab values including BUN and creatinine, hemoglobin, hematocrit for signs of worsening kidney function or bleeding

◆ Assess patient for signs of peritonitis: hard, rigid abdomen, distended abdomen, nausea and vomiting, and fever

◆ Administer other medications as ordered: antibiotics; diuretics; dopamine

◆ Insert an indwelling catheter unless the ureter is damaged; keep the catheter patent; carefully monitor intake and output; notify the physician immediately for a significant drop in urine output; and also monitor urine for signs of hematuria

◆ Monitor patient for signs of infection, including fever, increased pain at wound, chills

◆ Prepare patient for surgery if indicated

◆ Monitor vital signs

◆ If a nephrostomy tube if present, monitor tube for patentcy, bleeding, or leakage of urine; some bleeding is normal and should decrease after 24 to 48 hours

◆ Monitor patient for complications including ileus, renal failure, shock, hemorrhage, infection, sepsis, and hypertension

Review questions

1. A 72-year-old patient with a 30-year history of type 2 diabetes mellitus and hypertension is concerned that his kidneys aren't functioning as well as they did when he was younger. With regard to aging and normal renal function, the nurse should remember that:

○ **A.** the GFR declines sharply, but renal blood flow doesn't change.

○ **B.** renal blood flow declines sharply, but the GFR doesn't change.

○ **C.** nephrons decrease in number.

○ **D.** the GFR increases, leading to increased urine output.

Correct answer: B Renal blood flow declines sharply as a normal part of aging, but the GFR doesn't change.

2. A patient with CRF asks the nurse why he's anemic. The nurse explains that anemia accompanies CRF because of:

○ **A.** blood loss via the urine.

○ **B.** renal insensitivity to vitamin D.

○ **C.** inadequate production of erythropoietin.

○ **D.** inadequate retention of serum iron.

Correct answer: C Erythropoietin, responsible for the stimulation and production of red blood cells, is produced mainly by the kidneys.

3. The nurse is caring for a patient who's experiencing hematuria, with red blood cell casts and proteinuria exceeding 3 to 5 g per day and albumin as the major protein. The most probable medical diagnosis is:

○ **A.** cystitis.

○ **B.** chronic pyelonephritis.

○ **C.** glomerulonephritis.

○ **D.** nephrotic syndrome.

Correct answer: C The patient's signs are most commonly related to glomerulonephritis, resulting in an inability to retain large cellular products in the tubules (such as red blood cells and protein).

4. During a preemployment health history, a 28-year-old female tells the nurse that she had two bouts of pyelonephritis while a high school exchange student in Germany 11 years ago. She asks the nurse what caused the pyelonephritis. The nurse explains that pyelonephritis, an infection of the renal pelvis and interstitium, is usually caused by:

○ **A.** bacteria.

○ **B.** fungi.

○ **C.** viruses.

○ **D.** all of the above.

Correct answer: A Bacterial invasion of the renal system is the most common cause of pyelonephritis.

5. The nurse is teaching a 20-year-old college student how to prevent urinary tract infections (UTIs). Which of the following factors normally acts to prevent UTIs?

○ **A.** Unobstructed flow of urine

○ **B.** High pH of urine

○ **C.** Ureterovesical junction that's open during micturition

○ **D.** Normal flora of the urinary tract

Correct answer: A Unobstructed urine flow is a primary factor in UTI prevention. Other factors include low urine pH and closed ureterovesical junction during micturition.

Multisystem disorders

❖ Shock
- Description
  - ◆ In shock, an insufficient circulating blood volume results in less than adequate perfusion of cells and vital organs
  - ◆ Regardless of its cause, the result of prolonged shock is the same—cell death due to lack of adequate nutrition and lack of tissue oxygenation
  - ◆ The severely ill patient typically seen in the critical care unit (CCU) is always at risk for some type of shock
  - ◆ There are four types of shock: hypovolemic (discussed in Chapter 2), cardiogenic (discussed in Chapter 2), obstructive, and distributive
    - ▶ Obstructive shock may be due to impaired diastolic filling (such as occurs in pericardial tamponade, tension pneumothorax, constrictive pericarditis, or compression of great veins), increased right ventricular afterload (from pulmonary emboli, pulmonary hypertension, positive end-expiratory pressure), or from increased left ventricular afterload (as in aortic dissection, systemic embolization, aortic stenosis, or abdominal distention)
    - ▶ Causes of distributive shock include neurogenic, anaphylactic, and septic
  - ◆ Many of the nursing assessments and basic nursing care are similar for all types of shock
- Septic distributive shock
  - ◆ Sepsis occurs when large numbers of pathogenic microorganisms or their toxins are present in the blood or other tissues
  - ◆ Although it doesn't always lead to septic distributive shock, sepsis is almost always fatal if left untreated
  - ◆ Septic distributive shock results when massive vasodilation occurs secondary to the release of toxins by certain bacteria
  - ◆ Septic distributive shock is most common in patients with sepsis caused by gram-negative organisms (such as *Escherichia coli, Klebsiella, Proteus,* and *Pseudomonas*), some gram-positive organisms (such as *Streptococcus* and *Staphylococcus*), fungi, viruses, or *Rickettsiae*
  - ◆ Sepsis and septic distributive shock may be caused by peritonitis, urinary tract infection, toxic shock syndrome, food poisoning, lacerations, compound fractures, major burn injuries, and conditions that cause debilitation, such as cancer and stroke

Assessment findings in early and late septic distributive shock

In early septic distributive shock, the body's compensatory mechanisms attempt to fight the widespread systemic infection. As septic shock progresses, it's complicated by inadequate perfusion of cells and vital organs. Early septic shock can be characterized as the hyperdynamic phase of septic shock; late shock can be characterized as the hypodynamic phase. The assessment findings for each stage are shown below.

System	Early stage	Late stage
Respiratory	Tachypnea, deep breaths	Tachypnea, shallow breaths
Cardiovascular	Mild hypotension, decreased afterload, decreased preload, increased cardiac output, sinus tachycardia	Severe hypotension, increased afterload, decreased preload, decreased cardiac output, ventricular arrhythmias
Neurologic	Anxiety, alertness, mild confusion	Decreased level of consciousness, severe confusion to unconsciousness
Renal	Near-normal urine output	Decreased or absent urine output
Hematologic (as evidenced by blood pH)	Normal or respiratory alkalosis	Metabolic acidosis

◆ The clinical signs and symptoms of early septic distributive shock differ from those of late septic shock (see *Assessment findings in early and late septic distributive shock*)
■ Medical management
◆ Rapidly infuse I.V. solutions
◆ Administer I.V. antibiotics
◆ Maintain the patient on strict bed rest
◆ Use the shock position (place the patient in a supine position with his legs elevated 10 to 30 degrees) or modified Trendelenburg's position, as needed
◆ Administer volume expanders, plasma, dextran, and albumin, as indicated, and monitor for fluid overload
◆ Insert arterial and central venous lines for pressure monitoring
■ Nursing management
◆ Monitor for restlessness, anxiety, apprehension, and decreased level of consciousness (LOC); decreased cerebral perfusion secondary to the shock state causes changes in neurologic status
◆ Assess for changes in skin temperature and color
▶ Decreased oxygenation and the stress response lead to vasoconstriction, causing the skin to become cold, pale, and diaphoretic
▶ A gray color to the skin often indicates gram-negative sepsis; a ruddy color may indicate a gram-positive infection
◆ Monitor vital signs, including heart and respiratory rates, blood pressure, and temperature
▶ The shock state reduces the circulating blood volume and typically lowers the blood pressure (mean arterial pressure [MAP] less than 70 mm Hg) and increases the pulse rate (above 100 beats per minute) as a compensatory mechanism

Hemodynamic changes in shock

	Hypovolemic	Cardiogenic	Early Septic	Late Septic
HR	High	High	High	High
BP	Normal to low	Normal to low	Normal to low	Low
CO/CI	Low	Low	High	Low
PAWP	Low	High	Low	High but may be normal or low
SVR	High	High	Low	High

◗ The respiratory rate tends to increase to help maintain oxygenation

◗ Body temperature may increase as a result of the bacterial infection, although the temperature may remain normal in patients with overwhelming infection and in older patients

◆ Control the patient's temperature with hypothermia blankets, light covers, tepid soaks, and alcohol baths; high fever must be lowered to prevent brain damage

◆ Monitor for decreased urine output (less than 25 ml per hour); a MAP of less than 70 mm Hg can lead to inadequate renal perfusion and decreased urine output

◆ Monitor arterial blood gas (ABG) values for metabolic acidosis; many organisms produce toxins that cause lactic acidosis, thereby lowering the pH below 7.35 and bicarbonate below 22 mEq/L

◆ Assess for thirst; as the circulating fluid volume decreases, the hydration mechanism attempts to compensate by increasing the patient's need for oral fluid intake

◆ Check data from pulmonary artery catheters or central venous pressure lines every 1 to 4 hours; these are generally inserted in patients with septic shock and are useful for monitoring cardiac output, fluid volume, and hydration status (See *Hemodynamic changes in shock*)

◆ Monitor oxygenation with pulse oximetry, ABG measurements, or other means; the shock state decreases partial pressure of oxygen, oxygen saturation, and pH levels

◆ Observe and report changes in the patient's condition that indicate worsening infection

◗ Sepsis and septic distributive shock progress rapidly to overwhelming infection that is often irreversible

◗ Any deterioration in the patient's condition requires aggressive treatment

◆ Maintain a patent airway, and administer supplemental oxygen to lessen the effects of cerebral anoxia

◆ Monitor for potential complications, which include pulmonary edema, metabolic acidosis, disseminated intravascular coagulation (DIC), systemic inflammatory response syndrome (SIRS), and multiple organ dysfunction syndrome (MODS)

◆ Monitor the rapid infusion of I.V. solutions; large amounts of I.V. solution are needed to lessen the effects of hypovolemia caused by vasodilation and blood pooling

◆ Maintain the patient on strict bed rest to decrease cellular oxygen demands

◆ Monitor the patient closely if the shock position or modified Trendelenburg's position is used; elevating the foot of the bed 45 degrees with the head of the bed slightly elevated increases peripheral venous return and permits adequate respiratory exchange

◆ Reposition the patient every 2 hours or more frequently, if necessary, to reduce the risk of skin breakdown resulting from immobility

◆ Monitor the effects of I.V. antibiotic therapy

  ▶ The patient with septic shock will typically receive large doses of several broad-spectrum I.V. antibiotics

  ▶ Allergic reactions, renal failure, aplastic anemia, and other adverse effects may result from antibiotic therapy

◆ Monitor the effects of volume expanders, plasma, dextran, and albumin, if prescribed, and check for fluid overload

  ▶ Hypertonic volume expanders draw fluid from the tissues into the vascular system

  ▶ Heart failure is a potential adverse effect of volume expanders, particularly in elderly patients

◆ Administer and monitor the effects of other commonly used medications

  ▶ High doses of dopamine, epinephrine, norepinephrine, and metaraminol bitartrate are used as sympathetic stimulants

  ▶ Low doses of dopamine and nitroglycerin are used as vasodilators

  ▶ High doses of steroids may be used to decrease inflammation and stabilize cell membranes; long-term steroid use suppresses the immune system

❖ **Multiple organ dysfunction syndrome**

  ■ Description

    ◆ This syndrome occurs when two or more organs or organ systems are unable to function in their role of maintaining homeostasis

    ◆ MODS isn't an illness itself; it's a manifestation of another progressive underlying condition

    ◆ MODS occurs when widespread systemic inflammation, a condition known as SIRS, overtaxes the patient's compensation mechanisms

      ▶ SIRS is triggered by injury, infection, ischemia, or trauma; SIRS can progress and lead to organ inflammation and MODS

      ▶ Burns, surgical procedures, shock, pancreatitis, DIC, nosocomial infection, sepsis, cardiopulmonary arrest, and immunosuppression are also causes of MODS

    ◆ Primary MODS involves organ or organ system failure that is caused by a direct injury (trauma, aspiration) or a primary disorder (pneumonia, pulmonary embolism)

      ▶ The patient will develop acute respiratory distress syndrome (ARDS), followed by encephalopathy, coagulopathy, and other organ systems failure

◆ Secondary MODS involves organ or organ system failure due to sepsis; the infection source usually isn't the lungs; common infection sources include intra-abdominal sepsis, extensive blood loss, pancreatitis, or major vascular injury

▶ ARDS develops sooner and progressive involvement of other organ and organ systems occur more rapidly than in primary MODS

◆ Mortality associated with MODS increases as more organ systems fail; when there are four or more organ or organ systems involved, the mortality exceeds 80%

■ Clinical signs and symptoms

◆ Dysfunction of two or more organ or organ systems, including pulmonary, hematologic, renal, hepatic, or neurologic

◆ Early symptoms reflect a hypermetabolic state and include fever, tachycardia, narrow pulse pressure, tachypnea, and decreased pulmonary artery pressure (PAP), pulmonary artery wedge pressure (PAWP), and central venous pressure (CVP) and an increased carbon dioxide (CO)

◆ Symptoms progress to impaired organ and tissue perfusion and include decreased LOC, respiratory depression, decreased bowel sounds, jaundice, oliguria or anuria, increased PAP and PAWP and decreased CO

◆ The patient will progress from a decreased LOC into a coma as perfusion to the brain continues to decrease

◆ Crackles will be heard in the lung fields due to the increased water presence in ARDS

◆ The systemic vascular resistance (SVR) will decrease due to inflammatory mediator-induced vasodilation

◆ The patient may have increased bleeding tendencies, depending on the degree of involvement of the hematologic system

■ Diagnostic tests

◆ The tests performed will depend on the cause, such as trauma, aspiration, pulmonary embolism, or sepsis; findings will vary based on what systems are affected

◆ ABGs will reveal hypoxemia with respiratory or metabolic acidosis

◆ Complete blood count will show decreased hemoglobin and hematocrit levels and leukocytosis

◆ Chest X-ray will show pulmonary infiltrates and findings consistent with ARDS

◆ Fibrin split products will be more than 1:40 or a D-dimer greater than 200 ng/ml, prothrombin time and partial thrombin time prolonged consistent with DIC

◆ Elevated serum creatinine level and increased urinary sodium level due to acute tubular necrosis

◆ Increase in serum bilirubin, alkaline phosphate, alanine aminotransferase, aspartate aminotransferase, and gamma glutamyltransferase levels

◆ Increased serum glucose level due to gluconeogenesis and hepatic failure

■ Medical management

◆ The more aggressive that treatment is in the early stages, the better the outcome

◆ Provide oxygenation and mechanical ventilation; often positive end-respiratory pressure (PEEP) is needed to maintain arterial oxygen saturation (SaO_2) greater than 95%

◆ Place a pulmonary artery catheter and monitor hemodynamics; administer fluid and vasopressors as needed

◆ If patient has renal system involvement, begin hemodialysis

◆ Administer antimicrobial agents to prevent the spread of infection

◆ Administer blood and blood products

◆ Administer inotropes to increase CO

◆ Consider use of activated protein C (drotrecogin alfa) to reduce the inflammatory response

■ Nursing management

◆ The care for a MODS patient is mostly supportive

◆ Maintain a patent airway and breathing with mechanical ventilation and supplemental oxygenation

❱ Assess ABGs for acidosis, decreased partial pressure of arterial oxygen, and increased partial pressure of carbon dioxide

❱ Monitor patient for development or worsening of ARDS as evidenced by an increasing pulmonary inspiratory pressure, an increase in PEEP, and an increase in fraction of inspired oxygen needed to maintain an SaO_2 greater than 95%

◆ Monitor vital signs, hemodynamic parameter, and cardiac rhythm

❱ Keep systolic blood pressure equal to or greater than 95 mmHg to help maintain tissue perfusion

❱ PAWP should be 6 to 12 mm Hg, CO 4 to 7 L/min, and an SVR of 900 to 1,200 dynes/sce/cm-5 for optimal tissue and organ perfusion

  • If patient becomes acutely hypotensive, place him in Trendelenburg position to optimize cerebral perfusion

  • Give crystalloids and colloids to maintain the PAWP; assess lung sounds frequently during fluid administration to detect signs of fluid overload

  • Use vasopressors to keep MAP greater than 70 for organ perfusion

  • Use inotropes to increase cardiac output

◆ Monitor mixed venous oxygen saturation (SvO_2) to assess tissue perfusion. An SvO_2 less than 60% indicates impaired oxygen delivery or increased oxygen consumption

◆ Prepare to transfuse blood or blood products to increase fluid status or to increase to oxygen-carrying capacity of the blood

◆ Weigh patient daily and carefully monitor intake and output; notify physician immediately if the urine output decreases significantly; monitor serum blood urea nitrogen and creatinine; prepare patient for dialysis if indicated

◆ Monitor laboratory values and watch patient for signs of DIC; be prepared to administer fresh frozen plasma, platelets, or vitamin K to help correct coagulopathies

◆ Administer medications as ordered, including antibiotics and corticosteroids to help block the inflammation

◆ Provide emotional support to the family and patient; explain diagnostic tests and treatments

◆ Monitor neurological status and assess for signs of decreased cerebral perfusion, including decreased LOC, restlessness, or confusion

◆ Monitor patient for signs of hypoperfusion, including cool extremities, pallor, mottling, and decreased capillary refill

◆ Turn or reposition patient every 2 hours to prevent skin breakdown

◆ Provide enteral nutrition if GI system functioning; administer parenteral nutrition if GI or hepatic system involvement precludes the use of enteral feedings

❖ **Toxic ingestions**
  ■ Description
    ◆ Toxic ingestions include all types of drug overdoses, whether accidental or intentional; this category also encompasses accidental ingestion of common household chemicals and withdrawal from addictive substances, including alcohol and drugs such as cocaine and heroin
      ▶ These substances range from cleaning products—such as furniture polish, liquid detergents, and window cleaners—to industrial chemicals, including antifreeze, lye-based compounds, and petroleum products
      ▶ The care of children and adults who ingest these substances is similar
    ◆ Patients who have ingested toxic substances are often monitored and managed in the CCU
    ◆ Although each substance causes unique problems and complications, nursing care is similar for all types of toxic ingestion
    ◆ Another group of patients who may be cared for in the CCU are those who have accidentally overdosed on prescription medications
      ▶ Elderly patients are particularly susceptible to this type of poisoning
      ▶ Many of the medications that older patients are routinely prescribed have narrow therapeutic ranges and potential toxicity; even small overdoses of cardiac medications, such as digoxin (Lanoxin), diltiazem (Cardizem), propranolol, and disopyramide, can cause severe arrhythmias or even cardiac arrest
      ▶ Other categories of medications, including antibiotics, steroids, antihypertensive agents, and hypoglycemic agents, can be lethal in large doses for elderly patients
  ■ Medical management
    ◆ Contact the regional poison control center to determine how to counteract the effects of the substance or eliminate it from the body
    ◆ Dilute the substance by giving the patient milk or water—as indicated by the poison control center—unless the patient is unresponsive
    ◆ If indicated, perform gastric lavage using a large-bore orogastric tube; gastric lavage is particularly important in patients who have ingested caustic substances (strong bases) or hydrocarbons (petroleum products or cleaning solutions)
    ◆ Use a peristaltic pump to wash out the patient's gut with warmed electrolyte solutions
    ◆ If the substance is a drug or noncaustic substance, induce emesis with 30 ml of ipecac syrup followed by 240 ml of water; vomiting should occur within 15 to 30 minutes

◆ Administer 25 to 50 g of activated charcoal by evacuator tube after the ipecac syrup has induced vomiting
◆ Administer antidotes or antagonist medications, as appropriate
◆ Support the patient's cardiopulmonary status as his condition indicates (ventilator, cardiac bypass, vasopressors)
◆ Consider dialysis if the substance requires this for elimination or to support renal status

■ Nursing management
◆ Monitor vital signs at least every 15 minutes until the patient is stable; most drug overdoses produce significant changes in vital signs, including increased pulse rate and decreased blood pressure, respiratory rate, and temperature
◆ Assess neurologic signs with the Glasgow Coma Scale or another appropriate neurologic assessment tool every hour until the patient is stable; many drugs, particularly those that affect the central nervous system (CNS), alter neurologic signs
◆ Obtain as complete a history as possible concerning the type and amount of substance ingested, when it occurred, current medication use, and whether the patient has associated health problems or long-term health problems; many factors influence how substances act in the body, and a complete history can be valuable in determining appropriate treatment
◆ Maintain a patent airway; many medications can suppress the CNS and respiratory center
◆ Position the patient on his side, and keep suction equipment at the bedside; the side-lying position promotes drainage of secretions, and suction equipment may be needed if the patient vomits
◆ Monitor ABG values, as prescribed; changes in ABG values may be the first warning sign of alterations in the respiratory system
◆ Monitor urine output every hour; report outputs of less than 25 ml per hour or any sudden changes in output; changes in output may indicate impending renal failure or changes in hydration status
◆ Monitor and maintain invasive lines, such as those used for CVP and PAP monitoring, and arterial or subclavian I.V. lines; patients who are treated in the CCU often have one or more of these devices in place to maintain hydration and facilitate monitoring
◆ Monitor for complications of acetaminophen overdose, including hepatic failure, coagulation defects, renal failure, hepatic encephalopathy, and shock
◆ Monitor for complications of salicylate overdose, including respiratory failure, arrhythmias, acid-base imbalances, renal tubular necrosis, GI bleeding, hepatotoxicity, pulmonary edema, and shock
◆ Monitor for signs of alcohol toxicity, including respiratory depression, aspiration, hepatic failure, and GI bleeding
◆ Monitor for complications of barbiturate overdose, including arrhythmias, respiratory arrest, seizures, pulmonary edema, and shock
◆ Monitor for signs of benzodiazepine overdose, including respiratory depression, tachycardia, hypotension, and coma

◆ Monitor for cocaine toxicity, which can cause myocardial infarction, tachyarrhythmias, cerebral hemorrhage, respiratory arrest, and status epilepticus

◆ Monitor for opioid overdose, which can result in respiratory arrest, arrhythmias, and shock

◆ Monitor for complications of tricyclic antidepressant overdose, including arrhythmias, complete heart block, heart failure, paralytic ileus, and shock

◆ Initiate and maintain good therapeutic communication with patients who have attempted suicide

  ▶ After a suicide attempt, many patients feel shame, guilt, hopelessness, and helplessness

  ▶ Allowing these patients to express their feelings in a noncondemning environment can aid in their recovery

◆ Check the environment for items that could be used in future suicide attempts; although most patients don't make another suicide attempt while in the hospital, the CCU isn't an especially safe place for such patients

❖ **Asphyxia**
  ■ Description
    ◆ Asphyxia is a general term used to describe low oxygen level in the blood with a corresponding increase in carbon dioxide level
    ◆ Anything that interrupts normal gas exchange in the respiratory system can produce asphyxia
    ◆ Common causes of asphyxia include near drowning; trauma to the face, neck, larynx, or trachea; trauma to the lungs; foreign body obstruction of the airways; electric shock; inhalation of toxic gases or smoke; and any severe disease of the lungs
    ◆ Almost all patients who experience an episode of asphyxia are cared for in the CCU
    ◆ Because of the cerebral and general systemic anoxia resulting from asphyxia, these patients are in critical condition, commonly unresponsive, and develop MODS
  ■ Medical management
    ◆ Insert an endotracheal tube, if indicated
    ◆ Administer 100% oxygen until carbohemoglobin level is less than 10%
    ◆ Insert an arterial and a central line for pressure monitoring
    ◆ Administer appropriate vasoactive, cardiotonic, and bronchodilating medications, as indicated
  ■ Nursing management
    ◆ Monitor the patient's respiratory capabilities continuously or at least every hour; note the rate, depth, and spontaneity of respirations; and assess breath sounds; data provided by continual respiratory system assessment are essential for developing a care plan
    ◆ Determine whether the injury that caused the asphyxia has resulted in other complications; traumatic injuries commonly affect other body systems
    ◆ Check for conditions that contribute to asphyxia, such as lung disease, obesity, chest wall injuries, and neuromuscular dysfunction resulting

from fractures of the spine; the presence of these conditions can complicate attempts to maintain adequate respiration

◆ Continuously monitor vital signs, output, and hemodynamic pressures; the invasive monitoring techniques almost always used in these critically ill patients provide important information about changes in their status

◆ Assess neurologic function every hour until the patient is stable; the use of a neurologic assessment sheet or the Glasgow Coma Scale provides important information about cerebral tissue oxygenation

◆ Place the patient in Fowler's or semi-Fowler's position to facilitate full expansion of the lungs

◆ Change the patient's position every 1 to 2 hours to prevent skin breakdown and to help mobilize secretions

◆ Check the settings, function, and effect of the mechanical ventilator; the patient is mechanically ventilated until spontaneous respirations resume

◆ Check the position, cuff pressure, and patency of the endotracheal tube; aeration of the patient is impeded if the endotracheal tube isn't patent or is improperly positioned

◆ Suction the patient, as indicated, if dyspnea, coughing, rhonchi, or visible secretions in the tubing occur; secretion buildup in the endotracheal tube can cause airway obstruction

◆ During suctioning, monitor the patient's blood pressure, heart rate, and electrocardiogram; suctioning can cause a number of complications ranging from hypotension to bradycardia and ventricular tachycardia

◆ Obtain ABG samples immediately if the patient's condition significantly deteriorates; ABG analysis can identify subtle changes in oxygenation

◆ Monitor the patient for pulmonary infections; intubation and mechanical ventilation place the patient at increased risk for pulmonary infection

◆ Administer medications, as indicated, to maintain tissue perfusion, as asphyxia is commonly accompanied by generalized multiple organ dysfunction syndrome; such medications include vasoactive drugs, sympathetic stimulants, antibiotics, steroids, and plasma expanders

◆ Monitor the patient for related complications, such as ARDS, DIC, renal failure, hepatic failure, and heart failure; asphyxia has many potential complications that may prevent the patient's recovery

❖ **Burns**
■ Integumentary anatomy
   ◆ The epidermis is the outermost layer of the skin; it consists of the stratum corneum and the stratum lucidum
      ▶ The stratum lucidum is a thick layer of skin found only in the palms of the hands and soles of the feet
      ▶ The basement membrane lies beneath the stratum lucidum and connects the epidermis to the dermis
   ◆ The dermis is a layer of connective tissue that supports and separates the epidermis from the subcutaneous adipose tissue
      ▶ It has a rich vascular supply

◗ The dermis contains elastin, collagen, and reticulum fibers for strength and sensory nerve fibers for pain, touch, itch, pressure, and temperature

◗ It also contains the autonomic motor nerves for innervation of blood vessels, glands, and arrectores pilorum muscles

◆ The hypodermis is a subcutaneous layer that connects the dermis with underlying organs

◗ It's composed of loose connective tissue filled with fatty cells

◗ The fat cells provide insulation, absorb shocks, and store calories

◆ Appendages of the skin

◗ Eccrine sweat glands open directly on the surface of the skin and regulate body temperature by secreting water

◗ Apocrine glands are found only in the axillae, nipples, areolae, genital area, eyelids, and external ears; these glands secrete fluids in response to intense emotional or physiologic stimulation

◗ Sebaceous glands respond to sex hormones and secrete sebum to keep the skin and hair moist

■ Integumentary physiology

◆ The skin forms an elastic, rugged, self-regenerating, protective covering for the body

◆ It protects the internal structures of the body from invasive microorganisms and minor physical trauma

◆ It maintains internal fluid balance by preventing fluid loss

◆ The skin regulates body temperature through radiation, conduction, convection, and evaporation

◆ It conveys sensory input to the CNS through nerve endings and specialized receptors

◆ It helps regulate blood pressure through vasoconstriction and vasodilation

◆ It helps eliminate waste products from the body by excreting sweat, urea, lactic acid, bilirubin, and the metabolites of many medications

■ Integumentary assessment

◆ Patient history

◗ Note skin care habits, including the use of soaps, sunscreens, and lotions

◗ Note hair care habits, including the use of shampoos, coloring, and permanents, and changes in care procedures

◗ Note nail care habits, including instruments used, procedures used, and difficulties encountered in care

◗ Assess exposure to environmental or occupational hazards, chemicals, and sunlight

◆ Physical examination

◗ Inspect and palpate the skin for coloration, lesions, temperature, texture, turgor, and mobility

◗ Inspect the hair for texture, color, distribution, quantity, abnormal location, and abnormal destruction

◗ Inspect the nails for color, length, configuration, symmetry, and cleanliness

◗ Take culture samples from the skin and skin lesions to determine bacteria growth and sensitivity to medications

- **Description**
  - ◆ Burns are injuries to the skin caused by exposure to heat, chemicals, electricity, or radiation
  - ◆ The severity of the burn depends on the depth of the injury and the amount of body surface area (BSA) affected
  - ◆ There are three classifications of burns: first-degree, second-degree, and third-degree
    - ▶ In first-degree burns, damage is limited to the epidermis, causing erythema and pain; it's red and dry and rarely blisters and heals within 5 days
    - ▶ Second-degree burns are divided into two subcategories:
      - In second-degree partial-thickness burns, the epidermis and part of the dermis are damaged, producing moist, pink, or mottled red painful blisters; healing occurs within 21 days
      - In second-degree deep partial-thickness burns, the epidermis and dermis are damaged; the area appears pale, mottled, pearly white, mostly dry, and often insensate; it's difficult to differentiate from full-thickness injury and may take 3 to 6 weeks to heal
    - ▶ In third-degree burns, or full-thickness burns, destruction of the epidermis and underlying subcutaneous tissue is evident; it appears thick, leathery eschar, cherry-red or brown-black, insensate, and dry with thrombosed blood vessels; it requires skin grafting to heal; damage may also extend to fat, muscle, and bone
  - ◆ Burns also are classified according to the amount of BSA affected; they may be categorized as minor, moderate, or major
    - ▶ Minor burns are those that involve a full-thickness burn of less than 2% of BSA, partial-thickness burns on less than 15% of an adult's BSA, or partial-thickness burns on less than 10% of a child's BSA; patients with minor burns usually are treated as an outpatient at the hospital emergency department or may require hospitalization for 1 to 2 days
    - ▶ Moderate burns are those that involve full-thickness burns on 2% to 10% of BSA, partial-thickness burns on 15% to 25% of an adult's BSA, or partial-thickness burns on 10% to 20% of a child's BSA; patients with moderate burns may be treated in a specialized burn unit
    - ▶ Major burns include full-thickness burns on more than 10% of BSA; partial-thickness burns on more than 25% of an adult's BSA; partial-thickness burns on more than 20% of a child's BSA; burns of the hands, face, feet, or genitalia; electrical burns; and all burns in poor-risk patients
  - ◆ Burns over 30% of BSA produce significant changes in all body systems, including changes in temperature regulation, fluid volume shifts, increased susceptibility to infections, and loss of self-image
  - ◆ Recovery from a burn injury can take months or even years
- **Medical management**
  - ◆ Begin fluid replacement with appropriate I.V. colloid or crystalloid solutions
  - ◆ Administer appropriate antibiotic therapy
  - ◆ Determine the appropriate treatment method (open, closed, or semi-open)

▶ *Open treatment* involves the application of an antimicrobial cream (such as Silvadene) to the burn area and leaving it exposed to the air; this method allows for better detection of infection and improved ambulation

▶ *Closed treatment* uses an occlusive dressing to cover the burn, which is left on for several days; it's used for burns of the hands and feet

▶ *Semi-open treatment* involves the application of an antimicrobial cream and a fine-mesh gauze cover on the burn area

◆ Debride the injured area, and perform skin grafting and other surgical procedures, as indicated

◆ Order a diet that meets the patient's caloric needs

■ Nursing management

◆ Assess the patient's airway for patency, and check for signs of respiratory complications, such as wheezing, increased respiratory rate, smoke-colored sputum, hoarseness, stridor, and burned facial hairs, nostril hairs, or eyebrows

▶ Burns that occur in closed areas or affect the head and neck are likely to cause airway obstruction from edema of the respiratory tract passages

▶ Respiratory complications can occur several hours after the burn injury

◆ Assess the depth and extent of the burn; use the Rule of Nines to determine an adult's total BSA burned (see *Rule of Nines,* page 288); the more extensive the burn and the greater its depth, the more likely the patient will experience multisystem complications during recovery

◆ Assess the burned areas for blisters, edema, charring, and open tissue or exposed bone; burns with these characteristics promote loss of large amounts of fluid by way of evaporation, contribute to dehydration, and leave the patient vulnerable to infection

◆ Check the burn wound for contamination, including burned clothing, dirt, ash, soot, and other foreign matter; these substances can cause invasive infections

◆ Obtain a complete health history, including allergies, chronic health problems (including previous skin conditions), current medications, and recent operations or injuries; because burn injuries stress the whole body, preexisting diseases can complicate the recovery process

◆ Assess the patient's urine output hourly; burns are a leading cause of acute renal failure, and urine output also provides an indication of hydration status

◆ Monitor vital signs continuously during the immediate postburn period; sudden changes in vital signs may indicate impending shock

◆ Assess the location, type, and severity of pain; burns can be extremely painful, and pain is a stressor in all types of trauma

◆ Monitor the patient's neurologic status, noting agitation, memory loss, confusion, headache, and mental changes; changes in neurologic status are commonly the first indication of changes in oxygenation, tissue perfusion, and cardiac output

◆ Assess the abdomen for bowel sounds, distention, and tenderness; burn injuries commonly result in paralytic ileus, bowel obstruction, and sloughing of the intestinal lining

Rule of Nines

To quickly estimate the extent of an adult's burns, the nurse can use the Rule of Nines, which divides the body into percentages. To use this method, mentally transfer the patient's burns to the body chart shown here. Then add up the corresponding percentages for each burned body section. The total is a rough estimate of the extent of the patient's burns.

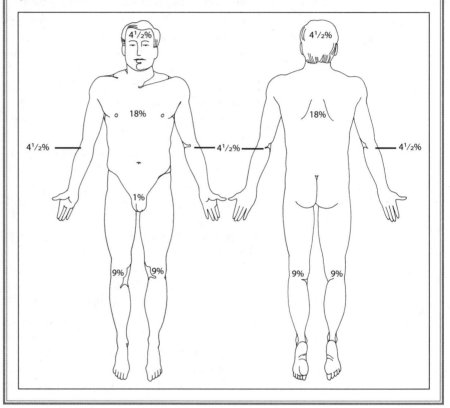

◆ Maintain a patent airway through intubation or tracheostomy, positioning, or mechanical ventilation; airway obstruction is a common complication in the immediate postburn period

◆ Identify vascular access sites, and start I.V. lines with large-gauge needles, or assist the practitioner with central lines; adequate hydration during the first 72 hours is essential for the survival of patients with severe burns

◆ Ensure that the patient receives the proper type and amount of fluids; both dehydration and fluid overload are potential problems in the early treatment period

◆ Administer tetanus prophylaxis; patients with burn injuries are at high risk for tetanus

◆ Maintain the patient on nothing-by-mouth status, and insert a nasogastric tube

▶ GI shutdown usually occurs after severe burns

▶ Giving the patient fluid or food by mouth can lead to vomiting and aspiration

◆ Administer medications, including antibiotics, plasma expanders, steroids, histamine$_2$-receptor antagonists, and analgesics, as prescribed; all medications should be given I.V.

◆ Check the data from invasive hemodynamic monitoring equipment; CVP, PAP, and cardiac output are commonly monitored to help regulate fluid administration in severely burned patients

◆ Assist with or perform burn wound care using strict aseptic technique

  ▶ Although reverse isolation is sometimes used, strict aseptic technique is effective in preventing infections from outside sources

  ▶ The patient's own body is the primary source of infective organisms

◆ Monitor for hypothermia, using a continuous temperature monitoring device; patients can lose large amounts of heat through open burn wounds

◆ Maintain the patient's room at 80° F (26.6° C) with 50% to 60% humidity; these measures help prevent hypothermia and reduce fluid loss through evaporation

◆ Begin active and passive range-of-motion exercises as soon as possible; the sooner physical therapy is started, the less likely that contractures and circulatory complications will develop

◆ Reposition the patient every 2 hours to prevent pressure ulcers and skin breakdown

◆ Use the Harris-Benedict formula to determine basal energy requirements, based on gender, height, weight, age, and stress associated with various injuries; provide a diet high in calories and protein; include vitamin supplements, especially B-complex vitamins and vitamin C; and provide frequent, small meals or supplemental feedings, if required

  ▶ Severe burns cause a negative nitrogen balance (catabolism)

  ▶ Extra calories (5,500 calories per day for an adult) are required to prevent muscle breakdown

  ▶ Vitamin supplements play an important role in the healing process

◆ Assess burn wounds for healing or signs of infection

  ▶ Healing is marked by the development of pink, healthy tissue

  ▶ Infection is characterized by redness, tenderness, and purulent drainage

  ▶ Obtain tissue culture samples from burn wounds, as prescribed, to determine bacterial growth and medication sensitivities

◆ Assist the patient during whirlpool debridement, dressing changes, and surgical procedures; the necrotic burned skin (eschar) must be removed before healing can take place

◆ Check skin grafts used on the burn wound for signs of infection

  ▶ Autologous skin grafts are taken from unburned areas of the patient's body; these grafts are surgically attached and will grow new skin

  ▶ Homologous skin grafts are taken from human cadavers; these grafts are surgically attached and don't grow, but they allow new skin to develop underneath; homologous grafts remain in place until they slough off

▶ Animal skin grafts form a type of biologic dressing, using the skin of cows (bovine grafts) or pigs (porcine grafts); these grafts remain on the wound for 3 to 4 days before they're changed

◆ Monitor the patient's psychological status and progression through the stages of grief

▶ Burn injuries produce profound changes in body image

▶ Patients who are severely burned commonly experience denial, anger, depression, and—ultimately—acceptance

◆ Teach the patient and family about the hospital care plan and about home care after discharge; this information allows the patient and family to participate in the recovery process, increases the patient's sense of security, and promotes continued family communication

◆ Contact social services to help the patient cope with financial and rehabilitation concerns; the prolonged recovery period of many burn patients often decimates their financial resources, may cause loss of employment, and stresses the family

◆ Monitor the patient for long-term complications of burn injuries

▶ Severe burn injuries can trigger numerous complications, which can develop at any time during the recovery period

▶ These complications include ARDS, DIC, heart failure, renal failure, hepatic failure, infection, pulmonary emboli, contractures, stress ulcers, pulmonary fibrosis, drug dependence, and depression

Review questions

1. The nurse is caring for a patient with a third-degree burn to the face and upper torso involving 25% of the BSA. Which initial admission assessment finding would require the nurse to notify the practitioner immediately?

○ **A.** Nausea

○ **B.** Heart rate greater than 100 beats/minute

○ **C.** Inability to speak

○ **D.** 2+ facial edema

Correct answer: C Suspect inhalation injury when there's the possibility of carbon monoxide inhalation, injury above the glottis (thermal), or injury below the glottis (chemical). Such an injury would require immediate medical attention. Nausea wouldn't require immediate treatment. Tachycardia is a normal finding in burns because of the loss of intravascular fluid. Facial edema results when sodium, water, and protein shift from intravascular to interstitial spaces, thereby decreasing oncotic pressure and increasing capillary permeability.

2. For optimal outcomes in patients with major burns, when should enteral feedings be started?

○ **A.** After the emergent phase of the injury

○ **B.** A few hours after the injury has occurred

○ **C.** Two to 3 days after the injury

○ **D.** Not until bowel sounds have returned

Correct answer: D Enteral feedings are started when bowel sounds return. Total parenteral nutrition may be administered before this to meet the patient's nutritional needs.

3. The nurse is assessing an elderly patient for signs of distributive shock. Why is hypotension not a reliable indicator?

   ○ **A.** Coronary blood flow increases with aging.

   ○ **B.** Reflux tachycardia occurs with aging.

   ○ **C.** Systemic vascular resistance decreases with aging.

   ○ **D.** Vasodilators may be part of an elderly patient's medical regimen.

Correct answer: D Hypertension is common in elderly patients because aging reduces the elasticity of the vascular system. Other effects of aging include bradycardia, decreased coronary blood flow, and increased systemic vascular resistance.

4. Hemodynamic values associated with the initial stage of septic distributive shock include:

   ○ **A.** cardiac output of 2.5 L per minute.

   ○ **B.** PAWP of 3 mm Hg.

   ○ **C.** right atrial pressure (RAP) of 10 mm Hg.

   ○ **D.** systemic vascular resistance of 1,600 dynes/sec/cm-5.

Correct answer: B During the initial stage of septic distributive shock, the PAWP is low and then progressively becomes high. Normal value for PAWP is 6 to 12 mm Hg; normal cardiac output is 4 to 8 L per minute. In the initial stage of septic shock, cardiac output is high. Normal RAP is 0 to 8 mm Hg, with low RAP in the initial stage. Normal systemic vascular resistance is 900 to 1,400 dynes/sec/cm-5, and in the initial stage, the systemic vascular resistance is low.

5. Why is it difficult for the nurse to obtain an accurate baseline vital sign assessment on a patient admitted for excessive cocaine use?

   ○ **A.** The patient has a heightened awareness of the environment.

   ○ **B.** Alcohol and drug abusers are usually uncooperative.

   ○ **C.** The sympathetic stimulation response is intensified.

   ○ **D.** Withdrawal symptoms make it difficult to obtain vital signs.

Correct answer: C Cocaine is a CNS stimulant that mimics and intensifies the sympathetic stimulation response. Notably, an increase in heart rate and blood pressure occur, along with vasoconstriction, dilated pupils, tremors, excitability, and restlessness. Heightened awareness of the environment is present but doesn't affect vital signs.

Professional caring and ethical practice

❖**Advocacy/moral agency**
- American Association of Critical-Care Nurses (AACN) definitions
  - ◆ An advocate represents the concerns of the patient, family, and community
  - ◆ A moral agent identifies and helps resolve ethical and clinical concerns within and outside the clinical setting
- Advocacy
  - ◆ Advocacy is based on the value of human dignity
  - ◆ Advocacy embraces certain nursing actions
    - ▶ Protect the patient's rights
    - ▶ Assist the patient and family to do what they can't do alone; negotiate for the patient
    - ▶ Keep the patient and family informed of the care plan, procedures, equipment in use, and medications
    - ▶ Encourage the presence of loved ones, as appropriate; advocate for flexible visitation
    - ▶ Enhance the patient's feelings of safety and security
    - ▶ Act in the patient's best interest
    - ▶ Respect and support the patient's and family's decisions
    - ▶ Serve as a liaison between the patient and other members of the health care team
    - ▶ Respect each patient's values, culture, and beliefs
  - ◆ Risks of patient advocacy can include conflicts
    - ▶ Conflict between the nurse and others (practitioner, hospital administration, family, and other nurses) involved with the patient
    - ▶ Conflict between the nurse's sense of professional duty and her personal values
- Moral agency
  - ◆ Morals are standards of behavior that distinguish between right and wrong
  - ◆ Agency is a concern for another's outcome
  - ◆ Ethics is the study of the standards of behavior and values to which we adhere
  - ◆ Moral and ethical dilemmas exist when conflicting principles exist
  - ◆ Nurses use codes of professional ethics to guide their behavior and decisions

- Ethical decision making
  - ◆ Assess: Gather information regarding the moral and ethical dilemma
  - ◆ Identify the problem: Determine if the problem is an ethical, legal, or communication issue
  - ◆ Establish alternatives and take action: Consider these ethical principles
    - ▶ Nonmaleficence (to do no harm)
    - ▶ Beneficence (to do good)
    - ▶ Respect for autonomy (self-determination)
    - ▶ Justice (fairness)
  - ◆ Evaluate: Assess the outcomes of actions, and take further action, if needed

❖ **Caring practice**
- AACN definitions
  - ◆ Caring practice is a constellation of nursing activities that are responsive to the uniqueness of the patient and family and that create a compassionate, supportive, and therapeutic environment, with the aim of promoting comfort and healing and preventing unnecessary suffering
  - ◆ These caring behaviors include, but are not limited to, vigilance, engagement, and responsiveness
- Appropriate nursing actions
  - ◆ Anticipate future needs of the patient and family
  - ◆ Base care on appropriate standards and protocols while individualizing them to the patient
  - ◆ Maintain a safe physical environment
  - ◆ Interact with patients and families in a compassionate manner
  - ◆ Support the patient and family in issues involving death and dying
  - ◆ Acknowledge your own feelings about death
  - ◆ Be familiar with the patient's wishes regarding end-of-life care, including advance directives
    - ▶ Living will: written instructions that specify the patient's wishes regarding treatment
    - ▶ Durable power of attorney: an individual designated to make health care decisions on behalf of a patient who can no longer do so
  - ◆ Withdraw treatment and limit further medical intervention when comfort, psychological care, and support become the priority
  - ◆ Continue to spend time with the dying patient and his family
  - ◆ Inform the family when death is near and provide privacy
    - ▶ Offer to contact a spiritual advisor, if desired
    - ▶ Contact the appropriate organ procurement agency
    - ▶ Allow the family to view the body after death
    - ▶ Explain any required procedures or paperwork

❖ **Collaboration**
- AACN definitions

◆ Collaboration involves patients, families, and health care providers working together to promote each person's contributions toward achieving optimal or realistic patient goals
◆ Collaboration involves intradisciplinary and interdisciplinary work with colleagues and the community
■ Additional characteristics
◆ Collaboration requires cooperative decision making, trust, and the sharing of goals and interventions among caregivers
◆ Nurses often fill the role of coordinator of services
■ Appropriate nursing actions
◆ Promote positive patient outcomes
◆ Serve as a mentor
◆ Participate in interdisciplinary team meetings regarding patient care and practice issues
◆ Use all appropriate resources to optimize patient outcomes
◆ Recognize that therapeutic goals are on a changing continuum in response to patient changes
◆ Examine methods of care delivery and processes of care
◆ Establish partnerships with other disciplines
■ Models of collaborative care
◆ Care management: integrating processes designed to coordinate patient care throughout the continuum of health care services
❱ Patient-focused
❱ Team approach
◆ Case management: coordinating and organizing patient care in collaboration with the primary care provider
◆ Outcomes management: using a quality improvement process and team approach to manage patient outcomes
■ Tools used in collaborative care
◆ Clinical pathways
❱ Overview of the multidisciplinary care plan
❱ Developed by the multidisciplinary team
❱ Focuses on critical elements involved in care
◆ Algorithms: decision-making flowcharts that outline disease management
◆ Practice guidelines
❱ Guidelines on which clinical pathways and algorithms are based
❱ Usually developed by a professional health organization
◆ Protocols: a set of rules by which the patient is treated

❖ Systems thinking
■ AACN definitions
◆ Systems thinking is a body of knowledge and tools that allow the nurse to manage resources for the patient's welfare
◆ These resources can exist for the patient and family within or across health care and non–health care systems
■ Appropriate nursing actions
◆ Use negotiation skills

        ◆ Develop strategies based on patient needs
        ◆ View the patient and family in a holistic manner
        ◆ Obtain thorough knowledge of health care systems
        ◆ Use pertinent models of collaborative care

❖ **Response to diversity**
  ■ AACN definitions
    ◆ Response to diversity refers to a sensitivity to recognize, appreciate, and incorporate differences into the provision of care
    ◆ These differences may include, but are not limited to, individuality, cultural differences, spiritual beliefs, gender, race, ethnicity, disability, family configuration, lifestyle, socioeconomic status, age, values, and alternative medicine involving patients, families, and members of the health care team
  ■ Appropriate nursing actions
    ◆ Recognize your own cultural beliefs
    ◆ Assess cultural diversity and recognize its impact on care
    ◆ Integrate cultural differences into the care plan
    ◆ Acknowledge, respect, and support patient and family cultural values

❖ **Clinical inquiry**
  ■ AACN definitions
    ◆ Clinical inquiry is the ongoing process of questioning and evaluating practice and providing informed practice
    ◆ The process also involves initiating beneficial changes in practice through research and experiential learning
  ■ Appropriate nursing actions
    ◆ Revise and formulate policies and standards of care based on current research and review of the literature
    ◆ Function as an innovator and evaluator
      ▶ Individualize the care plan for each patient
      ▶ Incorporate research findings in patient care (research-based practice)
      ▶ Participate in research
      ▶ Question current practice
      ▶ Compare and contrast alternatives to care

❖ **Clinical judgment**
  ■ AACN definitions
    ◆ Clinical reasoning that includes clinical decision-making, critical thinking, and a global grasp of the situation
    ◆ These are combined with nursing skills that have been acquired through integrating formal and experiential knowledge and evidence-based guidelines
  ■ Appropriate nursing actions
    ◆ Make appropriate decisions
      ▶ Collect information and identify the problem
      ▶ Identify a possible solution or solutions

▸ Analyze the consequences of the solutions, and select the best solution
▸ Carry out the solution
▸ Evaluate the results of the solution
◆ Learn from mistakes
◆ Seek new opportunities for learning both in the clinical setting and in education
◆ Compare and contrast alternatives
◆ Find out what you aren't sure of

❖ **Facilitator of learning**
  ■ AACN definition
    ◆ The ability to facilitate learning for patients, families, nursing staff, and other members of the health care team
  ■ Three domains of learning
    ◆ Cognitive: teaching that progresses from simple to complex
    ◆ Affective: teaching that requires changes in attitude or emotion or that involves patient values and feelings
    ◆ Psychomotor: teaching that involves technical skills
  ■ Appropriate nursing actions
    ◆ Function as a patient and family educator
    ◆ Develop patient and family education programs, and integrate them throughout care delivery
    ◆ Evaluate patient and family learning
    ◆ Become familiar with principles of adult learning
    ◆ Be aware of barriers to learning, particularly in the critically ill patient
    ◆ Assess learning needs
    ◆ Assess patient and family readiness to learn
    ◆ Determine teaching content and set goals or learning objectives when formulating the teaching plan
    ◆ Assess the environment for conduciveness to learning
    ◆ Present information clearly
    ◆ Gear teaching sessions toward appropriate levels of understanding for the patient and family
      ▸ Explain all procedures
      ▸ Teach during nursing care activities
      ▸ Use visual aids when appropriate
      ▸ Present information from simple to complex; avoid medical jargon
      ▸ Provide written information to reinforce teaching, when appropriate
      ▸ Use return demonstration techniques for skills the patient or family will need to perform; provide appropriate feedback
      ▸ Reinforce new knowledge and behaviors
      ▸ Ensure appropriate follow-up
      ▸ Teach toward transfer (Prepare the critically ill patient and his family for eventual transfer to the general floor)

Review questions

1. An 80-year-old patient with metastatic cancer has died, and the family wishes to donate tissue. The nurse should:

   ○ **A.** explain that the patient's condition is ineligible for tissue donation.

   ○ **B.** contact the organ procurement agency.

   ○ **C.** contact the primary care provider for orders to donate.

   ○ **D.** contact the ethics committee.

Correct answer: B Most state laws require the hospital to contact the appropriate organ procurement agency upon the donor's death. Neither the nurse nor the physician is supposed to determine whether a patient is appropriate for organ or tissue donation. This situation doesn't suggest an ethical dilemma. The caring practice of nursing requires the nurse to support the patient and family in issues of death and dying.

2. A stable patient with pancreatitis is to be transferred from the intensive care unit (ICU) to the floor. The patient expresses concern over the transfer and refuses to leave the ICU. The nurse should discuss with the patient:

   ○ **A.** the qualifications of the nursing staff on the floor.

   ○ **B.** the financial impact of remaining in the ICU.

   ○ **C.** the fact that other, sicker patients need the ICU bed.

   ○ **D.** the excellent progress that he has made.

Correct answer: D As a facilitator of learning, the nurse should use opportunities to "teach toward transfer"; that is, she should prepare the patient for eventual transfer to the floor as his condition improves. Reinforcing the patient's progress will assist him in moving toward independence.

3. The wife of a patient with multisystem organ dysfunction following major trauma is quiet and withdrawn. You haven't seen her cry during any of her visits. Today she seems particularly anxious. An appropriate response by the nurse would be:

   ○ **A.** "How are you feeling?"

   ○ **B.** "It's good that you are so strong and brave."

   ○ **C.** "Whatever happens is God's will."

   ○ **D.** "Why haven't you cried?"

Correct answer: A The caring practice of nursing requires the nurse to interact with family members in a compassionate manner and to support them in issues surrounding death and dying. Acknowledging the wife's feelings and letting her know it's appropriate to express her feelings is important.

4. To provide competent and efficient care to all patients, the nurse must:

○ **A.** develop and implement a structured routine care plan.

○ **B.** assign nurses with the same cultural backgrounds as their patients.

○ **C.** require family members to participate in patient care.

○ **D.** perform a cultural assessment of each patient and individualize care.

Correct answer: D The nurse's response to diversity should include incorporation of cultural differences into the care plan.

5. A nurse who's caring for a patient with a tracheostomy will be teaching his wife how to suction. When developing the teaching plan, the nurse must first:

○ **A.** assess the wife's knowledge and skills.

○ **B.** set up a schedule to demonstrate the technique.

○ **C.** provide the wife with written materials about the procedure.

○ **D.** establish goals and learning objectives.

Correct answer: A To develop an effective teaching plan, the nurse must first assess the wife's current knowledge of the procedure and her ability to carry it out properly. Setting up a schedule, providing written materials, and establishing learning goals and objectives are appropriate nursing actions that the nurse will perform after she has assessed the wife's knowledge and skills.

Appendices, Posttests, and Index

Common drugs used in critical care

This chart identifies drugs by class and summarizes their action, indications, and nursing implications.

Common drugs	Action	Indications	Nursing implications
Antihistamines			
cetirizine (Zyrtec), diphenhydramine (Benadryl), fexofenadine (Allegra), loratadine (Claritin)	These drugs compete with histamines for histamine$_1$-receptor sites.	• Allergic rhinitis, allergic reaction to drugs, sedation (diphenhydramine) • Pruritus	• Diphenhydramine commonly causes drowsiness, but may cause paradoxical agitation in children and elderly patients. Newer agents cause less drowsiness. • Evaluate therapeutic response and intake and output. • Implement oral care for dry mouth.
Anti-infectives			
Antibacterials *Aminoglycosides:* amikacin (Amikin), gentamicin (Garamycin), tobramycin (Nebcin)	Aminoglycosides inhibit protein synthesis in the susceptible bacteria.	• I.V. or I.M. antibiotic for aerobic gram-negative bacilli; bacteremia, peritonitis; complicated urinary tract infection (UTI)	• Dosage is reduced in renal impairment. Assess blood urea nitrogen (BUN) and creatinine levels. • Record time of dosage accurately if serum concentrations are monitored. • Monitor for signs and symptoms of superinfection. • Prolonged or excessive dosage may cause vertigo and hearing loss.
Cephalosporins: cefazolin (Ancef), cefotaxime (Claforan), cefotetan (Cefotan), ceftazidime (Fortaz), ceftriaxone (Rocephin), and others	Cephalosporins inhibit bacterial cell wall synthesis of actively dividing cells in susceptible bacteria.	• Antibacterial activity varies for each agent, ranging from narrow gram-positive activity to broad spectrum gram-negative coverage	• Dosage of most agents reduced in renal impairment. • Monitor closely for allergic reactions in patients with stated penicillin allergy.
Macrolides: azithromycin (Zithromax), clarithromycin (Biaxin), erythromycin	Macrolide antibiotics attach to the 50S subunit of the bacterial ribosome, preventing bacterial protein synthesis in susceptible bacteria.	• Active against many gram-positive bacterial and atypical pathogens; commonly used for pneumonia, skin or ear infections	• May cause nausea if given orally. Most drugs in this class may precipitate cardiac arrhythmias.

Common drugs	Action	Indications	Nursing implications
Anti-infectives (continued)			
Antibacterials (*continued*) *Penicillins:* amoxicillin, ampicillin, methicillin (Staphcillin), penicillin G, piperacillin (Pipracil)	Penicillins inhibit bacterial cell wall synthesis by binding to one or more of the penicillin-binding proteins in susceptible bacteria.	● Antibacterial activity varies for each agent, ranging from narrow gram-positive activity to broad spectrum gram-negative coverage ● Respiratory tract infections ● Otitis media ● Pneumonia	● Ask patient about possible penicillin allergy before first dose. ● Report hematuria to the physician. ● Monitor kidney and liver function test results. ● These drugs may cause diarrhea and superinfection.
Fluoroquinolones: ciprofloxacin (Cipro), gatifloxacin (Tequin), levofloxacin (Levaquin), moxifloxacin (Avelox), and others	Quinolones inhibit deoxyribonucleic acid (DNA) gyrase activity and prevent DNA replication in susceptible bacteria.	● Antibacterial activity varies for each agent, most agents useful for pneumonia and respiratory infections; some agents useful for cellulitis	● Don't give oral doses within 2 hours of aluminum or calcium antacids, or iron. ● Rarely, these drugs may cause headaches, dizziness, or diarrhea. ● Dosage is reduced in renal impairment.
Sulfonamides: co-trimoxazole (Bactrim), sulfadiazine (Coptin)	Sulfonamides inhibit bacterial synthesis of dihydrofolic acid by competition with para-amino benzoic acid.	● Prevention or treatment of *Pneumocystis carinii* pneumonia; nocardia; toxoplasmosis; bronchitis; ear infections; UTI	● Ask patient about possible sulfa allergy before first dose. ● Watch for rash, which is common in patients with human immunodeficiency syndrome. ● Monitor intake and output and serum creatinine.
Antifungals *Amphotericin B analogs:* amphotericin B (Fungizone), amphotericin B cholesteryl sulfate complex (Amphotec), amphotericin B liposomal (Abelcet, AmBisome) *Triazole derivatives:* fluconazole (Diflucan), itraconazole (Sporanox) *Glucan synthesis inhibitor:* caspofungin (Cancidas)	Amphotericin B–like drugs change cell membrane permeability; fluconazole and itraconazole directly damage the cell membrane phospholipids. Caspofungin inhibits cell wall formation.	● Severe systemic fungal infections	● Amphotericin B–like drugs may cause hypersensitivity, and may need premedication. ● Premedicate with anti-inflammatory drugs and antihistamines. ● Monitor liver enzyme values and intake and output. ● Amphotericin B–like drugs aren't stable in saline. Caspofungin is stable only in saline. ● Don't piggyback infusions. ● Monitor for nephrotoxicity, electrolyte imbalance, fever, and weight loss.
Antivirals acyclovir (Zovirax), foscarnet (Foscavir), ganciclovir (Cytovene), and others	These drugs interfere with viral replication.	● Prevention and treatment of herpes simplex viral infection ● Ganciclovir also active against cytomegalovirus	● Use with caution in a patient with a history of pancreatitis. ● Rapid infusion may cause renal impairment. ● Monitor fluid intake and output. ● Ganciclovir may cause neutropenia; monitor white blood cell (WBC) count. ● Foscanet may cause renal toxicity. ● These drugs may cause blood dyscrasias, coma, arrhythmias, hypotension, and hypertension.

Common drugs	Action	Indications	Nursing implications
Antidotes			
flumazenil (Romazicon)	This drug blocks benzodiazepine receptors and antagonizes the actions of benzodiazepine on the central nervous system (CNS).	• Complete or partial reversal of the sedative effects of benzodiazepine compounds	• Monitor the level of consciousness (LOC) and watch for respiratory depression during and after administration. • Because the half-life of many benzodiazepine drugs is longer than that of flumazenil, resedation may occur in 15 to 30 minutes. • This drug may not reverse the amnesia associated with benzodiazepine drugs. Patient teaching may need to be repeated after surgical procedures. • This drug may cause seizures in patients with multiple drug acidoses.
naloxone (Narcan), naltrexone (ReVia)	Opioid antagonists occupy opioid receptor sites and displace opioid (narcotic) drug molecules.	• Opioid (narcotic) drug overdose • Reversal of opioid-induced respiratory depression • Reversal of sedation from opioid drugs	• Duration of naloxone effects is almost always less than those of the opioid being reversed. • Periodically monitor for return of respiratory depression. • Excessive dosages in opioid-tolerant patients may cause extreme discomfort, hypertension, and pain.
acetylcysteine (Mucomyst)	Acetylesteine is believed to act as a glutathione substitute and directly combine with a toxic metabolite of acetaminophen.	• Treatment of acetaminophen overdose • May be used to reduce incidence of nephrotoxicity in some patients receiving contrast media	• Most effective if given soon after an acute acetaminophen overdose. May be sent in a form labeled for respiratory use. To mask foul taste and smell for oral use, dilute 20% solution with cola to 5% solution. • Follow dosage protocol.
fomepizole (Antizole)	Competitive inhibitor or alcohol dehydrogenase prevents initial metabolism of ethylene glycol and methanol to more toxic compounds.	• Ethylene glycol (antifreeze) overdose; methanol (wood alcohol) overdose	• Dosage increased if hemodialysis is used. • Need for dosage based on serum toxin concentration. • May cause headache, nausea, and dizziness.
Autonomics			
Anticholinergics atropine sulfate	This drug blocks cholinergic stimuli from the brain causing an increased heart rate (due to blocked vagal stimulation); also dries oral secretions.	• Bradyarrhythmias • Suppression of oral secretions • Urine retention	• May increase intraocular pressure in acute angle-closure glaucoma. • May cause respiratory depression in patients with myasthenia gravis. • Use with caution in a patient with heart failure, coronary artery disease, or Down syndrome. • Additive cholinergic effects may occur when this drug is administered concurrently with antiarrhythmics, meperidine, or antiparkinsonians. • Monitor intake and output and electrocardiogram (ECG). • This drug may cause dry mouth, headache, and tachycardia.

Common drugs	Action	Indications	Nursing implications
Autonomics (continued)			
Sympathetics (adrenergic drugs) albuterol sulfate (Proventil)	Beta-2 smooth muscle relaxant works primarily on smooth muscle in the lungs.	• Bronchospasm related to asthma	• Use with caution in a patient with a cardiovascular disorder, diabetes mellitus, or hyperthyroidism. • Monitor cardiovascular and pulmonary values. • This drug may cause arrhythmias (especially tachycardia, palpitations), hypertension, paradoxical bronchospasm, tremor, nervousness, and nausea. • Monitor serum potassium level for hypokalemia.
dobutamine (Dobutrex)	Increases cardiac contractility (through beta-1 stimulation) and causes vasodilation (through beta-2 stimulation), with little change in heart rate.	• Acute heart failure • Stabilization of cardiac function after coronary bypass graft surgery • Insufficient cardiac output	• Monitor the patient's ECG and blood pressure. • Use a pulmonary artery catheter to monitor cardiac parameters. • This drug may cause sinus or ventricular tachycardia and hypertension.
dopamine (Intropin)	Dopamine's effects are dose-related: low infusion rates improve renal blood flow; intermediate infusion rate increases heart rate and cardiac output; high infusion rate causes peripheral vasoconstriction and elevation of blood pressure.	• Acute renal failure • Hypotension caused by myocardial infarction (MI), trauma, sepsis, or open heart surgery • Shock	• Monitor ECG and blood pressure continuously. • Monitor hemodynamic parameters, if available. • Avoid soft tissue extravasation, which may cause skin necrosis.
epinephrine hydrochloride (Adrenalin Chloride)	This drug produces vasoconstriction and dilates bronchial smooth muscles.	• Hypotension • Cardiac arrest	• Use with caution in a patient with hyperthyroidism or bronchial asthma. • Monitor hemodynamic variables, including ECG, blood pressure, and fluid status. • This drug may cause tachyarrhythmias, hypertension, and vasoconstriction-induced tissue sloughing.
isoproterenol (Isuprel)	This catecholamine has positive inotropic and chronotropic effects; it increases atrioventricular (AV) node conduction.	• Bradycardia • Treatment of anaphylaxis • Bradycardia (due to AV node heart block)	• For infusion, use only an accurate infusion device. • This drug may cause tachycardia and hypotension. • Avoid use in acute MI as tachycardia may extend damage to the heart.

Common drugs	Action	Indications	Nursing implications
Autonomics (continued)			
Sympathetics (adrenergic drugs) *(continued)* norepinephrine bitartrate (Levophed)	This catecholamine increases cardiac contractility and causes vasoconstriction to increase blood pressure.	● Acute hypotension ● Septic shock	● Don't administer to a patient with peripheral vascular thrombosis. ● Monitor capillary refill because excessive dose may cause necrosis of extremities. ● Avoid extravasation, which may cause tissue necrosis, and infuse through central line, if possible. ● Monitor the patient's cardiovascular status, central venous pressure, pulmonary artery pressure, and intake and output. ● This drug may cause hypertension, arrhythmias, ventricular tachycardia, and ventricular fibrillation.
Sympatholytics (adrenergic-blocking) drugs esmolol (Brevibloc)	An ultra–short-acting beta-adrenergic blocker used to lower blood pressure and heart rate.	● Acute supraventricular tachycardia ● Control of ventricular rate in atrial flutter or fibrillation ● Short-term control of hypertension	● For infusion use only an accurate infusion device. ● The drug may precipitate bronchospasm in patients with asthma. ● Monitor cardiovascular status continuously. ● Compare liver and kidney function test results to baseline values, then monitor liver and kidney function daily. ● Excessive dose may cause profound bradycardia and hypotension.
labetalol (Normodyne)	Labetalol is a selective alpha-blocking and nonselective beta-adrenergic blocking agent.	● Mild, moderate, or severe hypertension	● The drug may precipitate bronchospasm in patients with asthma. ● Monitor patient's cardiovascular status (heart rate and blood pressure) to avoid excessive bradycardia and hypotension.
Skeletal muscle relaxants *Nondepolarizing blocking drugs:* atracurium (Tracrium), cisatracurium (Nimbex), pancuronium bromide (Pavulon), vecuronium bromide (Norcuron), and others	Nondepolarizing neuromuscular blocking agents cause flaccid paralysis due to blockade of skeletal muscles.	● Skeletal muscle relaxation during mechanical ventilation, surgery, or intubation	● Skeletal muscle relaxants don't change mentation or ability to feel pain. ● Patient may be fully conscious and able to hear and remember conversations. ● Ensure adequate sedation and pain control. ● Periodically reevaluate the need for use. ● Assess motor reflexes regularly. ● These drugs may cause bradycardia or tachycardia, increased or decreased blood pressure, and bronchospasm.
Depolarizing blocking drugs: succinylcholine (Anectine)	An ultra–short-acting neuromuscular blocker used only by trained individuals during intubation.	● Used to acutely relax patients and prevent resistance during mechanical ventilation intubation	● These drugs may cause hyperkalemia (in patients with renal impairment, crush or burn injuries). ● These drugs don't change mentation or ability to feel pain. ● These drugs have a rapid onset and short duration of action.

Common drugs	Action	Indications	Nursing implications
Drugs used in coagulation disorders			
Anticoagulants heparin	This anticoagulant enhances inhibitory effect of antithrombin III; it prevents clots from enlarging, but can't dissolve those already formed.	• Treatment or prevention of deep vein thrombosis (DVT) • Anticoagulant during cardiac procedures • Acute pulmonary embolism (PE)	• Watch for hematuria and other signs of bleeding. • Monitor partial thromboplastin time for therapeutic effect of drug. • Monitor platelets because drug may cause thrombocytopenia.
Low-molecular weight heparins: dalteparin (Fragmin), enoxaparin (Lovenox), fondeparinux (Arixtra), tinzaparin (Innohep)	Increases anti-Xa activity in blood to prevent new clot formation.	• DVT prevention following hip or knee replacement surgery • Disseminated intravascular coagulation • Atrial fibrillation	• Watch for hematuria and other signs of bleeding. • Monitor serum creatinine because dosage is reduced in renal impairment. • Monitor platelets because drug may cause thrombocytopenia.
warfarin (Coumadin)	An anticoagulant, this drug alters synthesis of vitamin K clotting factors in the liver.	• Treatment of chronic DVT • Intravascular blood clot prevention in patients with select clotting disorders • Stroke prevention in atrial fibrillation	• Monitor for therapeutic prothrombin time and international normalized ratio (INR) • This drug may cause bleeding, bruising, and allergic response.
Thrombolytics alteplase (Activase), reteplase (Retavase), streptokinase (Kabikinase, Streptase), tenecteplase (TNKase)	Thrombolytic drugs break down existing clots.	• Complicated DVT or PE • Lysis of coronary artery thrombi in acute MI • Treatment of acute thrombolytic stroke (alteplase only) • Lysis of arterial- and catheter-related clots	• Monitor cardiovascular, pulmonary, and neurologic status carefully. • Evaluate patient for signs of active bleeding, head trauma, recent surgery, recent history of GI bleeding, or uncontrolled hypertension before use. • In acute MI, drug should be given with aspirin; and give heparin, as ordered. (Heparin may not be needed with streptokinase.
Drugs that assist with coagulation			
desmopressin (DDAVP)	This drug increases plasma levels of factor XIII in patients with hemophilia. It also has antidiuretic properties.	• Hemophilia A in patients with factor VIII coagulant activity levels greater than 5% • von Willebrand's disease	• Monitor coagulation studies (for confirmed bleeding), and intake and output because drug has antidiuretic properties. • This drug may cause hypertension or hypotension. • Watch for signs of bleeding because drug isn't uniformly effective.
phytonadione [vitamin K_1] (AquaMEPHYTON)	These drugs stimulate hepatic synthesis of clotting factors that are depressed during warfarin therapy.	• Hypothrombinemia in patients taking warfarin • Overdose involving warfarin-like rat poisons	• Monitor INR and hematocrit to ensure effects. • Excessive dosage will make it difficult to restart warfarin. • Ineffective in advanced liver disease. • Infuse I.V. doses slowly to avoid hypotension.

Common drugs	Action	Indications	Nursing implications
Drugs that assist with coagulation (continued)			
protamine sulfate	This antidote binds with heparin, thus making heparin ineffective.	• Postoperative bleeding in situations when heparin was used • Heparin overdose	• Monitor coagulation studies (for continued bleeding) and vital signs. • This drug may cause bronchospasm, hypotension, and anaphylaxis.
Cardiovascular system drugs			
Antihypertensives *Angiotensin-converting enzyme (ACE) inhibitors:* captopril (Capoten), enalapril maleate (Vasotec), enalaprilat (Vasotec I.V.), ramipril (Altace), lisinopril (Prinivil, Zestril), and others	ACE inhibitors prevent conversion of angiotensin I to angiotensin II, resulting in dilation of arteries and veins.	• Hypertension • Treatment and prevention of heart failure • Treatment and prevention of diabetic neuropathy	• Monitor for angioedema, a swelling of the throat and airway that rarely occurs, commonly after the first few doses. • Monitor for persistent chronic cough, which typically develops about 1 month after starting therapy. • Monitor electrolytes for hyperkalemia. • Contraindicated in pregnancy after week 20. • May cause renal impairment; monitor serum creatinine and BUN.
nitroprusside (Nitropress)	A vasodilator, this drug directly relaxes arteriolar and venous smooth muscle, decreasing afterload and preload.	• Hypertensive emergencies • Acute decompensated heart failure • To produce controlled hypotension	• Titrated to effect; continuously monitor blood pressure, if possible. • Toxicity possible from accumulation of cyanide and thiocyanate metabolites, particularly if used in high doses or in patients with renal failure. • Monitor blood chemistries for acidosis, a sign of thiocyanate toxicity. • Monitor blood pressure and ECG continuously; also monitor pulmonary, kidney, and liver function. • This drug may cause severe hypotension and altered LOC.
Antiarrhythmics adenosine (Adenocard)	This drug slows electrical conduction in the AV node and interrupts the reentry circuit.	• Paroxysmal supraventricular tachycardia	• Given by rapid I.V. push over seconds into a free-flowing venous line. • Efficacy decreased. • Monitor the patient's ECG and blood pressure during administration to document effects of cardiac rhythm in patients taking theophylline. • This drug may cause bronchial constriction and chest tightness, which lasts seconds to minutes.

Common drugs	Action	Indications	Nursing implications
Cardiovascular system drugs (continued)			
Antiarrhythmics *(continued)*			
lidocaine (Xylocaine)	This antiarrhythmic decreases ventricular excitability and slightly decreases the force of ventricular contraction. If injected locally, it produces local anesthesia.	● Hemodynamically unstable premature ventricular contractions ● Ventricular tachycardia ● Ventricular fibrillation ● Useful as a local anesthetic during minor surgical procedures	● Drug may accumulate following long infusion, and in patients with liver disease; monitor closely. ● Monitor ECG and blood pressure. ● Watch for change in LOC (sedation, confusion, or excitability), which may indicate toxicity.
procainamide (Procanbid, Pronestyl)	This antiarrhythmic depresses atrial and ventricular excitability and slows conduction.	● Life-threatening ventricular arrhythmias ● Conversion of atrial fibrillation to sinus rhythm	● Monitor ECG (especially length of PR interval and QRS complex, excessive prolongation may predispose the patient to arrhythmias), blood pressure, electrolyte status, and serum drug level. ● Watch for hypotension. ● If used chronically, monitor for signs of joint pain and pericardial pain. ● Monitor WBC for neutropenia.
quinidine gluconate	This antiarrhythmic decreases atrial and ventricular excitability.	● Conversion of atrial fibrillation and atrial flutter to sinus rhythm ● Prevention and treatment of ventricular tachycardia	● Monitor ECG (especially length of PR interval and QRS complex), excessive prolongation may predispose patient to arrhythmias. ● Monitor blood counts for thrombocytopenia; may provoke arrhythmias.
Cardiac glycoside and bipyridines			
Bipyridines: inamrinone (Inocor), milrinone (Primacor)	Vasodilating drugs reduce preload and afterload, and may increase cardiac contractility.	● Acute decompensated heart failure	● Continuously monitor cardiovascular (blood pressure and ECG) and pulmonary status. ● Monitor electrolyte status and renal function. ● This drug may cause arrhythmias and hypotension. ● If inamrinone is used, monitor for fever and thrombocytopenia.
Cardiac glycoside: digoxin (Lanoxin)	Cardiac glycoside increases cardiac contractility actions (positive inotropic), and slows conduction in the AV mode (negative dromotropic effects).	● Chronic heart failure ● Ventricular rate control in atrial fibrillation and atrial flutter ● Prevention of paroxysmal atrial tachycardia	● Monitor and record apical (over the heart) and radial (from the wrist) pulses daily. ● Monitor for toxicity, which may present as rhythm disturbance, vision changes, nausea, and vomiting. ● Monitor serum creatinine and serum electrolytes, particularly serum potassium. ● Dose reduction needed in renal impairment.

Common drugs	Action	Indications	Nursing implications
Cardiovascular system drugs (continued)			
Antianginals *Calcium channel blockers:* amlodipine besylate (Norvasc), diltiazem (Cardizem), nifedipine (Adalat, Procardia), verapamil (Calan, Isoptin), and others	These drugs produce coronary vascular smooth muscle relaxation and lower blood pressure; verapamil and diltiazem slow heart rate and AV node conduction.	● Angina ● Hypertension ● Treatment or prevention of paroxysmal supraventricular tachycardia (diltiazem or verapamil)	● Use with caution in a patient with decompensated heart failure. ● Monitor ECG and blood pressure to avoid hypotension or bradycardia. ● These drugs may cause heart failure, arrhythmias, hypotension, and AV block.
nitroglycerin (Nitro-Bid, Nitrostat)	This coronary vasodilator decreases preload.	● Angina ● Pulmonary congestion from heart failure ● Short-term control of hypotension (if given by infusion)	● Monitor blood pressure for hypotension and orthostasis. ● This drug may cause postural hypotension, tachycardia, and headache; educate the patient that headache is a common adverse effect that usually improves with time. ● Ask patient about use of erectile dysfunction drugs before administration of nitroglycerin.
Central nervous system drugs			
Analgesics and antipyretics *Nonsteroidal anti-inflammatory drugs:* ibuprofen (Motrin), indomethacin (Indocin), naproxen (Naprosyn), and others	These drugs produce an antipyretic, analgesic, and anti-inflammatory effect by inhibiting prostaglandin activity.	● Analgesia ● Fever ● Pain and stiffness of osteoarthritis and rheumatoid arthritis	● Watch for signs and symptoms of renal impairment. ● Monitor daily weights and input and output. ● Watch for decreased effects from antihypertensives and heart failure drugs. ● Monitor stool color for signs of GI bleeding. ● Give with food to decrease GI upset. ● The most common adverse reactions to these drugs include GI disturbances and hepatotoxicity.
Para-aminophenol derivatives: acetaminophen (Tylenol)	Acetaminophen produces analgesic and antipyretic action by acting on the CNS.	● Pain ● Fever ● Osteoarthritis	● Monitor liver function test results. ● This drug may cause hepatotoxicity and anemia. ● Avoid overdose by limiting combination drugs that also contain acetaminophen (such as Darvocet, Lortab, and Percocet).
Salicylates: acetylsalicylic acid (aspirin)	Aspirin produces analgesic, antipyretic, and anti-inflammatory effects by inhibiting prostaglandin synthesis; it also irreversibly inhibits platelet aggregation in low doses.	● Prevention of arterial blood clots ● Prevention and treatment of acute MI ● Prevention of transient ischemic attacks ● Pain ● Fever	● Report tinnitus to the physician immediately, a sign of excessive dose. ● Monitor liver function test results. ● Monitor platelet count for thrombocytopenia. ● Watch for bleeding disorders. ● Ask patient about true allergy (not GI distress sensitivity) before administering.

Common drugs	Action	Indications	Nursing implications
Central nervous system drugs (continued)			
Opioid agonists codeine, fentanyl citrate (Sublimaze), hydrocodone bitartrate (Lortab, Vicodin), hydromorphone (Dilaudid), meperidine (Demerol), morphine sulfate, oxycodone (OxyContin, Percocet), sufentanil citrate (Sufenta), and others	These drugs reduce pain and anxiety through opioid receptors in the spinal cord and the CNS.	● Severe pain ● Antitussive therapy (codeine, hydromorphone) ● Premedicant for invasive procedures and primary anesthesia in surgery (fentanyl citrate, sufentanil citrate)	● Monitor for CNS changes and changes in respiratory or cardiovascular function. ● Evaluate pain level using a quantitative scale. ● Monitor for diminished bowel sounds and constipation, which may be severe.
Anticonvulsants *Barbiturates:* phenobarbital	Barbiturates limit seizure activity by increasing the threshold for motor cortex stimuli.	● Status epilepticus ● Partial, generalized tonic-clonic, and febrile seizures	● Excessive dose may cause tachycardia, palpitations, tremor, nervousness, and nausea. ● Monitor serum potassium level for hypokalemia.
Benzodiazepines: clonazepam (Klonopin), diazepam (Valium, Diastat), lorazepam (Ativan)	Its anticonvulsive effect is due to enhancement of the inhibitory neurotransmitter gamma-aminobutyric acid to neurons in the brain.	● Anxiety ● Insomnia ● Alcohol withdrawl ● Muscle spasm ● Epilepsy ● Status epilepticus	● Monitor patient for excessive sedation or confusion. ● Monitor the elderly patient who may be at risk for falls. ● Rapid I.V. administration may cause hypotension.
Hydantoins: fosphenytoin (Cerebyx), phenytoin (Dilantin)	These drugs inhibit the spread of seizure activity, possibly by promoting sodium efflux from neurons in the motor cortex.	● Complex partial (psychomotor, temporal lobe) and generalized tonic-clonic (grand mal) seizures	● Monitor serum drug level, blood studies, and pulmonary and cardiovascular status. ● Administer I.V. phenytoin in normal saline solution at a rate of no more than 50 mg/minute. ● Rapid administration may cause severe hypotension and can be fatal. ● Watch for a decrease in seizure activity.
magnesium sulfate	The benefit of magnesium in the treatment of preeclampsia may be a result of cerebral vasospasm relief. In the heart, magnesium acts as a calcium channel blocker.	● Preeclampsia and eclampsia ● Treatment of *torsade de pointes* (polymorphous ventricular tachycardia), and other arrhythmias	● Carefully monitor cardiovascular and pulmonary status and serum magnesium level. ● Watch for depressed reflexes. ● This drug may cause hypotension and AV heart block with bradycardia.
Antipsychotics haloperidol (Haldol), olanzapine (Zyprexa), risperidone (Risperdal) and others	These drugs produce antipsychotic effects by blocking CNS dopamine receptor sites.	● Psychotic disorders ● Sedation during mechanical ventilation ● Agitation associated with senile dementia	● Monitor QT interval on ECG for prolongation, which may predispose the patient to arrhythmias. ● Watch for extrapyramidal symptoms and movement disorders. ● Elderly patients may require lower dosage.

Common drugs	Action	Indications	Nursing implications
Central nervous system drugs *(continued)*			
Anxiolytics, sedatives, and hypnotics *Barbiturates:* pentobarbital sodium (Nembutal Sodium)	These drugs depress activity in the reticular activating system, located in the brain stem.	● Insomnia ● Sedation ● Preanesthetic medication ● Anticonvulsant	● Watch for respiratory depression and hypotension. ● Watch for skin rash, which may evolve to Stevens-Johnson syndrome. ● Monitor blood studies as well as cardiovascular, pulmonary, and neurologic status closely; immediately report changes to the practitioner.
Benzodiazepines: diazepam (Valium), lorazepam (Ativan), midazolam (Versed)	Benzodiazepines depress subcortical levels in the CNS and may act on the limbic and subcortical ends in the brain.	● Anxiety ● Acute alcohol withdrawal ● Muscle spasm ● Adjunct to anesthesia or endoscopic procedures ● Status epilepticus	● Monitor pulmonary and cardiovascular status; assess for therapeutic response. ● Watch for excessive sedation or confusion. ● Rapid infusion may cause hypotension. ● Monitor the elderly patient who may be at risk for falls.
Electrolyte replacement			
calcium chloride, calcium gluconate	It replaces calcium (the major cation in extracellular fluid [ECF]), which is necessary for normal maintenance of nervous, muscular, skeletal, and cardiac symptoms; and for cell membrane and capillary permeability.	● Acute hypocalcemia ● Reversal of cardiac ECG effects in hyperkalemia ● Hypermagnesemia (magnesium intoxication) ● Calcium channel blocker overdose	● Infuse drug slowly, according to facility policy. ● Infuse into a central I.V. line or large vein to avoid phlebitis and tissue necrosis. ● Monitor ECG (especially Q and T waves), therapeutic response, and signs and symptoms of hypercalcemia (nausea, vomiting, headache, mental confusion, anorexia).
magnesium sulfate	Magnesium has CNS and respiratory depressant effects; it prevents or controls seizures by blocking neuromuscular transmission.	● Hypomagnesemia ● Treatment or control of eclamptic seizures in pregnant women ● Treatment of *torsade de pointes* and life-threatening arrhythmias	● Infuse I.V. bolus dose slowly to avoid respiratory or cardiac arrest. ● Monitor ECG and serum magnesium level (for hypermagnesemia). ● This drug may cause hypotension, decreased cardiac function, heart block, and depressed reflexes or paralysis.
potassium chloride	Potassium is necessary for cellular function maintenance, adequate nerve impulse transmission, cardiac and skeletal muscle contraction, acid-base balance, and renal function.	● Treatment and prevention of hypokalemia (which may predispose to cardiac arrhythmias)	● Know and follow facility policy that limits rate of administration and concentration of I.V. solutions. ● Oral solutions are rapidly absorbed but have a poor taste. ● Don't crush sustained-release oral dose forms.

Common drugs	Action	Indications	Nursing implications
Electrolyte replacement (continued)			
concentrated sodium chloride solution (3% and 5%)	These solutions replace sodium (the major cation in ECF), which is necessary to maintain osmotic and water balance.	● Correction of severe sodium deficits (sodium level less than 120 mEq/L), which may predispose to seizures	● Infuse solutions slowly and cautiously to avoid pulmonary edema. ● Use a large vein or central line to prevent phlebitis. ● Assess for changes in LOC and balanced intake and output; monitor electrolyte status.
GI system drugs			
Antacids: aluminum hydroxide (Amphojel), aluminum and magnesium (Maalox), calcium carbonate (Tums)	Antacids neutralize gastric acid, increasing stomach pH.	● Acid indigestion ● Heartburn ● Dyspepsia	● Shake oral suspensions well before use. ● If given by nasogastric (NG) tube, flush after use to prevent obstruction. ● Constipation is common with calcium and aluminum antacids. ● Diarrhea is common with magnesium antacids.
Antiulcer drugs (histamine-2 [H_2] receptor antagonists): cimetidine (Tagamet), famotidine (Pepcid), nizatidine (Axid), ranitidine (Zantac)	These drugs inhibit histamine, and markedly inhibit basal and stimulated gastric acid secretion in the stomach.	● Gastric or duodenal ulcer ● Gastroesophageal reflux disease ● Prophylaxis of GI bleed ● Premedicant to procedures to reduce incidence of aspiration ● Zollinger-Ellison syndrome	● Intragastric pH monitoring may be useful in some settings. ● Therapeutic response may include a decrease in symptoms, such as daytime and nocturnal pain, GI bleeding, abdominal discomfort, postprandial fullness, acid regurgitation, and heartburn.
sucralfate (Carafate)	This antiulcer drug forms a complex that adheres to the ulcer site and protects it from gastric acid, pepsin, and bile erosion.	● Duodenal ulcer	● Oral suspension is available for patients with NG tubes. ● This drug may cause NG tube occlusion if mixed with tube feeds.
Antiulcer drugs (proton pump inhibitors): esomeprazole (Nexium)-lansoprazole (Prevacid), omeprazole (Prilosec), pantoprazole (Protonix), rabeprazole (Aciphex)	This class of drugs markedly inhibits basal and stimulated gastric acid secretion in the stomach.	● Treatment of duodenal and gastric ulcers ● Ulcerative peptic esophagitis ● Zollinger-Ellison syndrome	● Capsules are enteric coated. Don't crush. ● This drug may cause headache, dizziness, and diarrhea.

Common drugs	Action	Indications	Nursing implications
Xanthine bronchodilators			
aminophylline, theophylline (Theo-Dur)	Brochodilation is probably mediated by the inhibition of phosphodiestersase (PD) isoenzymes (PD111 and, to a lesser extent, PDV); which increases cyclic adenosine monophosphate production.	• Asthma (in some patients) • Prevention of neonatal apnea	• Monitor serum drug levels and ECG. • Assess for signs of drug toxicity (tachycardia, tremor, nausea, vomiting). • These drugs may cause refractory seizures. • Aminophylline must be given by slow infusion.
Immunosuppressants			
mycophenolate mofetil (CellCept)	Mycophenolate inhibits the proliferative responses to T- and B-lymphotcytes and suppresses antibody formation by B-lymphocytes.	• Rejection prophylaxis (in patients with heart and kidney transplants) • Rescue therapy (heart, kidney, and liver transplants)	• Monitor WBC for myelosuppression. • Monitor blood pressure for hypertension. • This medication may cause tremor, diarrhea, nausea, and vomiting.
cyclosporine (Neoral, Sandimmune) tacrolimus (FK506, Prograf)	Cyclosporine inhibits the antigenic response of helper T lymphocytes and suppresses production of interleukin-2 and interferon-gamma; it also inhibits production of the receptor site for interleukin-2 on T lymphocytes.	• Organ transplant rejection prophylaxis • Rheumatoid arthritis • Psoriasis	• Watch for signs of nephrotoxicity, including elevated serum creatinine and BUN. • Monitor blood pressure for hypertension. • Monitor serum electrolytes for hyperkalemia and hypomagnesemia. • Watch for coarse tremor, which may suggest excessive dose. • Watch for signs of infection.
Tacrolimus (FK506, Prograf)	This drug suppresses cell-mediated reactions and some types of humoral immunity. It prevents activation of T lymphocytes and selectively inhibits secretions of various cytokines (such as interleukin-a, interleukin-3, and interferon-gamma).	• Liver and kidney transplants	• Monitor for hypertension. • This medication may cause tremor, headaches, diarrhea, nausea, and vomiting.

Care of the bariatric patient

System	Pathophysiologic consequences	Potential problems	Nursing interventions
Pulmonary			
	• Decreased diaphragmatic excursion • Decreased vital capacity • Decreased alveolar ventilation • Decreased compliance • Decreased respiratory drive • Chronic carbon dioxide (CO_2) retention	• Increased respiratory rate • Ventilation/perfusion mismatch • Hypoxemia • Respiratory acidosis • Difficulty weaning from the ventilator • Obstructive sleep apnea • Increased risk of aspiration	• Try non-invasive positive pressure ventilation such as bilevel positive airway pressure (BiPAP) or continuous positive airway pressure (CPAP). • Be prepared for intubation. • Calculate tidal volume based on ideal weight, not actual weight. • Minimize time patient spends in a supine position. • Control secretions to prevent skin breakdown. • Reposition at least every 2 hours.
Cardiovascular			
	• Left ventricular hypertrophy • Increased total blood volume • Increased stroke volume • Increased cardiac output • Increased cardiac deconditioning	• Right and left heart failure • Hypertension • Myocardial infarction • Stroke • Chronic venous insufficiency • Deep vein thrombosis • Pulmonary embolism	• Encourage mobility as tolerated. • Watch for signs of fluid overload. • Monitor blood pressure. • Administer medications as ordered.
Endocrine			
	• Increased metabolic requirements • Increased insulin resistance	• Type 2 diabetes • Hyperlipidemia	• Carefully monitor blood glucose levels, especially if patient is receiving a steroid. • Work with dietitian to ensure metabolic needs are met.
Gastrointestinal			
	• Increased intra-abdominal pressure • Increased gastric volume	• Increased incidence of gastroesophageal reflux disease • Increased risk of aspiration, especially with enteral feedings • Increased constipation • Increased risk of pancreatitis	• Administer medications as ordered. • Keep head of bed at 30 degrees when possible. • Increase fluid and fiber intake. • Monitor amylase and lipase levels. • Be alert for altered pharmacokinetics for some drugs.

System	Pathophysiologic consequences	Potential problems	Nursing interventions
Immune			
	• Impaired immune response • Impaired cell-mediated immunity	• Impaired healing • Increased wound infections • Increased skin breakdown and pressure ulcers • Decreased resistance to infection	• Monitor wounds for early signs of infection. • Reposition patient at least every 2 hours. • Monitor skin folds for pressure ulcers or skin breakdown. • Work with dietician to ensure metabolic needs are met for proper healing.
Musculoskeletal			
	• Increased joint trauma • Decreased mobility • Increased atrophy from lack of use • Increased pain with movement	• Osteoarthritis • Rheumatoid arthritis	• Encourage mobilization. • Perform range-of-motion exercises with patient. • Provide non-pharmacological pain-relief measures.

Normal aging-related changes

Body system	Changes related to aging	Nursing implications
Sensory		
Eyes	• Decreased peripheral vision • Decreased pupil size • Decreased pupil response time • Decreased tear production • Opacification of the lens	• Keep glasses within reach. • Increase light. • Allow increased time for accommodation. • Use artificial tears as needed.
Ears	• Decreased speech discrimination ability	• If patient has a hearing aid, make sure it's functional, and keep it within reach for the patient. • Keep background noise to a minimum when possible.
Smell and taste	• Deterioration of taste buds • Decreased sense of smell—more than any other sense	• Offer the patient seasoning to increase palatability of food.
Neurologic		
Balance, gait, and proprioception	• Decreased reflexes • Increased sway in posture • Altered gait patterns • Decreased deep tendon reflexes	• Provide assistive devices and handrails. • Remove clutter and debris from floor and environment.
Sleep	• Decreased sleep time despite increased time spent in bed • Decreased stage 4 sleep	• Treat causes of insomnia when possible.
Tactile	• Decreased tactile sensitivity	• Use heating pads or ice packs cautiously. • Reposition patient at least every 2 hours if immobile to prevent skin breakdown.
Cognition	• Decreased brain mass, neurons, and neurotransmitters • Slowed processing • Decreased vocabulary • Increased forgetfulness (not dementia)	• Present teaching slowly to allow opportunities for questions. • Provide environmental cues for memory.
Cardiac		
Heart	• Increased mass • Decreased blood flow to coronary arteries • Decreased cardiac output • Decreased contractility • Decreased pulse rate • Increased frequency of systolic murmurs	• Benign fourth heart sound common. • Less responsive pulse rate stimuli, such as fever, blood loss, and anxiety.

Body system	Changes related to aging	Nursing implications
Cardiac (continued)		
Vasculature	• Decreased blood flow to extremities • Decreased blood vessel elasticity • Increased occurrence of systolic hypertension • Increased occurrence of atherosclerosis	• Monitor blood pressure carefully to avoid rapid decrease. • Extremities tend to have increased edema.
Pulmonary		
	• Weaker muscles of the chest wall • Increased anterior-posterior chest diameter • Decreased chest compliance • Decreased vital capacity • Decreased cough reflex • Increased susceptibility to hypoxia. • Decreased lung base ventilation.	• Carefully monitor oxygen status and be alert for rapid decompensation. • Montor patient for possible silent aspiration. • Provide ample rest time between activites.
Genitourinary		
	• Decreased renal function • Decreased perineal muscle tone leading to urgency or incontinence	• Provide adequate hydration. • Serum creatinine poor indicator of renal function due to decreased muscle mass. • Provide incontinence pads as needed.
Gastrointestinal		
	• Decreased secretion of saliva and hydrochloric acid • Decreased digestive enzymes • Impaired absorption of vitamins and nutrients • Decreased peristalsis and increased constipation	• Keep head elevated at least 30 degrees after meals. • Give patient small, frequent meals. • Provide vitamin replacement, as appropriate. • Increase dietary fiber and fluids.
Musculoskeletal		
Bones	• Decrease in height of 1″ to 3″ • Increased bone fragility	• Use hip protectors to reduce risk of fractures. • Follow fall risk precautions.
Muscles and soft tissue	• Decreased muscle mass • Decreased subcutaneous fat • Increased stiffness due to crosslinking of cartilage	• Provide warm environment as needed.
Endocrine		
	• Decreased insulin receptor sensitivity • Increased concentration of insulin	• Monitor patient for decreased glucose tolerance.
Integumentary		
	• Decreased rate of cell replacement • Decreased elasticity • Thinning skin	• Tissue friability increases risk for skin tears.
Immunologic		
	• Decreased cell-mediated immunity • Decreased T-cell function • Decreased antibody response	• Check for current vaccinations.

Physiologic adaptations to pregnancy

Cardiovascular system
- Increased blood volume
- Decreased systemic vascular resistance
- Increased cardiac output
- Decreased pulmonary vascular resistance
- Increased heart rate
- Orthostatic hypotension
- Systolic ejection murmur
- Increased fibrinogen levels
- Decreased hematocrit
- Increased hemoglobin level

Gastrointestinal system
- Delayed intestinal motility and gastric and gallbladder emptying time
- Constipation
- Increased tendency of gallstone formation

Endocrine system
- Increased basal metabolic rate (up 25% at term)
- Increased body temperature
- Increased production of prolactin
- Increased estrogen levels
- Increased cortisol levels
- Decreased maternal blood glucose levels
- Decreased insulin production in early pregnancy
- Increased production of estrogen, progesterone, and human chorionic somatomammotropin
- Increased levels of maternal cortisol

Pulmonary system
- Increased vascularization of the respiratory tract
- Shortening of the lungs
- Upward displacement of the diaphragm
- Increased tidal volume, causing slight hyperventilation
- Increased oxygen levels
- Increased chest circumference (by about $2^{3}/_{8}$" [6 cm])
- Altered breathing, with abdominal breathing replacing thoracic breathing as pregnancy progresses
- Slight increase (2 breaths/minute) in respiratory rate
- Increased pH; leads to mild respiratory alkalosis

Metabolic system
- Increased water retention
- Decreased serum protein levels
- Increased intracapillary pressure and permeability
- Increased protein retention

Genitourinary system
- Dilated ureters and renal pelvis
- Increased glomerular filtration rate and renal plasma flow early in pregnancy
- Increased clearance of urea and creatinine
- Decreased blood urea and nonprotein nitrogen values
- Glycosuria
- Decreased bladder tone

Musculoskeletal system
- Lumbosacral curve increases accompanied by a compensatory curvature in the cervicodorsal region
- The rectus abdominis muscles separate in the third trimester, allowing the abdominal contents to protrude at the midline

Crisis values of laboratory tests

The abnormal laboratory test values listed below have immediate life-and-death significance to the patient. Report these values to the patient's physician immediately.

Test	Critical Low value	Common causes and effects	Critical High value	Common causes and effects
Ammonia	< 15 mcg/dl	Renal failure	> 56 mcg/dl	Severe hepatic disease leading to hepatic coma, Reye's syndrome, GI hemorrhage, heart failure
Bicarbonate	< 10 mEq/L SI < 10 mmol/L	Complex pattern of metabolic and respiratory factors	> 40 mEq/L SI > 40 mmol/L	Complex pattern of metabolic and respiratory factors
Calcium, serum	< 6 mg/dl SI < 1.5 mmol/L	Hypoalbuminemia Vitamin D or parathyroid hormone deficiency: tetany, seizures	> 13 mg/dl SI > 3.2 mmol/L	Hyperparathyroidism: coma, tetany
Creatinine, serum	0.4 mg/dl SI 35 mcg mol/L	Severe liver disease	> 2.8 mg/dl SI > 247 mcg mmol/L	Dehydration, rhabdomyolosis Renal failure: coma
Creatine kinase isoenzymes	None	None	> 6%	Acute myocardial infarction, cardioversion, myocarditis
D-dimer, serum	None	None	> 250 mcg/ml SI > 1.37 mmol/L	Disseminated intravascular coagulation (DIC), pulmonary embolism, arterial or venous thrombosis, secondary fibrinolysis
Glucose, blood	< 70 mg/dl SI < 3.9 mmol/L	Insulin overdose, liver damage: brain damage	> 300 mg/dl SI > 16.6 mmol/L	Diabetes, pancreatitis, steroid administration: coma
Gram stain, cerebrospinal fluid (CSF)	None	None	Gram positive or gram negative	Bacterial meningitis

Test	Critical Low value	Common causes and effects	Critical High value	Common causes and effects
Hemoglobin	< 7 g/dl SI < 70 g/L	Hemorrhage, vitamin B_{12} or iron deficiency: heart failure	> 20 g/dl SI > 200 g/L	Chronic obstructive pulmonary disease, dehydration: thrombosis, polycythemia vera
International Normalized Ratio	None	None	> 3.0	DIC, uncontrolled oral anticoagulation
Partial pressure of carbon dioxide in arterial blood	< 20 mm Hg SI < 2.7 kPa	Complex pattern of metabolic and respiratory factors	> 77 mm Hg SI > 10.2 KPa	Complex pattern of metabolic and respiratory factors
Partial pressure of oxygen in arterial blood	< 40 mm Hg SI < 5.3kPa	Complex pattern of metabolic and respiratory factors	None	None
Partial thromboplastin time	None	None	> 40 sec (> 78 sec for patient taking heparin)	Anticoagulation factor deficiency: hemorrhage
pH, blood	< 7.20 SI < 7.20	Complex pattern of metabolic and respiratory factors	> 7.60 SI > 7.60	Complex pattern of metabolic and respiratory factors
Platelet count	40 × 10³/mm³ SI < 40,000/mm³	DIC Bone marrow suppression: hemorrhage	> 10,000 × 10³/mm³ SI > 1,000,000/mm³	Chronic myelogenous leukemia, reaction to acute bleeding: hemorrhage
Potassium, serum	< 2.8mEq/L SI < 2.8 mmol/L	Vomiting and diarrhea, diuretic therapy: cardiotoxicity, arrhythmia, cardiac arrest	> 6.5 mEq/L SI > 6.5 mmol/L	Burns, diabetic ketoacidosis Renal disease, diuretic therapy: cardiotoxicity, arrhythmia
Prothrombin time	None	None	> 14 sec (> 20 sec for patient taking warfarin)	Anticoagulant therapy, anticoagulation factor deficiency: hemorrhage
Sodium, serum	< 120 mEq/L SI < 120 mmol/L	Burns, GI suction Diuretic therapy: weakness, neurologic changes	> 160 mEq/L SI > 160 mmol/L	Dehydration: cardiac failure
Troponin I	None	None	> 1.5 ng/mL SI > 1.5 mcg/L	Acute MI
White blood cell (WBC) count	2 × 10³/mm³ SI < 2,000 mm³	Bone marrow suppression: infection	> 30 × 10³/mm³ SI > 30,000/mm³	Leukemia, infection
WBC count, CSF	None	None	> 20/μl	Meningitis, encephalitis, infection

JCAHO pain management standards

In 2000, the Joint Commission on Accreditation of Healthcare Organizations (JCAHO) issued new standards for pain assessment, management, and documentation. These standards require that patients be asked about pain when admitted to a JCAHO-accredited facility. Any patient who reports pain must be assessed further by licensed personnel. Facility policies must identify a standard pain screening tool to be used for all patients able to use it.

If you work in a JCAHO-accredited facility, check policies and procedures for information on which screening tool to use, how often to assess pain, and which pain level warrants further assessment and action.

Pain is commonly called the fifth vital sign because pain assessment scores must be monitored and recorded regularly—and at least as vigilantly as you monitor and record vital signs. To meet JCAHO standards, you must record pain assessment data in a way that promotes reassessment.

JCAHO standards also mandate that health care facilities plan and support activities and resources that assure pain recognition and use of appropriate interventions. These activities include:
- initial pain assessment
- regular reassessment of pain
- education of health care workers about pain assessment and management
- development of quality improvement plans that address pain assessment and reassessment.

Pain assessment tools

When the patient is admitted, ask him if he's currently in pain or has ongoing problems with pain. If he has ongoing pain, find out if he has an effective treatment plan. If so, continue with this plan if possible. If he doesn't have such a plan, use an assessment tool, such as a pain rating scale, to further assess his pain.

Pain rating scales

Pain rating scales quantify pain intensity—one of pain's most subjective aspects. These scales offer several advantages over semistructured and unstructured patient interviews:

- They're easier to administer.
- They take less time.
- They can uncover concerns that warrant a more thorough investigation.
- When used before and after a pain control intervention, they can help determine if the intervention was effective.

Pain rating scales come in many varieties. When choosing an appropriate scale for the patient, consider his visual acuity, age, reading ability, and level of understanding.

Pain intensity rating scale

You can evaluate pain in a nonverbal manner for pediatric patients ages 3 and older or for adult patients with language difficulties. One common pain rating scale consists of six faces with expressions ranging from happy and smiling to sad and teary.

To use a pain intensity rating scale, tell the patient that each face represents a person with progressively worse pain. Ask him to choose the face that best represents how he feels. Explain that although the last face has tears, he can choose this face even if he isn't crying.

Visual analog scale

The visual analog scale is a horizontal line, 10 cm long, with word descriptors at each end—"no pain" on one end, "pain as bad as it can be" on the other. The scale also may be used vertically.

Ask the patient to place a mark along the line to indicate the intensity of his pain. Then measure the line in millimeters up to his mark. This measurement represents the patient's pain rating. Be aware that this scale may be too abstract for some patients to use.

Numerical rating scale

The numerical rating scale is perhaps the most commonly used pain rating scale. Simply ask the patient to rate his pain on a scale from 0 to 10, with 0 representing no pain and 10 representing the worst pain imaginable. Instead of giving a verbal rating, the patient can use a horizontal or vertical line consisting of descriptive words and numbers.

Although most patients find the numerical rating scale quick and easy to use, it may be too abstract for some patients.

Verbal descriptor scale

With the verbal descriptor scale, the patient chooses a description of his pain from a list of adjectives, such as "none," "annoying," "uncomfortable," "dreadful," "horrible," and "agonizing."

Like the numerical rating scale, the verbal descriptor scale is quick and easy, but it does have drawbacks:

- It limits the patient's choices.
- Patients tend to choose moderate rather than extreme descriptors.
- Some patients may not understand all the adjectives.

Overall pain assessment tools

Overall pain assessment tools evaluate pain in multiple dimensions, providing a wider range of information. These tools are time-consuming and may be more practical for outpatient use. Still, you might want to use one for a hospitalized patient with hard-to-control chronic pain.

Pain assessment guide

Although lengthy, a pain assessment guide can help you collect important information about the patient's overall pain experience. These guides may vary from one facility to the next.

Brief pain inventory

The brief pain inventory (BPI) focuses on the patient's pain during the past 24 hours. The patient or health care provider can complete it in about 15 minutes. It comes in several languages besides English, including Chinese, French, and Vietnamese.

To use the BPI, have the patient rate the least and worst pain he's experienced over the past 24 hours and at the present time. Have him point to the location of his pain on a body map.

The BPI also asks questions that focus on:
● whether the patient has had pain other than common types (such as a headache or toothache)
● whether pain has interfered with his activities (such as walking, work, and sleep) in the past 24 hours, and if so, to what extent
● whether the patient's current pain management plan is effective.

McGill pain questionnaire

The McGill pain questionnaire assesses the multiple dimensions of neuropathic pain (a tingling, burning, or shooting pain generated by nerves). It provides word descriptors to measure sensory, affective, and evaluative pain domains.

This tool is available in a short and long form. The short form has 15 word descriptors and takes less than 5 minutes. The long form consists of 78 word descriptors and takes about 20 minutes.

The McGill questionnaire can be used for baseline and periodic assessments. However, it doesn't quantify the patient's pain and isn't useful for frequent assessments.

Self-monitoring record

If your patient has chronic or recurrent pain, consider giving him a self-monitoring record to help him accurately describe pain occurrence and severity.

Documenting pain assessment findings

Be sure to document baseline pain assessment findings so that you and other team members can use them for later comparison. You may want to use a standardized documentation form such as the pain assessment guide mentioned earlier.

If the patient has unrelieved pain, you'll need to conduct frequent assessments. To make pain assessment findings more visible, consider using a graphic sheet that lets you document pain severity next to vital signs.

Using pain assessment flow sheets

A pain assessment flow sheet provides a convenient way to track the patient's pain level and response to interventions over time. On a typical flow sheet, you record information about the patient's pain severity rating, therapeutic interventions, effects of each intervention, and adverse effects of treatments (such as nausea or sedation).

A pain assessment flow sheet is useful inside and outside the hospital. After discharge, the patient and his family may want to use the flow sheet along with a pain diary, in which the patient records his activities, pain intensity, and pain interventions. The diary can reveal the extent to which pain management measures and activities affect his pain level.

Analgesic infusion flow sheet

If the patient is receiving an analgesic infusion, you may use an analgesic infusion flow sheet to speed documentation and track his progress. Information to record on the flow sheet includes the:
- medication name and dosage
- date and time of each dose
- concentration and dose
- volume infused and volume remaining.

Oral medication flow sheet

An oral medication flow sheet can be a valuable tool for:
- patients who will receive analgesics after discharge
- home-care patients with pain caused by progressive illness
- patients with chronic nonmalignant pain.
  These flow sheets should be brief and simple to use.

Posttest 1

This posttest has been designed to evaluate your readiness to take the certification examination for critical care nursing. Similar in form and content to the actual examination, the posttest consists of 50 questions based on brief clinical situations. The questions will help sharpen your test-taking skills while assessing your knowledge of critical care nursing theory and practice.

Allow yourself 50 minutes to complete this posttest. To improve your chances for performing well, consider these suggestions:

- Read each clinical situation closely. Weigh the four options carefully, and then select the option that best answers the question. (*Note:* In this posttest, options are lettered A, B, C, and D to aid in later identification of correct answers and rationales. These letters don't appear on the certification examination.)

- If you have difficulty understanding a question or are unsure of the answer, mark it and, if time permits, return to it later. (For the actual examination, the computer tutorial will provide complete instructions on how to take the examination, including how to select an answer, change it, or mark it for later review.)

- If you have no idea of the correct answer, make an educated guess. (Only correct answers are counted in scoring the certification examination.)

After you complete the posttest, or after the 50-minute time limit expires, check your responses against the correct answers and rationales provided on pages 338 to 344.

Now, select a quiet room where you'll be undisturbed, set a timer for 50 minutes, and begin.

Questions

1. A patient is admitted to the surgical intensive care unit (SICU) with a suspected bowel obstruction. In performing the initial assessment, the nurse knows that auscultation of the abdomen:

○ **A.** should be performed after palpation.

○ **B.** is best done with the bell of the stethoscope.

○ **C.** should reveal hyperactive sounds above the obstruction and absent sounds below the obstruction.

○ **D.** should be performed after percussion.

2. A 36-year-old man who has had hypertension for 4 years was brought by family members to the emergency department (ED). The patient complains of chest pain that is unrelieved by nitroglycerin. He states that he has had the pain for 3 hours and rates the pain at 8 on a scale of 1 to 10. His blood pressure is 178/98 mm Hg; heart rate, 116 beats/minute; respiratory rate, 26 breaths/minute; and temperature, 98.9° F (37.2° C). A 12-lead electrocardiogram (ECG) shows an elevated ST segment in leads II, III and AV_F. The medical diagnosis is myocardial infarction (MI). The physician orders O_2 by nasal cannula at 4 L/minute nitroglycerin I.V. infusion titrated to a systolic blood pressure of 90 mm Hg and pain relief, tissue plasminogen activator (TPA) 100 mg over 3 hours (60 mg in the first hour, 20 mg/hour for the next 2 hours) followed by a heparin I.V. infusion to run at 1,000 U/hour, and morphine sulfate 2 mg slow I.V. push every 2 hours as needed for chest pain. Which of the following indicates that the TPA therapy is effective?

○ **A.** Prothrombin time/partial thromboplastin time ratio (PT/PTT) 2.5 times greater than normal

○ **B.** Relief of chest pain

○ **C.** Few premature ventricular contractions and a return of the ST segment to normal

○ **D.** Blood pressure 120/85 mm Hg and heart rate 86 beats/minute

3. During an initial assessment, the nurse notices that the patient's arterial systolic blood pressure decreases by 14 mm Hg on inspiration. When documenting this change, the nurse should note this drop as:

○ **A.** pulsus magnus.

○ **B.** pulsus alternans.

○ **C.** pulsus parvus.

○ **D.** pulsus paradoxus.

4. An unconscious patient is brought to the ED, and the nurse suspects an upper airway obstruction. What is the best initial action for the nurse to take?

○ **A.** Perform deep tracheal suctioning.

○ **B.** Begin mechanical ventilation.

○ **C.** Tilt the patient's head and do a chin lift.

○ **D.** Perform 6 to 10 upward abdominal thrusts.

5. A 67-year-old woman is admitted to the ntensice care unit (ICU) in a severely obtunded state. She withdraws from painful stimuli and exhibits random movement of all extremities. Her potassium level is 4.6 mEq/L; sodium, 135 mEq/L; hematocrit (HCT), 46%; blood urea nitrogen (BUN)–creatinine ratio, 46:2.1; and plasma glucose, 1,099 mg/dl. Arterial blood gas (ABG) values include pH, 7.31; partial pressure of oxygen (Pa_{O_2}). 92 mm Hg; partial pressure of arterial carbon dioxide (Pa_{CO_2}), 30 mm Hg; and HCO_3^-, 20 mEq/L. A medical diagnosis of hyperglycemic hyperosmolar nonketotic syndrome (HHNS) is made. Which underlying diagnosis places the patient at greatest risk of developing HHNS?

○ **A.** Insulin-dependent (type I) diabetes mellitus

○ **B.** Non-insulin-dependent (type II) diabetes mellitus

○ **C.** Long-term exogenous corticosteroid use

○ **D.** Chronic renal failure

6. A female patient is placed on oxygen via nasal cannula at a rate of 5 L/minute, with orders for repeat ABG sampling and serum glucose and electrolyte measurements in 1 hour. Urine output has dropped to 30 ml for the past hour, and the patient's current blood pressure is 94/48 mm Hg. Which intervention should the nurse plan for this patient?

○ **A.** Potent diuretic therapy to increase urine flow

○ **B.** Administration of large volumes of I.V. hypertonic solutions to increase urine flow

○ **C.** Administration of large volumes of I.V. isotonic solutions, hypotonic solutions, or plasma expanders to increase circulating volume

○ **D.** Administration of large volumes of hypotonic solutions to reverse hyperosmolality

7. A 66-year-old woman is transferred to the ICU from the surgery unit after developing disseminated intravascular coagulation (DIC). The nurse develops a care plan, knowing that the care of a patient with a bleeding disorder usually includes:

○ **A.** close monitoring of body temperature.

○ **B.** ambulation twice daily.

○ **C.** strict bed rest.

○ **D.** avoidance of blood products that may cause reactions.

8. A 55-year-old man with chest pain is admitted to the ED. On the 12-lead ECG, the ED nurse notes ST-segment elevation and large Q waves in leads II, III, and aV$_F$ and ST-segment depression in leads I and aV$_L$. What's the diagnosis?

   ○ **A.** Angina attack

   ○ **B.** Normal ECG

   ○ **C.** Inferior wall MI

   ○ **D.** Subendocardial MI

9. A patient post–cardiac arrest has an implantable cardioverter defibrillator (ICD) inserted. His wife is concerned about what to do if her husband collapses again. The nurse's best response would be:

   ○ **A.** "Now that your husband has the ICD you need not worry."

   ○ **B.** "Do you know how to access the emergency medical service (EMS) system?"

   ○ **C.** "Would you like to be taught cardiopulmonary resuscitation (CPR) to help ease your concern?"

   ○ **D.** "I'll have the physician talk to you."

10. A 38-year-old man is admitted to the ICU with a diagnosis of acute pancreatitis. When assessing his condition, the nurse notes that he has a positive Trousseau's sign. This sign is associated with what condition?

   ○ **A.** Hypomagnesemia

   ○ **B.** Hypophosphatemia

   ○ **C.** Hyponatremia

   ○ **D.** Hypocalcemia

11. A woman is admitted to the ICU with a diagnosis of hepatic coma. She's lethargic and responds only to painful stimuli. Which therapy would probably be used to lower her serum ammonia level?

   ○ **A.** Provide a high-protein diet, and increase fluid intake.

   ○ **B.** Administer lactulose and neomycin.

   ○ **C.** Administer opioid analgesics and sedatives.

   ○ **D.** Administer digoxin (Lanoxin) and furosemide (Lasix).

12. A patient is diagnosed with acute transmural MI. While analyzing the patient's ECG strip, the nurse would find that the ST segment is:

○ **A.** isoelectric.

○ **B.** elevated.

○ **C.** prolonged.

○ **D.** depressed.

13. A patient's ECG pattern changed from sinus rhythm, rate 80, to junctional escape rhythm, rate 46. Of the following medications available to the nurse, which would be the most appropriate to use to correct this pattern change?

○ **A.** Digoxin (Lanoxin) 0.25 mg I.V.

○ **B.** Atropine 1 mg I.V.

○ **C.** Lidocaine 100 mg I.V.

○ **D.** Verapamil 60 mg P.O.

14. A 78-year-old man with a diagnosis of dementia who has just undergone lung resection is admitted to the SICU. He's intubated, connected to a mechanical ventilator, and agitated. His blood pressure is 158/96 mm Hg; heart rate, 135 beats/minute; respiratory rate, 40 breaths/minute; and temperature, 97.8° F (36.6° C). The ventilator settings are fraction of inspired oxygen (FIO_2), 0.40; synchronized intermittent mandatory ventilation, 8; and tidal volume, 800 ml. Other assessment data include pH, 7.5; $Paco_2$, 30 mm Hg; Pao_2, 80 mm Hg; HCO_3^-, 24 mEq/L; and arterial oxygen saturation, 94%. Vecuronium, a nondepolarizing neuromuscular blocker, is prescribed to induce skeletal muscle relaxation during ventilation and to decrease oxygen consumption. What other medication would the nurse expect to administer in conjunction with vecuronium?

○ **A.** Adenosine

○ **B.** Neostigmine

○ **C.** Diazepam

○ **D.** Furosemide

15. A patient is admitted with actively bleeding duodenal ulcers. What's the most important goal of treatment for this condition?

○ **A.** Stabilizing the patient to prepare for surgery as soon as possible

○ **B.** Administering I.V. vasopressin to decrease blood flow to the area

○ **C.** Replacing fluid volume loss to prevent shock

○ **D.** Administering I.V. histamine inhibitors to decrease the acid level

16. The family of a critically ill patient in the trauma unit wishes to visit more frequently than policy allows. The nurse's best action is to:

   ○ **A.** insist on adherence to the visiting policy.

   ○ **B.** allow only one family member to visit frequently.

   ○ **C.** allow the family to visit frequently, and evaluate the patient's response.

   ○ **D.** discourage any discussion with the family about visiting policy.

17. A rhythm strip from a patient's ECG shows the following pattern:

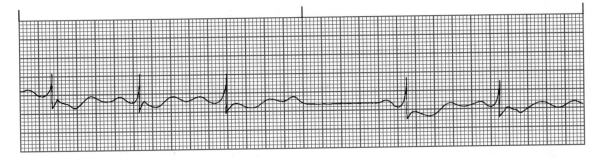

How should the nurse interpret this pattern?

   ○ **A.** Sinus bradycardia

   ○ **B.** Junctional escape rhythm

   ○ **C.** Second-degree atrioventricular (AV) block, Mobitz type II

   ○ **D.** Ventricular escape rhythm

18. A man is admitted to the ICU with acute MI. Which nursing goal would have the highest priority in planning the patient's care?

   ○ **A.** Maintain normal fluid and electrolyte balance.

   ○ **B.** Maintain adequate nutrition.

   ○ **C.** Prevent invasive infections.

   ○ **D.** Provide physical and psychological rest.

19. A patient with DIC has a severe reaction to a unit of packed cells and develops a humoral immunity. The nurse knows that humoral immunity:

   ○ **A.** is produced by T-cell activity.

   ○ **B.** involves immunoglobulins.

   ○ **C.** occurs only in anaphylactic reactions.

   ○ **D.** involves the thymus.

20. A man attending a stressful business meeting complains of severe substernal chest pain. He rates the pain as 12 on a scale of 1 to 10. After his third sublingual nitroglycerin tablet, the man states that his pain has decreased to 3. His blood pressure is 146/90 mm Hg; heart rate, 113 beats/minute; respiratory rate, 28 breaths/minute; and temperature, 98.6° F (37° C). The patient is admitted to the cardiac care unit to rule out MI. Orders include MI profile, nitroglycerin I.V. infusion titrated for relief of pain, oxygen at 2 L via nasal cannula, and one enteric-coated aspirin every day. The monitoring of which vital sign should receive the highest priority?

○ **A.** Blood pressure

○ **B.** Heart rate

○ **C.** Respiratory rate

○ **D.** Temperature

21. A man who is having continuous, seizurelike movements is brought to the ED by the police. The patient has no identification, and his history is unknown. Which medication should the nurse administer first?

○ **A.** Naloxone

○ **B.** Sodium bicarbonate

○ **C.** Glucose

○ **D.** Diazepam

22. A patient in the ICU is intubated and connected to a mechanical ventilator. She becomes extremely anxious, and the pressure alarm sounds with each inspiration. What's the best nursing intervention for this situation?

○ **A.** Increase the tidal volume.

○ **B.** Increase the oxygen concentration.

○ **C.** Disconnect the ventilator and manually ventilate the patient using a ventilator bag for a few breaths.

○ **D.** Administer the prescribed diazepam or morphine sulfate as needed.

23. A patient is admitted to the ICU with a diagnosis of acute upper GI bleeding. Which nursing diagnosis would have the highest priority?

○ **A.** Deficient fluid volume related to bleeding

○ **B.** Impaired tissue integrity related to mucosal damage

○ **C.** Disturbed sensory perception (visual) related to increased blood ammonia levels

○ **D.** Anxiety related to critical illness

24. Which laboratory values are most consistent with a medical diagnosis of HHNS?

   ○ **A.** Glucose, 600 mg/dl; plasma osmolality, 300 mOsm/kg; serum potassium, 4.2 mEq/L

   ○ **B.** Glucose, 800 mg/dl; plasma osmolality, 365 mOsm/kg; pH, 7.3

   ○ **C.** Glucose, 450 mg/dl; pH, 7.2; potassium, 5.2 mEq/L

   ○ **D.** Glucose, 600 mg/dl; pH, 7.2; anion gap, 16

25. A patient in the ICU has just undergone surgery to remove a large brain tumor. He's attached to an intracranial pressure (ICP) monitoring system using a subarachnoid screw. What's the most important nursing responsibility when caring for this patient?

   ○ **A.** Periodically obtain samples of cerebrospinal fluid.

   ○ **B.** Keep the transducer below the level of the foramen of Monro.

   ○ **C.** Open the system to air to zero-balance it.

   ○ **D.** Use a continuous low-flow flush device to maintain patency.

26. When preparing to teach a patient about his illness, the nurse needs to realize that learning is most likely to occur under which condition:

   ○ **A.** Anxiety is mild and acceptance is congruent with the illness.

   ○ **B.** Anxiety is moderate and the patient is motivated.

   ○ **C.** Anxiety is high and the patient is highly motivated.

   ○ **D.** Anxiety is low and the patient denies the severity of the illness.

27. A 47-year-old woman is admitted to the ICU with a diagnosis of syndrome of inappropriate antidiuretic hormone (SIADH) after treatment for oat cell adenocarcinoma of the lung. What's the most likely reason for the onset of SIADH in this patient?

   ○ **A.** Ectopic secretion of antidiuretic hormone (ADH) by the tumor cells.

   ○ **B.** Ingestion of large amounts of water after chemotherapy.

   ○ **C.** Inappropriate secretion of ADH by the posterior pituitary gland secondary to the prolonged nausea and vomiting caused by chemotherapy.

   ○ **D.** Diminished ADH secretion secondary to brain metastasis.

28. Laboratory values for a patient with SIADH would probably reflect which of the following?

- ○ **A.** Elevated serum sodium level, decreased urine osmolality, and elevated plasma osmolality

- ○ **B.** Decreased serum sodium level, decreased urine sodium level, and elevated plasma osmolality

- ○ **C.** Decreased serum sodium level, elevated urine sodium level, and elevated urine osmolality

- ○ **D.** Elevated serum sodium level, elevated urine sodium level, and elevated urine specific gravity

29. A patient with DIC is receiving I.V. albumin. The nurse knows that albumin:

- ○ **A.** is isotonic.

- ○ **B.** decreases the intravascular volume.

- ○ **C.** increases the interstitial volume.

- ○ **D.** increases the intravascular volume.

30. A 34-year-old man is admitted to the ICU with severe respiratory difficulty and a diagnosis of *Pneumocystis carinii* pneumonia secondary to acquired immunodeficiency syndrome. Which of the following is the most important factor in planning the patient's care?

- ○ **A.** Pacing nursing care to avoid patient fatigue

- ○ **B.** Placing an "HIV positive" sign on the door so that laboratory and nursing personnel take appropriate precautions when handling blood and body fluids

- ○ **C.** Ensuring that the patient wears a mask and gloves outside the room to prevent the spread of infection

- ○ **D.** Restricting visitors to the immediate family to prevent contamination

31. A patient is admitted to the ICU with a blood pressure of 76/38 mm Hg and a diagnosis of septic shock. Which assessment finding would best confirm this diagnosis?

- ○ **A.** Hot, dry skin with poor skin turgor

- ○ **B.** ABG analysis revealing metabolic alkalosis

- ○ **C.** Temperature of 105° F (40.6° C) and a pulse rate of 122 beats/minute

- ○ **D.** Urine output of 30 ml/hour and central venous pressure of 8 cm H_2O

32. A patient with head trauma is admitted to the ICU for observation and exhibits the following signs: decreased level of consciousness (LOC), altered respiratory pattern with frequent yawns, small but reactive pupils, and positive bilateral Babinski's reflex. Shortly after admission, Cheyne-Stokes respirations, decorticate posturing, and coma occur. What's the most likely cause of this deterioration?

○ **A.** Uncal herniation

○ **B.** Central herniation

○ **C.** Transcranial herniation

○ **D.** Nucleus pulposus herniation

33. For a patient with an acute, uncomplicated MI, the nurse should question which of the following physician's orders?

○ **A.** Morphine 5 mg I.V. push every 2 hours as needed for chest pain

○ **B.** Isoproterenol (Isuprel) infusion at 20 mcg/minute

○ **C.** Heparin 5,000 units subcutaneous every 12 hours

○ **D.** Diltiazem (Cardizem) 60 mg by mouth every 8 hours

34. A 53-year-old woman with a history of coronary artery disease and alcohol abuse is in the ICU with a diagnosis of bleeding esophageal varices. Her blood pressure is 105/60 mm Hg; heart rate, 130 beats/minute; respiratory rate, 28 breaths/minute; and temperature, 98° F (36.7° C). Significant laboratory values are hemoglobin 8 g/dl and HCT 26%. Burgundy-colored aspirate appears in the nasogastric (NG) tube. The patient is receiving cimetidine I.V. at a rate of 42 ml/hour, dextrose 5% in water in combination with 0.9% normal saline solution, and 20 mEq potassium chloride I.V. at a rate of 150 ml/hour. After 1 hour, the nurse notices that NG tube drainage has changed from burgundy to bright red, the blood pressure has decreased to 90/50 mm Hg, and the heart rate is 142 beats/minute. The physician is notified and gives a verbal order to start a vasopressin infusion at 0.3 U/minute. After initiating the infusion, the nurse instructs the patient to notify the nurse immediately if she experiences which of the following?

○ **A.** Increase in urinary urgency

○ **B.** Numbness or tingling

○ **C.** Metallic taste in the mouth

○ **D.** Chest pain

35. A patient experiencing transient confusion and drowsiness is scheduled for a lumbar puncture. Knowing that the spinal subarachnoid space is continuous with the cerebral subarachnoid space, the nurse discusses her concern with the physician about performing lumbar puncture when the patient's LOC changes. In what circumstances is lumbar puncture contraindicated?

○ **A.** If the patient's blood pressure is 100/60 mm Hg

○ **B.** If the patient's family reports that the patient recently had a severe viral cold

○ **C.** If the patient shows signs of increasing ICP

○ **D.** All of the above

36. A 30-year-old pregnant woman who is admitted to the ED has a history of sudden onset of severe headaches followed by seizures. Bruits are heard over the patient's carotid arteries and eyeballs. Nuchal rigidity is present. What's the most likely diagnosis, and what test can be used to confirm this diagnosis?

○ **A.** Guillain-Barré syndrome and electromyography

○ **B.** Meningitis and lumbar puncture

○ **C.** Autonomic dysreflexia and spinal series

○ **D.** Arteriovenous malformation and computed tomography (CT) scan

37. An 84-year-old man is diagnosed with septic shock. Aggressive treatment is started in the ICU. Which is the most important action for the nurse to take during this therapy?

○ **A.** Placing the patient in the shock position to increase blood pressure

○ **B.** Keeping the patient on strict bed rest

○ **C.** Controlling the patient's temperature by placing him on a hypothermia blanket

○ **D.** Monitoring the patient's vital signs and urine output every 4 hours for changes

38. A 24-year-old man has accidentally ingested about 200 ml of a lye-based liquid drain cleaner. Which of the following should the nurse be prepared to administer when the patient arrives at the ED?

○ **A.** A cathartic to promote elimination of the caustic substance

○ **B.** 30 ml of ipecac syrup followed by 240 ml of water to induce vomiting

○ **C.** 150 ml of milk or water to dilute the caustic substance

○ **D.** 75 g of activated charcoal to absorb the ingested chemical

39. A 29-year-old man is brought to the ED by EMS personnel after he was found sitting in his car in an enclosed garage with the motor running. He's unresponsive and hypotensive, and his skin is bright red. Which nursing diagnosis is of the highest priority for this patient?

○ **A.** Ineffective coping related to depression

○ **B.** Ineffective cardiopulmonary tissue perfusion related to decreased cardiac output

○ **C.** Ineffective cerebral tissue perfusion related to depressed neurologic functioning

○ **D.** Ineffective breathing pattern related to suppressed respirations

40. A patient with burns on the face and neck is at risk for airway obstruction. Which of the following would be most indicative of a potential airway obstruction?

○ **A.** Singed nasal hairs

○ **B.** Neck and face pain

○ **C.** Pao_2 of 80 mm Hg

○ **D.** Coughing up large amounts of thick, white sputum

41. A 63-year-old man is admitted to the ICU with a diagnosis of a dissecting thoracic aneurysm. His blood pressure is 180/110 mm Hg; heart rate, 110 beats/minute; respiratory rate, 12 breaths/minute; and temperature, 99° F (37.2° C). The patient is anxious, and several family members are present. What medications will probably be ordered to lower the patient's blood pressure and decrease his anxiety level?

○ **A.** Meperidine (Demerol) and propranolol (Inderal)

○ **B.** Midazolam (Versed) and nifedipine (Procardia)

○ **C.** Morphine and digoxin (Lanoxin)

○ **D.** Lorazepam (Ativan) and nitroprusside sodium

42. A 50-year-old woman comes to the ED complaining of "fluttering" in her chest, dyspnea, lethargy, and syncope. She's barrel-chested, has a history of schizophrenia, and smokes two packs of cigarettes per day. Her blood pressure is 99/50 mm Hg; heart rate, 220 beats/minute; respiratory rate, 38 breaths/minute; and temperature, 98.6° F (37° C). An ECG shows that she's experiencing atrial fibrillation with a rapid ventricular response. Verapamil 2.5 mg I.V. is administered twice. To determine the desired therapeutic response, the nurse should watch for which of the following?

○ **A.** Decrease in blood pressure

○ **B.** Decrease in respiratory rate

○ **C.** Decrease in hallucinations

○ **D.** Decrease in heart rate

43. A patient with a closed head injury begins to show a decreased LOC and increased ICP. His arms extend and adduct, his wrists are hyperpronated, and his lower extremities extend stiffly, with the feet in plantar flexion. His ABG values show a Pao_2 of 90 mm Hg and a $Paco_2$ of 50 mm Hg. He's on a ventilator with a tidal volume of 800 ml; Fio_2, 0.40; and respiratory rate, 14 breaths/minute. What type of posturing is the patient displaying, and what can be done to correct this?

○ **A.** Opisthotonic posturing, increase tidal volume

○ **B.** Decorticate posturing, increase Fio_2

○ **C.** Decerebrate posturing, increase ventilation rate

○ **D.** Temporary posturing, no changes necessary

44. A patient has suffered deep partial-thickness and full-thickness burns over 35% of his body. In what ambient environment would the patient be most comfortable?

○ **A.** Room temperature is lower than skin surface temperature and humidity at 25% or lower.

○ **B.** Room temperature is lower than skin surface temperature and humidity at 50% or higher.

○ **C.** Room temperature is slightly higher than skin surface temperature and humidity at 25% or lower.

○ **D.** Room temperature is slightly higher than skin surface temperature and humidity at 40% to 50%.

45. A patient with myasthenia gravis arrives in the ED. Based on the presenting symptoms, she appears to be in cholinergic crisis. The administration of which drug and which response to the drug would confirm the diagnosis?

○ **A.** Edrophonium (Tensilon); worsening of symptoms

○ **B.** Ambenonium (Mytelase); worsening of symptoms

○ **C.** Edrophonium; improvement of symptoms

○ **D.** Ambenonium; improvement of symptoms

46. A patient with chronic bronchitis requires tracheobronchial suctioning. Which of the following nursing actions would best help prevent the potential complications of this procedure?

○ **A.** Hyperoxygenating the patient with 100% oxygen

○ **B.** Keeping the patient in a supine position

○ **C.** Inserting the suction catheter no farther than 4¾" (12 cm)

○ **D.** Giving an I.V. bolus dose of lidocaine to prevent ventricular ectopic beats

47. A patient is in the ED. His pH is 7.36; Pao_2, 88 mm Hg; $Paco_2$, 62 mm Hg; and HCO_3^-, 35 mEq/L. Which condition is reflected by these values?

○ **A.** Respiratory acidosis

○ **B.** Compensated respiratory acidosis

○ **C.** Metabolic alkalosis

○ **D.** Compensated metabolic alkalosis

48. A 35-year-old man with bacterial meningitis is at risk for increasing ICP. Which measure is appropriate for preventing increased ICP?

○ **A.** Encouraging the patient to avoid straining or performing maneuvers similar to the Vasalva maneuver

○ **B.** Avoiding hyperoxygenation before and after suctioning by limiting suctioning to 5 to 10 seconds each time

○ **C.** Keeping the head of the bed flat

○ **D.** Encouraging hyperextension or hyperflexion of the neck and extremities

49. A patient suffered deep partial-thickness and full-thickness burns over 40% of his body about 12 hours ago. Urine output is 22 ml/hour, and the hematocrit is 50%. ABG values show pH, 7.32; Pao_2, 95 mm Hg; $Paco_2$, 35 mm Hg; and HCO_3^-, 18 mEq/L. Based on this data, the nurse would assume that the patient:

○ **A.** is dehydrated, developing renal failure, and in metabolic acidosis.

○ **B.** is in the early stages of heart failure caused by overhydration.

○ **C.** is adequately hydrated, but in acute renal failure and respiratory acidosis.

○ **D.** has developed a polycythemia as his body attempts to compensate for metabolic acidosis and renal failure.

50. After an insulin infusion is initiated, serial fingerstick blood glucose tests reveal a progressive decrease in the patient's serum glucose level. At which of the following plasma glucose levels will the nurse probably begin adding dextrose to the maintenance I.V. infusion?

○ **A.** 250 mg/dl

○ **B.** 200 mg/dl

○ **C.** 150 mg/dl

○ **D.** 100 mg/dl

Answers and rationales

1. Answer: C In a patient with bowel obstruction, bowel sounds are typically hyperactive above the obstruction and absent below the obstruction. Palpation and percussion tend to increase bowel sounds. The diaphragm, not the bell, of the stethoscope is best for hearing high-pitched bowel sounds.

2. Answer: C As the clot dissolves, and the myocardium is perfused, a few arrhythmias may occur; these are known as reperfusion anomalies. After these initial events, the ST segment slowly returns to baseline value or within normal limits as a result of the decreased pain and increased oxygen levels. Heparin therapy, not TPA therapy, will increase the PT/PTT to 2 to 2.5 times greater than normal. Although chest pain may be relieved by TPA, pain relief may also result from administration of nitroglycerin or morphine sulfate. Vital signs aren't used to evaluate the effectiveness of TPA therapy.

3. Answer: D A small decrease in systolic blood pressure normally occurs during inspiration, but decreases greater than 10 mm Hg are abnormal. Pulsus paradoxus (paradoxical pulse) is the correct term for describing this decrease in systolic blood pressure. Pulsus magnus refers to a large or strong pulse. Pulsus alternans describes an alternating strong and weak heartbeat. Pulsus parvus is a small or weak pulse.

4. Answer: C The most common cause of airway obstruction in an unconscious person is the tongue blocking the airway. Opening the airway by tilting the patient's head will relieve the obstruction. Deep tracheal suctioning is unnecessary, unless some other blockage is present. Mechanical ventilation should be used only if the patient isn't breathing after the airway is opened. Upward abdominal thrusts are performed only if an obstruction is present in the airway.

5. Answer: B Patients with non-insulin-dependent diabetes mellitus are most at risk for developing HHNS because low levels of circulating endogenous insulin are thought to inhibit glycogenolysis and gluconeogenesis in the liver. Patients with insulin-dependent diabetes mellitus tend to develop diabetic ketoacidosis. Long-term exogenous corticosteroid use can lead to the development of insulin-dependent diabetes. Chronic renal failure isn't indicated by the laboratory values reported for this patient.

6. Answer: C Isotonic solutions (such as normal saline solution) are administered initially. As fluid volume approaches normal, hypotonic fluids (such as half-normal saline solution or 0.225% sodium chloride solution) are administered until blood pressure and serum electrolyte and glucose values approach normal. Plasma expanders may be required in the presence of hypovolemic shock. Diuretic therapy would be detrimental to this patient because her urine output has dropped due to severe osmotic diuresis. Serum osmolality should be increased, not decreased.

7. Answer: C Bed rest is important to prevent further injury and, possibly, bleeding. Body temperature isn't a critical consideration. Ambulation should be avoided until the patient is stable. Blood products are commonly used to treat DIC.

8. Answer: C The ECG changes noted by the ED nurse clearly aren't normal. They are classic signs of an inferior (diaphragmatic) MI. Attacks of angina typically don't cause ECG changes. A subendocardial MI is a type of MI, not a location.

9. Answer: B Early access of the EMS system quickly alerts EMS providers who can respond with a defibrillator. Knowing how to access the system is the first priority. An implantable cardioverter defibrillator may not always be successful. It's appropriate to offer CPR education, but not the first priority. It isn't necessary to refer to her husband's physician.

10. Answer: D The carpal spasm caused by compressing the upper arm is an indication of a low calcium level. Trousseau's sign isn't an indication of hypomagnesemia, hypophospatemia, or hyponatremia.

11. Answer: B Neomycin kills bacteria in the intestine to diminish protein breakdown, whereas lactulose eliminates protein from the GI tract. Appropriate therapy for this patient includes a low-protein diet and fluid restrictions. Opioid analgesics and sedatives are inappropriate for a patient who is lethargic. Digoxin and furosemide are prescribed for heart failure, not hepatic coma.

12. Answer: B The ECG of a patient with transmural MI most commonly shows an elevated ST segment. An isoelectric ST segment is the normal configuration. A prolonged ST segment indicates hypocalcemia. A depressed ST segment is a sign of angina, right ventricular hypertrophy, or digoxin toxicity.

13. Answer: B Atropine is used for most slow arrhythmias. It blocks the parasympathetic system and directly increases the rate of the AV node and the atria and indirectly increases the rate of the ventricles. Digoxin slows the rate and increases the force of contraction. Lidocaine is used exclusively for ventricular arrhythmias. Verapamil is used to slow atrial arrhythmias.

14. Answer: C Because skeletal muscle relaxants don't inhibit the patient's awareness, a sedative or anxiolytic agent, such as diazepam, would also be administered. Adenosine is used to treat supraventricular tachycardia, neostigmine is used to treat myasthenia gravis or an overdose of a nondepolarizing blocking agent, and furosemide is used to induce diuresis.

15. Answer: C The best way to stabilize the patient is to maintain fluid volume, blood pressure, and pulse rate. Preparing for surgery may not be necessary because many patients stop bleeding on their own. Administering I.V. vasopressin would be an ineffective treatment. Administering I.V. histamine inhibitors is a long-term treatment after recovery from active bleeding.

16. Answer: C Research has indicated that critically ill patients prefer more flexible visiting. Studies have supported the need for individualized, less restrictive visiting for patients and families.

17. Answer: C An ECG pattern of two P waves for each QRS complex and a PR interval that's uniform across the strip indicates second-degree AV block, Mobitz type II. The pattern for sinus bradycardia is one P wave for each QRS complex. Junctional escape rhythm wouldn't have P waves, or P waves after the QRS complex. The QRS complexes on this strip are too narrow for a ventricular escape rhythm.

18. Answer: D Resting the heart is a major goal of treatment after an acute MI. The other options all have lower priorities.

19. Answer: B B lymphocytes initiate the development of immunoglobulins and the antigens. Only helper T cells play a small role in the development of humoral immunity, which usually occurs in conjunction with hemolytic, not anaphylactic, reactions. The bone marrow and lymph cells, not the thymus, are involved in humoral immunity.

20. Answer: A Hypotension is one of the most common adverse effects of nitroglycerin. Although the heart rate may be increased, it usually acts as a compensatory mechanism for the hypotension. Respiratory rate and temperature aren't generally affected.

21. Answer: C Hypoglycemia is a common cause of seizurelike movements. It's easily corrected but can be fatal if left untreated. Given the situation, the nurse could safely administer glucose. Naloxone is inappropriate because the patient's condition isn't consistent with an opioid overdose. Sodium bicarbonate is inappropriate because there's no evidence of acidosis. Diazepam would be appropriate after glucose has been administered.

22. Answer: C Disconnecting the ventilator and manually ventilating the patient enables the nurse to evaluate whether the endotracheal tube or the patient's airway is blocked. Increasing the tidal volume may cause pneumothorax. Increasing the oxygen concentration or administering prescribed medications won't help the underlying problem.

23. Answer: A According to Maslow's hierarchy of needs, a fluid volume deficit has the highest priority.

24. Answer: B In HHNS, the glucose level usually is higher than that seen in diabetic ketoacidosis. Plasma osmolality greater than 350 mOsm/kg is the most significant finding in HHNS. Because ketoacidosis doesn't occur in HHNS, pH should be normal or slightly decreased.

25. Answer: C This type of monitoring system needs to be balanced against atmospheric pressure, usually every 8 hours. Cerebrospinal fluid (CSF) can't be obtained through this device. The transducer should be level. A flush device should never be used with an ICP monitoring system.

26. Answer: A Learning readiness depends on the patient's anxiety level and the level of adaptation to his illness. The best time to teach the patient is when his anxiety level is mild, and physical and psychological adaptation to illness are congruent.

27. Answer: A Ectopic production of ADH is the most common cause of SIADH. There's no evidence that excessive fluid intake or dehydration contributes to the inappropriate release of ADH by the posterior pituitary gland. SIADH is associated with increased, not decreased, levels of ADH.

28. Answer: C Hyponatremia, elevated urine sodium level, and elevated urine osmolality are consistent with the clinical findings of SIADH. Elevated serum sodium level, decreased urine osmolality, and elevated plasma osmolality are indicative of diabetes insipidus.

29. Answer: D Albumin consists of large protein molecules that help draw and hold fluid in the vascular system. Albumin is hypertonic and helps to decrease fluid volume in the tissues.

30. Answer: A The patient's generalized weakened condition can lead to severe dyspnea even with minimal activity. An "HIV positive" sign isn't necessary and would be an invasion of privacy. The patient need not wear a mask and gloves, nor must visitors be restricted to immediate family, because HIV isn't spread through airborne organisms or casual contact.

31. Answer: C In response to an infection, body temperature rises and pulse rate increases. In a patient in septic shock, the skin is cold and diaphoretic. ABG analysis would reveal metabolic acidosis caused by lactic acid buildup. A urine output of 30 ml/hour and a central venous pressure (CVP) of 8 cm H_2O are normal parameters; in septic shock, urine output is likely to be lower and CVP is likely to be decreased.

32. Answer: B Central herniation causes bilateral rostral-caudal deterioration. Uncal herniation causes unilateral signs. Transcranial herniation is related to herniation of cerebral tissue through the skull. Nucleus pulposus herniation involves the spinal canal and spinal cord.

33. Answer: B Isoproterenol is a powerful cardiac stimulant used for heart blocks and heart failure. In uncomplicated MI, it isn't needed and would increase the workload of the heart. Morphine typically is prescribed for pain relief. Heparin is administered to prevent clots while the patient is on bed rest. Diltiazem reduces the workload of the heart.

34. Answer: D Caution must be used when administering vasopressin to patients with coronary disease due to the drug's constrictive effects on the coronary arteries. Vasopressin causes urine retention and reabsorption by the kidneys. Although numbness and tingling may be experienced in the extremities, chest pain is a more ominous sign. Vasopressin usually doesn't cause a metallic taste in the mouth.

35. Answer: C A decreasing LOC is possibly a sign of increasing ICP. If a lumbar puncture is performed in the presence of increased ICP, brain stem herniation may occur. As the lumbar puncture needle enters the spinal subarachnoid space, pressure is released and the brain stem is forced down through the foramen magnum. A blood pressure of 100/60 is normal and doesn't preclude lumbar puncture. A viral infection may precipitate sterile meningitis but isn't a contraindication for lumbar puncture.

36. Answer: D The presence of bruits over the eyes with nuchal rigidity suggests a leaking arteriovenous malformation, which can be confirmed with a CT scan. Most arteriovenous malformations are present at birth but are asymptomatic until the third decade of life. The likelihood of hemorrhage is increased during pregnancy. Seizures and headaches are common presenting symptoms. Guillain-Barré syndrome is a neuromuscular demyelination disease characterized by progressive ascending paralysis. Although nuchal rigidity, headache, and seizures are signs and symptoms of meningitis, this disease doesn't cause bruits. Autonomic dysreflexia is a syndrome associated with spinal cord injuries below the level of T6 and is characterized by loss of sympathetic inhibition.

37. Answer: B Bed rest reduces the energy and oxygen demands on the circulatory system. The shock position may be unnecessary or contraindicated. Hypothermia blankets may be unnecessary because body temperature is commonly normal in early septic shock. Vital signs should be checked every 15 minutes and urine output every hour.

38. Answer: C If the patient is alert and can swallow, he should drink milk or water to dilute the caustic substance. The use of ipecac syrup isn't advisable because caustic and corrosive substances shouldn't be vomited to prevent further damage to the esophagus. Activated charcoal and a cathartic aren't effective in decreasing the caustic properties of the ingested chemical.

39. Answer: D   Respiratory diagnoses are always of the highest priority.

40. Answer: A   Singed nasal hairs indicate that the patient has inhaled hot toxic gases or flames that may cause respiratory problems. A patient can have facial burns without airway damage. A Pa_{O_2} of 80 mm Hg is a normal laboratory value. White sputum is normal; black sputum would indicate possible respiratory problems.

41. Answer: D   Lorazepam is used to decrease anxiety. Nitroprusside sodium is used to quickly lower the blood pressure in an attempt to prevent rupture of the aneurysm. The other drugs don't effectively lower the patient's blood pressure or decrease anxiety.

42. Answer: D   The priority for this patient is to slow the heart rate. Verapamil interrupts the reentry pathway to effectively decrease the heart rate. Verapamil may also decrease the blood pressure which, in this case, is an undesirable effect because of the patient's already low blood pressure. Although the respiratory rate may decrease, it isn't the priority in this case. Verapamil has no effect on hallucinations.

43. Answer: C   Decerebrate posturing, or abnormal extension, is an ominous sign, indicating rostral-caudal deterioration. A Pa_{CO_2} of 50 mm Hg is slightly high, but can be lowered by increasing the rate of ventilation. A decreasing Pa_{CO_2} causes cerebral vessels to constrict, thereby decreasing ICP. Opisthotonic posturing is characterized by rigid spinal hyperextension. It's seen in tetanus and some acute cases of meningitis and is indicative of meningeal irritation. A tidal volume of 800 ml is normal for an adult. Decorticate posturing, or abnormal flexion, is characterized by rigid flexion of the arms and extension of the legs. Decorticate posturing commonly precedes decerebrate posturing in cases of neurologic deterioration. An F_{IO_2} of 0.40 is normal.

44. Answer: D   Patients with burns over a large area of the body lose heat and moisture through the open wounds. An environment in which the temperature is slightly higher than the skin surface temperature, with the humidity at 40% to 50% helps prevent heat and fluid loss.

45. Answer: A   Edrophonium is a short-acting anticholinesterase agent. It's the drug of choice for differentiating between the two types of crisis in a patient with myasthenia gravis. Administration of edrophonium to a patient in myasthenic crisis resulting from inadequate anticholinesterase would improve the symptoms. Ambenonium is a long-acting anticholinesterase agent. Administration of ambenonium to a patient who has been overmedicated with anticholinesterase drugs would intensify or worsen the symptoms.

46. Answer: A   Hypoxia is one of the most common complications of tracheo-bronchial suctioning and can cause arrhythmias and changes in heart rate. An upright position is best for suctioning. The catheter must be inserted approximately 7½″ (19 cm). Ventricular ectopic beats that occur during suctioning are best treated by reoxygenating the patient.

47. Answer: B   The pH is in the normal range, but the $Paco_2$ value indicates acidosis.

48. Answer: A   Maneuvers that are similar to the Valsalva maneuver increase central venous and central thoracic pressures, thereby hindering outflow of venous return from the cerebral vessels and possibly causing increased ICP. Hypercapnia and hypoxemia cause vasodilation, which increases ICP. Lengthy suctioning times can cause a sympathetic response of increased heart rate and blood pressure, leading to increased cerebral blood flow and cerebral edema. Keeping the head of the bed elevated 15 to 30 degrees, and avoiding hyperextension or hyperflexion of the neck and extremities, facilitates drainage of blood and CSF from the head and decreases impedance.

49. Answer: A   The elevated HCT indicates insufficient fluids, the low urine output is an early sign of renal failure, and the ABG values indicate metabolic acidosis. A patient with heart failure would have edema and crackles on auscultation of lungs. A patient who is adequately hydrated would have an HCT lower than 50%. Polycythemia takes longer than 12 hours to develop.

50. Answer: A   Dextrose is added to the I.V. infusion at a glucose level of 250 mg/dl to prevent hypoglycemia and to accelerate the resolution of ketone bodies by decreasing lipolysis. The other values listed are too low and increase the risk of hypoglycemia.

Analyzing the posttest

Total the number of incorrect responses to posttest # 1. A score of 1 to 9 indicates that you have an excellent knowledge base and that you're well prepared for the certification examination; a score of 10 to 14 indicates adequate preparation, although more study or improvement in test-taking skills is recommended; a score of 15 or more indicates the need for intensive study before taking the certification examination.

For a more detailed analysis of your performance, complete the self-diagnostic profile.

Self-diagnostic profile for posttest

In the top row of boxes, record the number of each question you answered incorrectly. Then beneath each question number, check the box that corresponds to the reason you answered the question incorrectly. Finally, tabulate the number of check marks on each line in the right-hand column marked, "Totals." You now have an individualized profile of weak areas that require further study or improvement in test-taking ability before you take the Critical Care Nursing Certification Examination.

Question number																				Totals
Test-taking skills																				
1. Misread question																				
2. Missed important point																				
3. Forgot fact or concept																				
4. Applied wrong fact or concept																				
5. Drew wrong conclusion																				
6. Incorrectly evaluated distractors																				
7. Mistakenly filled in wrong circle																				
8. Read into question																				
9. Guessed wrong																				
10. Misunderstood question																				

Posttest 2

This posttest has been designed to evaluate your readiness to take the certification examination for critical care nursing. Similar in form and content to the actual examination, the posttest consists of 50 questions based on brief clinical situations. The questions will help sharpen your test-taking skills while assessing your knowledge of critical care nursing theory and practice.

Allow yourself 50 minutes to complete this posttest. To improve your chances for performing well, consider these suggestions:

● Read each clinical situation closely. Weigh the four options carefully, and then select the option that best answers the question. (*Note:* In this posttest, options are lettered A, B, C, and D to aid in later identification of correct answers and rationales. These letters don't appear on the certification examination.)

● If you have difficulty understanding a question or are unsure of the answer, mark it and, if time permits, return to it later. (For the actual examination, the computer tutorial will provide complete instructions on how to take the examination, including how to select an answer, change it, or mark it for later review.)

● If you have no idea of the correct answer, make an educated guess. (Only correct answers are counted in scoring the certification examination.)

After you complete the posttest, or after the 50-minute time limit expires, check your responses against the correct answers and rationales provided on pages 359 to 365.

Now, select a quiet room where you'll be undisturbed, set a timer for 50 minutes, and begin.

Questions

1. The nurse is preparing to discharge a 75-year-old patient who has experienced a myocardial infarction (MI). Which of the following evaluation outcomes would be inappropriate for this patient?

○ **A.** The patient will be free from arrhythmias.

○ **B.** The patient will have no signs of infection at the invasive line sites.

○ **C.** The patient will gain no more than 4 lb (1.8 kg) per week.

○ **D.** The patient will remain alert and oriented.

2. A 46-year-old teacher with advanced cirrhosis is being examined by the emergency department (ED) nurse. What can the nurse expect to find when palpating the patient's liver?

○ **A.** Rebound tenderness

○ **B.** Enlarged, soft, painful mass

○ **C.** Enlarged, hard, painless mass

○ **D.** Enlarged, soft mass

3. A 21-year-old man is admitted to the intensive care unit (ICU) after suffering a traumatic injury to the left side of his neck. The patient has flaccid paralysis of the upper and lower extremities on the left side but retains the sensations of pain and temperature on the left side. He has some movement of his upper and lower extremities on the right side but no sensations of pain or temperature on the right side. What type of spinal cord injury should the nurse suspect when doing an assessment?

○ **A.** Posterior spinal cord injury associated with hyperextension

○ **B.** Central spinal cord compression

○ **C.** Brown-Séquard syndrome associated with intervertebral disk rupture

○ **D.** Anterior spinal cord injury associated with dislocation

4. A 21-year-old man is admitted to the ICU complaining of polydipsia, polyuria, nocturia, and weight loss. He reports that he has been voiding large amounts of clear, colorless urine about 20 times per day. His blood pressure is 96/48 mm Hg; heart rate, 124 beats/minute; and respiratory rate, 22 breaths/minute. His laboratory test values are potassium, 4.1 mEq/L; sodium, 146 mEq/L; serum osmolality, 306 mOsm/kg; serum glucose, 122 mg/dl; urine specific gravity 1.004; hemoglobin, 13.2 g/dl; and hematocrit, 48%. Based on the clinical evidence, what's the most likely medical diagnosis?

○ **A.** Diabetic ketoacidosis (DKA)

○ **B.** Hyperglycemic hyperosmolar nonketotic syndrome (HHNS)

○ **C.** Syndrome of inappropriate antidiuretic hormone (SIADH)

○ **D.** Diabetes insipidus

5. A patient is admitted with a diagnosis of diabetes insipidus. Which nursing interventions should be planned for this patient?

○ **A.** Administration of vasopressin, administration of I.V. hypertonic sodium chloride solution, and hourly intake and output measurement

○ **B.** Administration of insulin, administration of I.V. normal saline solution, and hourly intake and output measurement

○ **C.** Administration of vasopressin, administration of I.V. and oral fluid replacements, and hourly intake and output measurement

○ **D.** Administration of furosemide, administration of I.V. hypertonic sodium chloride solution, and hourly intake and output measurement

6. A woman has been admitted with acute upper GI bleeding. She's receiving I.V. aqueous vasopressin (Pitressin) at a rate of 0.4 U/minute. Which other medication would be used concurrently with vasopressin?

○ **A.** I.V. dopamine infusion

○ **B.** I.V. nitroglycerin infusion

○ **C.** I.M. vitamin K

○ **D.** I.V. lidocaine infusion

7. A patient is admitted to the ICU with heart failure. He is 5′4″ tall, weighs 125 lb, and has a cardiac output of 6 L/minute. What is the correct cardiac index for this patient?

○ **A.** 4.4 L/minute/m²

○ **B.** 4 L/minute/m²

○ **C.** 3.8 L/minute/m²

○ **D.** 2.8 L/minute/m²

8. A patient with severe head trauma is monitored for Cushing's triad, which results when pressure is exerted on the brain stem by intracranial hypertension or a herniation syndrome. What are the three signs of Cushing's triad?

○ **A.** Increased blood pressure with widening pulse pressure, bradycardia, and abnormal respiratory pattern

○ **B.** Hypertension, seizures, and cluster breathing pattern

○ **C.** Pinpoint pupils, unilateral paresthesia, and Wernicke's aphasia

○ **D.** Contralateral loss of vision in the same side of each eye, diplopia, and loss of contralateral sensation

9. A 62-year-old man has been in the ICU for 2 weeks after an acute MI. His activity level has been increased to include bathroom privileges. While in the bathroom, he calls out that he doesn't feel well. Simultaneously, the monitor technicians report a decrease in heart rate. The nurse finds the patient unresponsive and slumped against the wall. After lowering him to the floor and calling for help, the nurse notes the patient's blood pressure is 60/36 mm Hg; heart rate, 38 beats/minute; and respiratory rate, 12 breaths/minute. The physician orders 1 mg atropine by I.V. push to be administered immediately. What's the minimum time the nurse should allow before suggesting that the dose be repeated?

○ **A.** 1 to 2 minutes

○ **B.** 3 to 5 minutes

○ **C.** 15 to 30 minutes

○ **D.** 1 to 2 hours

10. The primary purpose of the Patient Self-Determination Act is to:

○ **A.** make patients aware of their right to accept or refuse medical treatments so that they can make choices while they're still capable.

○ **B.** require patients to complete an advance directive.

○ **C.** give the patient's surrogate the power to make decisions for him.

○ **D.** ensure treatment for the terminally ill patient.

11. Which treatment is appropriate for a patient with pancreatitis?

○ **A.** Administering codeine to control the pain

○ **B.** Giving an anticholinergic or antienzyme agent to suppress pancreatic function.

○ **C.** Administering antibiotics to prevent abscess formation

○ **D.** Placing the patient on nothing-by-mouth status during the acute phase, and a low-fat diet during the recovery phase

12. The nurse has noticed that a patient's electrocardiogram (ECG) pattern has changed. There are now erratic, undulating waveforms in place of identifiable QRS complexes. What does this change in pattern indicate?

○ **A.** Atrial fibrillation

○ **B.** Junctional tachycardia

○ **C.** Ventricular fibrillation

○ **D.** Agonal rhythm

13. A 19-year-old patient with insulin-dependent (type I) diabetes is admitted to the ED complaining of nausea, vomiting, abdominal cramping, and fever. Her blood pressure is 132/74 mm Hg; heart rate, 118 beats/minute; and respiratory rate, 32 breaths/minute. Her breath has a fruity odor, and she appears lethargic and has slurred speech. A diagnosis of DKA is made. Which admission laboratory values would the nurse expect to find for this patient?
    (1) pH less than 7.3
    (2) Serum osmolality greater than 350 mOsm/kg
    (3) Serum potassium less than 3.5 mEq/L
    (4) Acetone present in serum and urine

○ **A.** 2 and 3

○ **B.** 1 and 3

○ **C.** 1 and 4

○ **D.** 2 and 4

14. The nurse is caring for a patient who had a heart transplant 2 weeks ago. Which sign would indicate that the patient is experiencing a rejection episode?

○ **A.** Chest pain and low blood pressure

○ **B.** Abnormally low temperature and renal failure

○ **C.** Dizziness and weakness

○ **D.** Bounding pulses and flushed skin

15. A 56-year-old man is scheduled for bypass surgery. His critical care nurse notes that his platelet count is 28,000/mm³. What's the best course of action for the nurse to take?

○ **A.** Complete the preoperative checklist, and administer the preoperative medication as prescribed.

○ **B.** Call the laboratory to have the complete blood count redone.

○ **C.** Delay preoperative preparations and call the physician.

○ **D.** Check the patient's blood pressure, heart rate, and respiratory status.

16. A 68-year-old man is admitted with an acute MI. A thermodilution catheter and arterial line are in place. The nurse notes that the patient's mean arterial pressure is 106 mm Hg; diastolic blood pressure, 90 mm Hg; systolic blood pressure, 140 mm Hg; cardiac output, 5.2 L/minute; mean pulmonary artery pressure, 20 mm Hg; and mean right arterial pressure, 16 mm Hg. What's the patient's systemic vascular resistance (SVR)?

○ **A.** 1,730 dynes/second/cm²

○ **B.** 1,384 dynes/second/cm²

○ **C.** 1,323 dynes/second/cm²

○ **D.** 1,138 dynes/second/cm²

17. A patient has just been intubated. The nurse auscultates his lungs soon after intubation and notes normal breath sounds on the right side and diminished breath sounds on the left side. What's the best action for the nurse to take?

○ **A.** Increase the tidal volume on the ventilator.

○ **B.** Pull the endotracheal tube back 1" (2.5 cm).

○ **C.** Suction the patient to remove the mucus plug.

○ **D.** Leave the tube alone because this is a normal finding.

18. A patient is admitted with a diagnosis of hepatocellular damage. In reviewing his laboratory values, the nurse would consider which of the following most relevant to his diagnosis?

○ **A.** Prothrombin time (PT) and partial thromboplastin time (PTT)

○ **B.** Alkaline phosphatase level

○ **C.** Alanine aminotransferase and aspartate aminotransferase levels

○ **D.** Amylase level

19. A 20-year-old college student develops toxic shock syndrome. Assuming that all of the following are appropriate, which nursing diagnosis has the highest priority for this patient?

○ **A.** Deficient knowledge related to use of tampons

○ **B.** Ineffective (cerebral) tissue perfusion related to low cardiac output

○ **C.** Infection related to streptococcal organisms

○ **D.** Impaired gas exchange related to depressed respirations

20. A 44-year-old man is admitted to the ICU. He attempted suicide by ingesting about 30 tablets of clorazepate dipotassium (each tablet contains 7.5 mg). What are the toxic effects of this drug?

○ **A.** Tachycardia and cerebral hemorrhage

○ **B.** Respiratory depression and hypotension

○ **C.** Complete heart block and paralytic ileus

○ **D.** Liver failure and GI bleeding

21. A patient is receiving nitroglycerin by I.V. infusion at a rate of 20 mcg/minute. The nurse notes that the nitroglycerin is mixed in a glass I.V. bottle of dextrose 5% in water (D_5W), and being administered through normal I.V. tubing using an infusion pump. What should be the nurse's first action?

○ **A.** Decrease the rate of the infusion.

○ **B.** Change the dilution solution to normal saline solution because the medication will precipitate in D_5W.

○ **C.** Change the normal I.V. tubing to nonabsorbent tubing.

○ **D.** Remove the infusion pump because it will cause the medication to crystallize.

22. A patient has been taking quinidine for an arrhythmia. Which of the following would indicate that the patient is experiencing quinidine toxicity?

○ **A.** Frequent diarrhea

○ **B.** Slow, irregular pulse rhythm

○ **C.** Tinnitus and rash

○ **D.** Widening QRS complex

23. A 22-year-old woman is brought to the ED by her mother, who states that her daughter has just ingested 50 iron tablets. Treatment is started. The nurse knows that activated charcoal should:

○ **A.** be administered after ipecac syrup has been administered and after vomiting has stopped.

○ **B.** be administered first to help absorb the iron.

○ **C.** not be administered to patients who have ingested iron.

○ **D.** be mixed with ipecac syrup and water to increase its effectiveness.

24. A 33-year-old firefighter is admitted to the ICU with burns on his face and neck after fighting a fire at a plastics factory. During her assessment, the nurse would give highest priority to which of the following actions?

○ **A.** Noting signs of increased intracranial pressure (ICP)

○ **B.** Obtaining an accurate weight

○ **C.** Assessing psychological status

○ **D.** Assessing changes in the circumference of the neck

25. A 31-year-old woman is admitted to the ICU after a motor vehicle accident during which she sustained a head injury. She's lethargic, but responsive to tactile stimulation. Several hours later, her level of consciousness (LOC) deteriorates, and she can't be aroused. Her blood pressure is 108/55 mm Hg; heart rate, 45 beats/minute; respiratory rate, 8 breaths/minute; and temperature, 101.5° F (38.6° C). Other assessment data include pH, 7.31; partial pressure of arterial carbon dioxide ($Paco_2$), 70 mm Hg; partial pressure of arterial oxygen (Pao_2), 75 mm Hg; HCO_3^-, 26 mEq/L; arterial oxygen saturation (Sao_2), 88%; and ICP, 20 mm Hg. The physician intubates the patient to correct the respiratory acidosis. The patient also receives 75 ml of a 20% solution of mannitol. The nurse knows that the patient is responding to the mannitol when which of the following occurs?

○ **A.** The patient spontaneously opens her eyes.

○ **B.** The patient experiences diuresis.

○ **C.** The patient has a decreased heart rate.

○ **D.** The patient has diarrhea.

26. In monitoring a patient for adverse reactions to vasopressin therapy, the nurse should check for which of the following signs and symptoms?

○ **A.** Headache, decreased LOC, decreased urine output, nausea, and vomiting

○ **B.** Pallor, diaphoresis, tremor, and seizures

○ **C.** Hemoconcentration, increased urine output, and complaints of thirst

○ **D.** Hyperglycemia, hyperkalemia, and increased urine output

27. A patient is admitted to the ICU with a temperature of 105.6° F (40.9° C). In reviewing the laboratory data, the nurse notices a leukocyte shift to the left, evidenced by an increased number of immature neutrophils. This is an indication of which condition?

○ **A.** Anemia

○ **B.** Thrombocytopenia

○ **C.** Acute infection

○ **D.** Leukemia

28. A patient was burned on the face, head, and neck while trying to light a barbecue grill. Which measure would be most effective in preventing pulmonary congestion for this patient?

○ **A.** Encourage the patient to increase his oral fluid intake.

○ **B.** Administer high-flow oxygen therapy.

○ **C.** Encourage the patient to cough.

○ **D.** Use tracheal suctioning to remove burn residue.

29. In developing a care plan for a patient with a severe burn, the nurse establishes a goal to monitor for bleeding to detect stress ulcers. To achieve this goal, the nurse should also monitor for:

○ **A.** renal failure.

○ **B.** hepatic failure.

○ **C.** disseminated intravascular coagulation (DIC).

○ **D.** increased ICP.

30. A 44-year-old man who suffered an MI 2 days ago is being transferred out of the critical care unit. He says, "I don't feel strong enough yet. Why can't I stay a few more days?" Which is the most appropriate response?

○ **A.** "There's a very sick patient who needs this bed."

○ **B.** "Most people do just fine after transfer."

○ **C.** "You sound concerned about leaving the ICU."

○ **D.** "Your insurance limits the time you can stay in the ICU."

31. A patient arrives in the ED after having been burned with boiling water over the lower anterior trunk and the anterior thigh to the knee. Which of the following would the nurse expect to find during the assessment?

○ **A.** Third-degree burns over 20% of the body

○ **B.** First-degree burns over 12% of the body

○ **C.** Second-degree deep partial thickness burns over 33% of the body

○ **D.** Second-degree superficial partial-thickness burns over 22% of the body

32. A patient with diabetes mellitus was discharged from the hospital 3 months ago. Which laboratory data would indicate that the patient complied with the ICU nurse's instructions about postdischarge care?

○ **A.** Fasting serum glucose, 125 mg/dl

○ **B.** Glycosylated hemoglobin (Hb A_{1C}), 6%

○ **C.** Serum potassium, 4.2 mEq/L

○ **D.** Arterial pH, 7.38

33. A 60-year-old man underwent a heart transplant 4 days ago. He's to be transferred out of the ICU tomorrow. The nurse will know that her teaching about posttransplant care has been successful when the patient states:

○ **A.** "I can stop taking these immunosuppressants after I feel better."

○ **B.** "I need to avoid crowds and people with colds."

○ **C.** "I can never kiss my wife again because I will get an infection."

○ **D.** "I will never be able to go hunting again."

34. A patient is admitted with septic shock. His pH is 7.23; Pao_2, 82 mm Hg; $Paco_2$, 44 mm Hg; and HCO_3^-, 18 mEq/L. What would be the best initial action for the nurse to take?

○ **A.** Administer one ampule of sodium bicarbonate by I.V. push.

○ **B.** Intubate and hyperventilate the patient.

○ **C.** Have the patient breathe into a paper bag.

○ **D.** Start oxygen therapy by nasal cannula.

35. A 20-year-old patient is admitted to the ICU with a severe closed head injury. He was riding a bicycle when he collided with an automobile. Intracranial monitoring shows an ICP of 23 mm Hg, and uncal herniation is occurring. During the assessment, the nurse would look for which eye signs and would expect which cranial nerves to be affected?

○ **A.** Hippus; cranial nerve III

○ **B.** Absent doll's eyes; cranial nerves III, VI, and VIII

○ **C.** Anisocoria; cranial nerve III

○ **D.** All of the above

36. A 42-year-old woman is in the early recovery period after a heart transplant. She's receiving immunosuppressants, including cyclosporine. Which of the following signs or symptoms are considered to be the most serious adverse reactions to this medication?

○ **A.** Gastritis and development of peptic ulcers

○ **B.** Paresthesia and headache

○ **C.** Elevated blood urea nitrogen (BUN) and serum creatinine levels

○ **D.** Decreased HCO_3^- level and hypertension

37. A patient with myasthenia gravis is in crisis and about to be admitted to the ICU. The patient has bradycardia and is complaining of blurred vision, nausea, and vomiting. What type of crisis is this patient experiencing, and what drug might be needed?

○ **A.** Myasthenic crisis; atropine

○ **B.** Cholinergic crisis; atropine

○ **C.** Myasthenic crisis; neostigmine bromide (Prostigmin)

○ **D.** Cholinergic crisis; neostigmine bromide

38. A 49-year-old man is brought to the unit with a diagnosis of status epilepticus. He's having generalized tonic-clonic seizures every 5 minutes, with each seizure lasting 30 to 90 seconds. He received a total of 50 mg of diazepam before arriving at the ICU. In accordance with accepted safety precautions, the nurse should ensure that which drug is at the patient's bedside?

○ **A.** Phenobarbital

○ **B.** Flumazenil (Mazicon)

○ **C.** Naloxone (Narcan)

○ **D.** Phenytoin (Dilantin)

39. A 56-year-old man has severe, chronic lung disease related to heavy smoking. In planning his care, which of the following would the nurse rank as most important?

○ **A.** Administering prophylactic antibiotics

○ **B.** Performing a thorough psychological assessment

○ **C.** Increasing the patient's level of exercise

○ **D.** Planning large, high-protein meals to maintain the patient's energy

40. A 50-year-old man with a diagnosis of cerebral aneurysm and subarachnoid hemorrhage is admitted to the surgical ICU. The patient has progressed through the first few days without increased neurologic deficits. What intervention is important on the 7th postoperative day and why?

○ **A.** Discharge planning, because 7 days is the usual length of stay for these patients

○ **B.** Neurologic checks and assessment of LOC, because the incidence of vasospasm or rebleeding is highest 7 to 10 days after surgery

○ **C.** Elevation of the head of the bed, because the development of Brudzinski's sign is seen after 7 postoperative days

○ **D.** Increasing the dose of osmotic diuretics because this action decreases transient cerebral edema

41. A 65-year-old man is admitted to the ICU after undergoing coronary artery bypass graft. He has a history of angina, coronary artery disease, and insulin-dependent diabetes mellitus. The effects of the anesthesia haven't yet reversed, and the patient's blood pressure is labile. His systolic blood pressure is 98 mm Hg (using Doppler flow probe); heart rate, 135 beats/minute; respiratory rate, 14 breaths/minute; and temperature, 96.8° F (36° C); pulmonary artery diastolic pressure, 32 mm Hg; pulmonary artery wedge pressure, 18 mm Hg; central venous pressure, 12 mm Hg; $Paco_2$, 4.5 mm Hg; and SVR, 700 dynes/second/cm². The physician orders vital signs assessment per ICU protocol, dopamine 800 mg in 500 ml D_5W titrated to keep the systolic blood pressure between 90 and 120 mm Hg, and nitroprusside (Nipride) 50 mg in 250 ml D_5W. The physician is to be notified if the systolic blood pressure is less than 90 or greater than 120 mm Hg. As the hours pass, the nurse notices that frequent increases in the dose of dopamine are required to maintain the blood pressure within the ordered parameters. At what dosage should the nurse initially notify the physician of the amount of dopamine being administered?

○ **A.** 5 mcg/kg/minute

○ **B.** 10 mcg/kg/minute

○ **C.** 15 mcg/kg/minute

○ **D.** 20 mcg/kg/minute

42. To help the family develop a sense of control, the nurse may:

○ **A.** refer family members to a grief counselor or clergy.

○ **B.** offer choices to family members whenever possible.

○ **C.** offer reassurance that the patient is receiving the best care possible.

○ **D.** increase their sense of understanding of the illness.

43. A 29-year-old woman arrives in the ED exhibiting audible wheezes and complaining of dyspnea and anxiety. The physician's diagnosis is status asthmaticus. The patient's blood pressure is 165/94 mm Hg; heart rate, 120 beats/minute; respiratory rate, 44 breaths/minute and labored; and temperature, 97.8° F (36.6° C); pH, 7.32; SaO_2, 87%; $PaCO_2$, 62 mm Hg; PaO_2, 74 mm Hg; HCO_3^-, 24 mEq/L; and hemoglobin, 14.4 g/dl. Auscultation reveals coarse crackles and wheezes. Inspection reveals forceful exhalation, diaphoresis, use of accessory muscles, and pale skin color. The physician orders epinephrine 0.1 mg subcutaneously and an aminophylline I.V. loading dose of 5 mg/kg infused over 20 minutes, followed by I.V. infusion at a rate of 0.5 mg/kg/hour. When the patient's heart rate increases to 170 beats/minute, what should the nurse do?

○ **A.** Stop the aminophylline infusion and notify the physician.

○ **B.** Increase the aminophylline infusion and notify the physician.

○ **C.** Teach the patient to do pursed-lip breathing.

○ **D.** Provide a quiet atmosphere to promote relaxation.

44. A patient suffered an acute head injury after a head-on motor vehicle accident. He's displaying cerebrospinal fluid (CSF) rhinorrhea. What would be a high priority of nursing care for this patient?

○ **A.** Inserting a nasogastric tube to eliminate swallowed CSF

○ **B.** Repacking the nasal passages every 4 hours and as needed

○ **C.** Administering prophylactic antibiotics

○ **D.** Testing the pH of the CSF every 2 hours

45. A patient suffered a major burn injury and is diagnosed with adult respiratory distress syndrome (ARDS). The nurse is formulating a care plan to reflect ARDS and knows that the goals with the highest priority should include:

○ **A.** improving the patient's nutritional status and decreasing his pulmonary compliance.

○ **B.** administering steroids and antibiotics to combat infection.

○ **C.** lowering the patient's blood pressure and increasing his $PaCO_2$ level.

○ **D.** maintaining adequate oxygenation and eliminating the underlying cause of ARDS.

46. A 51-year-old man is admitted to the ED complaining of dyspnea, weakness, poor appetite, and headache. He has no drug allergies but had an MI 3 years ago, and has a history of atrial fibrillation and flutter. Current medications include enteric-coated aspirin, furosemide (Lasix), quinidine, and digoxin. His blood pressure is 98/58 mm Hg; heart rate, 54 beats/minute; respiratory rate, 28 breaths/minute; and temperature, 99.2° F (37.3° C). ED personnel inserted two I.V. lines, sent admitting blood samples to the laboratory, and performed a 12-lead ECG that showed ST-segment depression. A report is called to ICU, and the patient will be arriving in approximately 30 minutes, after a chest X-ray is done. After preparing the patient's room, what's the first thing the nurse should do?

○ **A.** Anticipate that the patient will require additional digoxin, and ensure that the admitting orders include an order for digoxin administration.

○ **B.** Anticipate that the patient may be agitated, and ensure that the admitting orders include an antianxiety medication.

○ **C.** Check the patient's laboratory test results.

○ **D.** Order a late dinner tray because the other patients' dinner trays have already been delivered.

47. A patient is intubated with a low-pressure-cuff endotracheal (ET) tube. Which measure is most important for the nurse to include in the care plan for this patient?

○ **A.** Maintaining 30 mm Hg pressure in the cuff at all times

○ **B.** Deflating the cuff every shift for 10 minutes to prevent pressure necrosis

○ **C.** Monitoring the cuff pressure every 4 hours

○ **D.** Changing the ET tube every 2 days

48. A patient is intubated and connected to a mechanical ventilator. The nurse would recognize an accumulation of secretions that alter the patient's airway resistance by which response?

○ **A.** Sudden decrease in the positive end-expiratory pressure (PEEP)

○ **B.** Gradual decrease in the inspired tidal volume

○ **C.** Increase in the amount of pressure required to deliver the selected tidal volume

○ **D.** Increase in the tidal volume without pressure changes

49. A 42-year-old woman who fell from the back of a pickup truck was admitted to the ICU with a diagnosis of basilar skull fracture. The patient has ecchymosis over the mastoid bone and around the eyes. She also has clear fluid draining from her nose and ears. What should the nurse do first?

    O **A.** Test the clear fluid for sugar.

    O **B.** Test the patient for cardinal signs of vision.

    O **C.** Send the clear fluid for culture.

    O **D.** Raise the head of the bed.

50. An 89-year-old woman suffers respiratory arrest at a nursing home. She's rushed to the ED, where she's breathing on her own. The nurse knows that before treatment, the patient's oxyhemoglobin dissociation curve is:

    O **A.** normal.

    O **B.** shifted to the right.

    O **C.** shifted to the left.

    O **D.** flattened out.

Answers and rationales

1. Answer: C Rapid weight gain in a patient who has had an MI is commonly a sign of fluid retention, and the development of heart failure. All the other goals are appropriate for this patient.

2. Answer: C In advanced cirrhosis, the liver has turned into scar tissue and is hard; palpation doesn't cause pain. Rebound tenderness is found in acute appendicitis. An enlarged, soft, painful mass is seen in hepatitis. An enlarged, soft mass usually indicates some type of cancer or tumor.

3. Answer: C Brown-Séquard syndrome should be suspected, because of the presence of ipsilateral loss of motor function with contralateral loss of pain and temperature sensations. The nurse can assume that laceration or hemisection of the spinal cord has occurred in this patient. The corticospinal (motor) tracts cross at the level of the medulla. Thus, the decussation is above the site of injury, which leads to motor loss on the same side. Trauma to the left side of the spinal cord below the level of decussation results in left-sided motor deficits. However, the spinothalamic (sensory) tracts cross at the level of entry into the spinal cord. Trauma to the left side of the spinal cord results in right-sided sensory deficits.

    Posterior cord injuries are rare and generally occur with hyperextension. Damage affects the posterior horns of the spinal cord; proprioception and light touch would be impaired bilaterally, but motor function would remain intact bilaterally. Anterior cord damage affects the anterior horns of the spinal cord; motor function, pain, and temperature sensations would be lost at the level of injury.

4. Answer: D Diabetes insipidus is characterized by symptoms of dehydration, such as hemoconcentration, tachycardia, and hypotension. The glucose level is too low to consider DKA or HHNS as possible medical diagnoses, although the elevated plasma osmolality is consistent with osmotic diuresis. Syndrome of inappropriate antidiuretic hormone is characterized by low serum osmolality, high urine specific gravity, and urine output less than 30 ml/hour.

5. Answer: A Administration of vasopressin and I.V. hypertonic sodium chloride solution is an appropriate intervention for diabetes insipidus. I.V. normal saline solution is inappropriate because the plasma sodium level is already elevated. Vasopressin administration and I.V. and oral fluid replacement is an appropriate intervention for DKA and HHNS. Furosemide and I.V. hypertonic sodium chloride solution administration are appropriate for SIADH.

6. Answer: B Nitroglycerin counteracts the adverse vasoconstricting effects of vasopressin and helps maintain coronary perfusion. Dopamine will exacerbate the vasoconstriction. Vitamin K may be given, but it has no effect on vasopressin. Lidocaine isn't indicated for GI bleeding.

7. Answer: C The cardiac index is calculated as follows: cardiac index equals cardiac output divided by body surface area. For this patient, $6 \div 1.57 = 3.82$ L/minute/m^2.

8. Answer: A The brain stem provides parasympathetic control to the heart, and controls respiration. As the centers for autoregulation lose control and parasympathetic stimulation from the compressing medulla occurs, a hyperdynamic state ensues with hypertension and decreased heart and respiratory rates. Cluster respirations are seen in lesions of the upper medulla and may be part of Cushing's triad, but seizures aren't. Pinpoint pupils are seen in medullary compression caused by parasympathetic innervation, but Wernicke's (receptive) aphasia is seen in patients with cerebrovascular accidents (CVAs), not those with head trauma. Homonymous hemianopsia, double vision, and hemiparesis are also seen in patients suffering from CVAs.

9. Answer: B Atropine can be repeated every 3 to 5 minutes, up to a maximum total dose of 3 mg. If the total dose is more than 3 mg, atropine has a vagolytic effect and doesn't have a positive effect. Atropine may take up to 5 minutes to be effective. If the desired effect isn't achieved within 5 to 10 minutes, atropine isn't likely to work within 30 minutes. Crisis intervention should be completed within 1 to 2 hours.

10. Answer: A The Patient Self-Determination Act requires health care facilities to provide patients with information about their rights under state law to make decisions regarding medical care, including the right to accept or refuse care, and information about advance directives. The act doesn't require advance directives or give the patient's surrogate power to make decisions. It applies to all patients, not just the terminally ill.

11. Answer: D The pancreas stops producing secretions when the patient receives nothing by mouth. A low-fat diet is necessary, because fat is poorly digested by patients with pancreatitis. Codeine is inappropriate, because it causes spasms of the biliary tract. Anticholinergic and antienzyme agents haven't proved effective in pancreatic disease. Antibiotics are unnecessary.

12. Answer: C In ventricular fibrillation, the ventricles quiver and produce no distinct QRS complexes. In atrial fibrillation, there are no distinct P waves, but the QRS complexes are normal. In junctional tachycardia, P waves may be hidden, but the QRS complexes are normal. Agonal rhythm is marked by wide, slow, semiregular QRS complexes.

13. Answer: C Metabolic acidosis and the presence of serum and urine ketones are indicators of ketogenesis, a hallmark of DKA. Serum osmolality greater than 350 mOsm/L H_2O is seen in HHNS, but is normal or slightly elevated in patients with DKA. The serum potassium level is typically normal or elevated in DKA. A decreased potassium level on admission indicates severe potassium depletion and constitutes a medical and nursing emergency.

14. Answer: A Most rejected organs begin to swell or enlarge, causing pain and poor functioning. Temperature would be elevated during a rejection episode. Dizziness and weakness aren't associated with rejection. Rejection causes weak pulses and pale skin.

15. Answer: C A normal platelet count is 150,000 to 400,000/mm^3. Platelet counts below 30,000/mm^3 place the patient at increased risk for bleeding, and most physicians wouldn't operate on such patients. Laboratory tests could be redone only with the physician's approval. Checking the patient's vital signs is appropriate but not of the highest priority.

16. Answer: B Systemic vascular resistance is calculated as follows:

$$SVR = \frac{\text{mean arterial pressure} - \text{right arterial pressure}}{\text{cardiac output}} \times 80$$

SVR is the same as afterload. Normal SVR is 800 to 1,500 dynes/second/cm^2.

17. Answer: B These findings indicate that the ET tube has been inserted too far and has entered the right bronchus. Increasing the tidal volume may cause pneumothorax. The patient isn't likely to have a mucus plug immediately after intubation.

18. Answer: C Alanine aminotransferase and aspartate aminotransferase are most likely to be elevated in patients with liver disease, although other diseases may also cause increases in these laboratory values. PT and PTT may be elevated indirectly. Alkaline phosphatase and amylase levels are elevated in pancreatic disease.

19. Answer: D Nursing diagnoses related to the airway and breathing have the highest priority. Ineffective (cerebral) tissue perfusion diagnoses have the next highest priority, followed by the nursing diagnoses relating to infection and knowledge deficit.

20. Answer: B Respiratory depression and hypotension are toxic effects of clorazepate dipotassium, which is a benzodiazepine. Tachycardia and cerebral hemorrhage are toxic effects of cocaine. The toxic effects of tricyclic antidepressants include complete heart block and paralytic ileus. Liver failure and GI bleeding result from aspirin toxicity.

21. Answer: C The plastic in I.V. bags and normal I.V. tubing will absorb the nitroglycerin, thereby reducing its effectiveness. The infusion rate need not be decreased; the normal dosage range is 5 to 100 mcg/minute. Nitroglycerin can be diluted in D_5W or normal saline solution. An infusion pump should always be used; no crystallization problem exists with nitroglycerin administration.

22. Answer: D Quinidine works by slowing electrical conduction through the ventricles. Quinidine toxicity commonly widens the QRS complex. Frequent diarrhea is an adverse effect that may occur long before toxicity occurs. Quinidine tends to increase the heart rate. Tinnitus and rash usually aren't seen in quinidine toxicity.

23. Answer: A Activated charcoal works in the intestine to absorb medications and toxic substances. It would be vomited if administered after ipecac syrup. Mixing activated charcoal with ipecac syrup and water reduces its effectiveness.

24. Answer: D Changes in neck size indicate edema and potential airway problems. The other options have a lower priority.

25. Answer: B Mannitol is an osmotic diuretic used to reduce cerebral edema. Diuresis will occur before a change in the LOC is noted. Mannitol will increase, not decrease, the heart rate. Diarrhea is an adverse effect of the medication, but doesn't indicate that the patient is responding to the drug.

26. Answer: A Water intoxication, which is characterized by the signs and symptoms listed in option A, is the most serious adverse effect of exogenous antidiuretic hormone (vasopressin) therapy. Pallor, diaphoresis, tremor, and seizures are signs of severe hypoglycemia. Hemoconcentration, increased urine output, and complaints of thirst are signs and symptoms of dehydration, which would be observed if the patient didn't respond to vasopressin therapy. Hyperglycemia, hyperkalemia, and increased urine output are presenting symptoms of DKA and HHNS.

27. Answer: C A shift to the left usually indicates an acute infection. Anemia is indicated by a low blood count. Thrombocytopenia is indicated by a low platelet count. Leukemia is indicated by a shift to the right.

28. Answer: C Coughing increases lung expansion and tends to eliminate burn residue without damaging the trachea. Increasing oral fluid intake could induce vomiting. High-flow oxygen therapy doesn't prevent pulmonary congestion. Suctioning may further damage the tracheal lining.

29. Answer: C DIC is a generalized bleeding disorder in which microembolisms deplete clotting factors. Renal failure, hepatic failure, and increased ICP are possible complications of burns, but aren't related to bleeding problems.

30. Answer: C Validating the patient's concern initiates the opportunity for the patient to discuss his concerns.

31. Answer: D Boiling water usually produces second-degree superficial partial thickness burns. According to the Rule of Nines, the anterior chest makes up 18% of the body surface area and the thigh makes up 4%, for a total of 22% of the body.

32. Answer: B Hb A_{1C} measures glucose levels over 120 days (the life span of an erythrocyte). The results of this test provide the most accurate indication of long-term glucose control. A fasting serum glucose level of 125 mg/dl, although considered acceptable for a patient with insulin-dependent diabetes, reflects a one-time measurement—not a span of days—of glucose control. The other measurements, although helpful in determining clinical status, don't provide information about glucose control.

33. Answer: B Patients who have undergone organ transplantation receive immunosuppressants and need to avoid crowds and people with infections. Immunosuppressants are needed indefinitely to prevent organ rejection. Although kissing his wife presents a small risk for infection, it shouldn't be a problem. After an extended recovery period, the patient should be able to resume most normal activities, including hunting.

34. Answer: A The patient has metabolic acidosis, which can be reversed by administering sodium bicarbonate. Intubation and hyperventilation are useful for respiratory acidosis. Having the patient breathe into a paper bag is an appropriate action for respiratory alkalosis. Oxygen therapy is used to treat hypoxia.

35. Answer: D Options A, B, and C describe pathologic pupil signs indicative of brain herniation. Hippus is the term given to a pupil that constricts to light but, because of oculomotor nerve involvement, can't sustain constriction and dilates. Absent doll's eyes is a pathologic condition in which the sensory acoustic nerve fails to accept stimuli, and the oculomotor and acoustic nerves fail to respond. This results in a fixed midline position of the pupils when the head is turned to the side. Anisocoria refers to unequal pupil size. It may be pathologic or a normal finding. When pathologic, it signifies dysfunction of the oculomotor nerve and occurs in early brain herniation.

36. Answer: C   Elevated BUN and serum creatinine levels are indicative of nephrotoxicity, which can lead to renal failure. The other adverse reactions are of a less serious nature.

37. Answer: B   Cholinergic crisis is caused by an excess of acetylcholine, which most commonly results from overmedication. Atropine may be needed to increase sympathetic responses. Myasthenic crisis is characterized by tachycardia, hypertension, and an absence of GI symptoms. Treatment includes the administration of an anticholinesterase such as neostigmine bromide.

38. Answer: B   Flumazenil is a benzodiazepine that reverses the effects of diazepam. It should be administered if respiratory distress secondary to an overdose of diazepam is noted. Although phenobarbital can effectively control seizure activity, the nurse must be aware of the amount of medication that has already been given because this medication may further suppress respiration. Naloxone is used to reverse the effects of opioids. Phenytoin won't reverse the effects of a benzodiazepine.

39. Answer: B   Chronic lung disease has a significant psychological component, and psychological support is an essential part of the treatment and recovery process. Prophylactic antibiotics may be used, depending on the underlying disease. Exercise levels should be increased in the later rehabilitative stages of treatment. Patients with lung disease respond better to small, high-calorie meals.

40. Answer: B   Neurologic checks and assessment of LOC are needed to detect a rebleeding episode. Because the bleeding has been sealed by a clot, normal fibrinolysis increases the chances for rebleeding during this period. The incidence of vasospasm is thought to be related to the breakdown of blood products in the subarachnoid space. Erythrocytes and platelets produce spasmogenic substances as they degrade. The usual length of stay for patients with cerebral aneurysm and subarachnoid hemorrhage is much longer than 7 days. Brudzinski's sign is the involuntary flexion of the hips and knees in response to passive flexion of the neck and is a sign of meningeal irritation. Osmotic diuretics are used during the early stages of treatment and gradually tapered off.

41. Answer: B   Once the dosage of dopamine rises above 10 mcg/kg/minute, the drug has strictly alpha-stimulating effects. Prolonged use at this or higher levels can lead to temporary or permanent renal damage because of vasoconstriction of the renal vasculature. A dosage of 5 mcg/kg/minute produces a mixture of beta- and alpha-receptor stimulation and doesn't decrease kidney perfusion. At 20 mcg/kg/minute, renal perfusion is severely decreased, and the patient may be at risk for renal failure. Although 15 mcg/kg/minute can be administered, it should be given only under a physician's order.

42. Answer: B   Offering choices will help the patient's family members achieve a sense of control.

43. Answer: A   Aminophylline commonly increases the heart rate. A rate of 170 beats/minute, however, can be harmful to the patient and must be evaluated by the physician before the infusion is continued. Increasing the aminophylline infusion rate would exacerbate the problem. During a crisis situation, the patient wouldn't be receptive to teaching. Although a quiet environment may be beneficial, it won't alleviate the crisis or decrease the patient's heart rate.

44. Answer: C   Patients with CSF leakage are at high risk for infection. An NG tube shouldn't be used because it may enter the brain through the tear. Packing isn't needed; CSF should drain freely. Frequent testing of pH isn't required.

45. Answer: D   Decreased compliance of the lungs in ARDS reduces the body's ability to oxygenate tissues. Patients are intubated and mechanically ventilated, with PEEP used to maintain oxygenation. The other nursing goals have lower priority.

46. Answer: C   The nurse should check the patient's admitting laboratory test results first. Digoxin is commonly used to treat atrial arrhythmias, and approximately 20% of patients who take digoxin experience toxic effects. The signs and symptoms of digoxin toxicity include dyspnea, bradycardia, nausea, vomiting, vision disturbances, and weakness. Additional digoxin shouldn't be administered unless a subtherapeutic level is verified by laboratory test results. The other options—relieving anxiety and ordering a meal—have lower priority.

47. Answer: C   Low-pressure cuffs are designed to prevent necrosis as long as the pressure is at or below 20 mm Hg. A pressure of 30 mm Hg is too high. Deflating the cuff isn't required and can cause aspiration and respiratory problems. Changing the ET tube isn't necessary unless there's a problem with the tube.

48. Answer: C   Secretions block the airway, necessitating a higher pressure to obtain the same tidal volume. A sudden decrease in the PEEP required isn't an indication of a blocked airway. A gradual decrease in the inspired tidal volume doesn't occur with a volume-cycled ventilator. Increasing the tidal volume almost always requires pressure increases.

49. Answer: A   The nurse should first test the clear fluid for sugar. If sugar is present, the fluid is CSF. Testing the cardinal signs of vision and elevating the head of the bed have lower priority. Although the fluid may be sent for culture, a sterile sample would need to be obtained, and this isn't an initial intervention.

50. Answer: B   A shift to the right indicates that more oxygen is being delivered and released to the tissues, which is caused by acidosis and an elevated $Paco_2$ level. A normal oxyhemoglobin curve wouldn't require treatment. A shift to the left occurs with alkalosis. A flattening of the curve never occurs.

Analyzing the posttest

Total the number of *incorrect* responses to posttest 2. A score of 1 to 9 indicates that you have an excellent knowledge base and that you're well prepared for the certification examination; a score of 10 to 14 indicates adequate preparation, although more study or improvement in test-taking skills is recommended; a score of 15 or more indicates the need for intensive study before taking the certification examination.

For a more detailed analysis of your performance, complete the self-diagnostic profile.

Self-diagnostic profile for posttest

In the top row of boxes, record the number of each question you answered incorrectly. Then beneath each question number, check the box that corresponds to the reason you answered the question incorrectly. Finally, tabulate the number of check marks on each line in the right-hand column marked, "Totals." You now have an individualized profile of weak areas that require further study or improvement in test-taking ability before you take the Critical Care Nursing Certification Examination.

Question number																		Totals
Test-taking skills																		
1. Misread question																		
2. Missed important point																		
3. Forgot fact or concept																		
4. Applied wrong fact or concept																		
5. Drew wrong conclusion																		
6. Incorrectly evaluated distractors																		
7. Mistakenly filled in wrong circle																		
8. Read into question																		
9. Guessed wrong																		
10. Misunderstood question																		

Selected references

Alberti, K.G.M.M. "Diabetic Acidosis, Hyperosmolar Coma, and Lactic Acidosis," in *Principles and Practice of Endocrinology and Metabolism,* 3rd ed. Edited by Becker, K.L., et al. Philadelphia: Lippincott, Williams & Wilkins, 2001.

American Association of Critical Care Nurses, Alspach, J., ed. *Core Curriculum for Critical Care Nursing,* 6th ed. Philadelphia: W.B. Saunders Co., 2006.

American Association of Critical Care Nurses, Wiegand, D., and Carlson, K.K., eds. *AACN Procedure Manual for Critical Care,* 5th ed. Philadelphia: W.B. Saunders Co., 2005.

American Diabetes Association. "Hyperglycemic Crises in Patients with Diabetes Mellitus," *Diabetes Care* 24(1):154-61 (Suppl 1):S83-S90, January 2001.

Baird, M., et al. *Manual of Critical Care Nursing,* 5th ed. St. Louis: Mosby, 2005.

Bayliss, P.H., and Thompson, C.J. "Diabetes Insipidus and Hyperosmolar Syndromes," in *Principles and Practice of Endocrinology and Metabolism,* 3rd ed. Edited by Becker, K.L., et al. Philadelphia: Lippincott, Williams & Wilkins, 2001.

Bendich, A., and Deckelbaum, R.J. *Preventive Nutrition: The Comprehensive Guide for Health Professionals,* 2nd ed. Totowa, NJ: Humana Press Co., 2001.

Braunwald, E., et al., eds. *Harrison's Principles of Internal Medicine,* 16th ed. New York: McGraw-Hill Book Co., 2005.

Burns, S.M., et al. "Development of the American Association of Critical-Care Nurses' Sedation Assessment Scale for Critically Ill Patients," *American Journal of Critical Care* 14(6):531-544, December 2005.

Craven, R.F., and Hirnle, C.J. *Fundamentals of Nursing: Human Health and Function,* 4th ed. Philadelphia: Lippincott, Williams & Wilkins, 2005.

Critical Care Nursing Made Incredibly Easy. Philadelphia: Lippincott, Williams & Wilkins, 2004.

Dennison, R. *Pass, CCRN!* 2nd ed. St. Louis: Mosby, 2000.

Diseases, 4th ed. Philadelphia: Lippincott, Williams & Wilkins, 2006.

Ferri, F. *Ferri's Clinical Advisor 2006.* St. Louis: Mosby, 2006.

Fink, M.P., et al. *Textbook of Critical Care,* 5th ed. Philadelphia: W.B. Saunders Co., 2005.

Gonder-Frederick, L.A. "Management: Hypoglycemia," in *A Core Curriculum of Diabetes Education,* 4th ed. Edited by American Association of Diabetes Educators. Chicago: American Association of Diabetes Educators, 2001.

Ignatavicius, D.D., et al. *Medical-Surgical Nursing: Critical Thinking for Collaborative Care,* 5th ed. Philadelphia: W.B. Saunders Co., 2006.

Jarvis, C. *Pocket Companion for Physical Examination and Health Assessment,* 4th ed. Philadelphia: W.B. Saunders Co., 2004.

Johnson, K. "Diagnostic Measures to Evaluate Oxygenation in Critically Ill Adults: Implications and Limitations," *AACN Clinical Issues: Advanced Practice in Acute and Critical Care* 15(4):506-524, October/December 2004.

Kreitzer, M.J., and Jensen, D. "Healing Practices: Trends, Challenges, and Opportunities for Nurses in Acute and Critical Care," *AACN Clinical Issues* 11(1):7-16, February 2000.

Professional Guide to Signs & Symptoms, 5th ed. Philadelphia: Lippincott, Williams & Wilkins, 2007.

Rakel, R., and Bope, E. *Conn's Current Therapy 2006.* Philadelphia: W.B. Saunders Co., 2006.

Smeltzer, S.C., and Bare, B.G. *Brunner and Suddarth's Textbook of Medical-Surgical Nursing,* 11th ed. Philadelphia: Lippincott, Williams & Wilkins, 2007.

Sole, M.L., et al. *Introduction to Critical Care Nursing,* 4th ed. Philadelphia: W.B. Saunders Co., 2005.

Verbalis, J.G. "Inappropriate Antidiuresis and Other Hypo-osmolar States," in *Principles and Practice of Endocrinology and Metabolism,* 3rd ed. Edited by Becker, K.L., et al. Philadelphia: Lippincott, Williams & Wilkins, 2001.

Zipes, D.P., et al., eds. *Braunwald's Heart Disease: A Textbook of Cardiovascular Medicine,* 6th ed. St. Louis: Elsevier Health Sciences, 2005.

Index

---

i refers to an illustration; t refers to a table.

i refers to an illustration; t refers to a table.

---

i refers to an illustration; t refers to a table.